SITE-SPECIFIC CANCER SERIES

Genitourinary Cancers

Edited by
Jeanne Held-Warmkessel, MSN, RN, AOCN®, ACNS-BC

Oncology Nursing Society
Pittsburgh, Pennsylvania

ONS Publishing Division

Publisher: Leonard Mafrica, MBA, CAE

Director, Commercial Publishing: Barbara Sigler, RN, MNEd

Managing Editor: Lisa M. George, BA

Technical Content Editor: Angela D. Klimaszewski, RN, MSN

Staff Editor: Amy Nicoletti, BA

Copy Editor: Laura Pinchot, BA

Graphic Designer: Dany Sjoen

Site-Specific Cancer Series: Genitourinary Cancers

Library of Congress Control Number: 2009933336

ISBN: 978-1-890504-85-4

Publisher's Note

This book is published by the Oncology Nursing Society (ONS). ONS neither represents nor guarantees that the practices described herein will, if followed, ensure safe and effective patient care. The recommendations contained in this book reflect ONS's judgment regarding the state of general knowledge and practice in the field as of the date of publication. The recommendations may not be appropriate for use in all circumstances. Those who use this book should make their own determinations regarding specific safe and appropriate patient-care practices, taking into account the personnel, equipment, and practices available at the hospital or other facility at which they are located. The editors and publisher cannot be held responsible for any liability incurred as a consequence from the use or application of any of the contents of this book. Figures and tables are used as examples only. They are not meant to be all-inclusive, nor do they represent endorsement of any particular institution by ONS. Mention of specific products and opinions related to those products do not indicate or imply endorsement by ONS. Web sites mentioned are provided for information only; the hosts are responsible for their own content and availability. Unless otherwise indicated, dollar amounts reflect U.S. dollars.

ONS publications are originally published in English. Publishers wishing to translate ONS publications must contact the ONS Publishing Division about licensing arrangements. ONS publications cannot be translated without obtaining written permission from ONS. (Individual tables and figures that are reprinted or adapted require additional permission from the original source.) Because translations from English may not always be accurate or precise, ONS disclaims any responsibility for inaccuracies in words or meaning that may occur as a result of the translation. Readers relying on precise information should check the original English version.

Printed in the United States of America

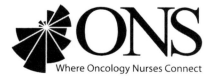

Oncology Nursing Society

Integrity • Innovation • Stewardship • Advocacy • Excellence • Inclusiveness

Contributors

Editor

Jeanne Held-Warmkessel, MSN, RN, AOCN®, ACNS-BC
Clinical Nurse Specialist
Fox Chase Cancer Center
Philadelphia, Pennsylvania
Chapter 1. Introduction to Genitourinary Cancers;
Chapter 3. Pathophysiology; Appendix

Authors

Jeffrey Albaugh, PhD, APRN, CUCNS
Advanced Practice Urology Clinical Nurse Specialist
Jesse Brown VA Medical Center and Memorial CIM
    Northwestern Wellness Institute, Sexual Health Program
Chicago, Illinois
Chapter 9. Sexual Function and Sexual Rehabilitation With
    Genitourinary Cancer

Tara S. Baney, RN, MS, AOCN®
Clinical Nurse Specialist
Mount Nittany Medical Center
State College, Pennsylvania
Chapter 4. Prevention, Screening, and Early Detection for
    Genitourinary Malignancies; Chapter 8. Treatment of
    Testicular Cancer

Maryann Carousso, MSN, RN, AOCNP®
Nurse Practitioner, Genitourinary Service
Memorial Sloan-Kettering Cancer Center
New York, New York
Chapter 3. Pathophysiology

Jennifer Cash, ARNP, MS, OCN®
Advanced Registered Nurse Practitioner
Dattoli Cancer Center
Sarasota, Florida
Chapter 5. Treatment of Bladder Cancer; Chapter 8. Treat-
    ment of Testicular Cancer

Frances Crighton, RN, PhD
Adjunct Faculty
Palm Beach Community College
Wellington, Florida
Chapter 10. Evidence-Based Practice for Urology Oncol-
    ogy Nursing Care

Anne Marie Flaherty, RN, MS, AOCNS®
Clinical Nurse Specialist
Memorial Sloan-Kettering Cancer Center
New York, New York
Chapter 3. Pathophysiology

Susan Kellogg-Spadt, PhD, CRNP
Director, Sexual Medicine
The Pelvic and Sexual Health Institute
Philadelphia, Pennsylvania
Chapter 9. Sexual Function and Sexual Rehabilitation With
Genitourinary Cancer

Denise Kramer-Levien, BA, CURN
CURN for Incontinence/Sexual Dysfunction Urology Clinic
of Southwest Washington
Vancouver, Washington
Chapter 9. Sexual Function and Sexual Rehabilitation With
Genitourinary Cancer

Linda U. Krebs, PhD, RN, AOCN®, FAAN
Associate Professor
University of Colorado Denver, College of Nursing
Aurora, Colorado
Chapter 9. Sexual Function and Sexual Rehabilitation With
Genitourinary Cancer

Jean H. Lewis, BSN, APRN-C, ANP
ED Clinic Nurse Practitioner
Veterans Affairs Medical Center
Minneapolis, Minnesota
Chapter 9. Sexual Function and Sexual Rehabilitation With
Genitourinary Cancer

Maureen E. O'Rourke, RN, PhD
Clinical Professor
School of Nursing
University of North Carolina at Greensboro
Greensboro, North Carolina
Adjunct Assistant Professor of Medicine
Hematology/Oncology
Wake Forest University
Winston-Salem, North Carolina
Chapter 2. Anatomy and Physiology of the Genitourinary
System

Dana Overstreet, RN, MSN, FNP-BC
Nurse Practitioner, Urology
University of Virginia Health System
Charlottesville, Virginia
Chapter 5. Treatment of Bladder Cancer

Albert A. Rundio Jr., PhD, DNP, APRN-BC
Associate Professor of Nursing
Felician College
Lodi, New Jersey
Chapter 6. Treatment of Penile Carcinoma

Terran W. Sims, MSN, CNN, ACNP-C, COCN
Nurse Practitioner
Genitourinary Oncology
University of Virginia, Health Services Foundation
Charlottesville, Virginia
Chapter 5. Treatment of Bladder Cancer

Laura S. Wood, RN, MSN, OCN®
Renal Cancer Research Coordinator
Cleveland Clinic Taussig Cancer Center
Cleveland, Ohio
Chapter 7. Treatment of Renal Cell Carcinoma

Hong Zhao, MSN, ACNP-BC, CCRN
Acute Care Nurse Practitioner
University of Virginia, Department of Urology
Charlottesville, Virginia
Chapter 5. Treatment of Bladder Cancer

Barbara H. Zoltick, MSN, CRNP, CURN
Oncology Nurse Practitioner
Division of Hematology/Oncology
University of Pennsylvania Health System
Philadelphia, Pennsylvania
Chapter 8. Treatment of Testicular Cancer

Field Reviewers

Christine Bradway, PhD, CRNP
Assistant Professor of Gerontological Nursing
Director, Gerontology Nurse Practitioner Program
University of Pennsylvania School of Nursing
Philadelphia, Pennsylvania

Peggy Ward-Smith, PhD, RN
Associate Professor
School of Nursing
University of Missouri at Kansas City
Kansas City, Missouri

Disclosure

Editors and authors of books and guidelines provided by the Oncology Nursing Society are expected to disclose to the participants any significant financial interest or other relationships with the manufacturer(s) of any commercial products.

A vested interest may be considered to exist if a contributor is affiliated with or has a financial interest in commercial organizations that may have a direct or indirect interest in the subject matter. A "financial interest" may include, but is not limited to, being a shareholder in the organization; being an employee of the commercial organization; serving on an organization's speakers bureau; or receiving research from the organization. An "affiliation" may be holding a position on an advisory board or some other role of benefit to the commercial organization. Vested interest statements appear in the front matter for each publication.

Contributors are expected to disclose any unlabeled or investigational use of products discussed in their content. This information is acknowledged solely for the information of the readers.

The contributors provided the following disclosure and vested interest information:

Jeffrey Albaugh, PhD, APRN, CUCNS, Pfizer, TIMM Medical, speakers bureaus

Jeanne Held-Warmkessel, MSN, RN, AOCN®, ACNS-BC, Novartis, TopoTarget, speakers bureaus

Denise Kramer-Levien, BA, CURN, Eli Lilly Corporation, speakers bureau

Laura S. Wood, RN, MSN, OCN®, Bayer, Onyx Pharmaceuticals, Pfizer Oncology, Novartis Oncology, Wyeth Pharmaceuticals, speakers bureaus

Contents

CHAPTER 1

Introduction to Genitourinary Cancers

Jeanne Held-Warmkessel, MSN, RN, AOCN®, ACNS-BC

Introduction

The purpose of this text is to provide nurses with the information necessary to care for patients and families who are affected by genitourinary (GU) malignancies, which comprise cancers of the bladder, kidney (renal), penis, and testicle. Prostate cancer is the most common malignancy diagnosed in males in the United States and is presented in detail in a separate text in this *Site-Specific Cancer Series*. Of the top 10 causes of *newly diagnosed* cancers in men, bladder cancer is the fourth most common, and renal cancer is the seventh most common. In women, renal cancer is the ninth most common cancer (Jemal et al., 2008). In a review of the top 10 causes of death in men, bladder cancer is eighth and renal cancer is tenth. None of these cancers are a top 10 cause of death in women. From 1990 to 2004, the death rate from both bladder cancer and renal cancer has decreased for both men and women (Jemal et al.).

The incidence of GU cancers is higher in men than in women, and in the case of bladder cancer, it is as much as three times higher (Lin et al., 2006). In addition, North American natives and African Americans have a higher incidence of renal cancer than other races. Most patients with bladder cancer are diagnosed with localized disease, but African Americans have a higher incidence of diagnosis with regional disease (Jemal et al., 2008). Clearly, GU malignancies affect a large number of patients each year, and because of the organs affected, these cancers have a significant impact on patients, as well as their spouses and other family members.

The risk factors for GU cancers have been studied extensively. This introductory section briefly reviews the most common risk factors.

Risk Factors for Bladder Cancer

In 2008, approximately 68,810 patients in the United States were diagnosed with bladder cancer (Jemal et al., 2008).

A number of risk factors have been identified for this disease. Controllable and environmental risk factors include cigarette smoking, occupation, exposure to radiation therapy for the treatment of another malignancy, exposure to cyclophosphamide, and exposure to the infectious organism *Schistosoma haematobium*. Uncontrollable risk factors include age (Borden, Clark, & Hall, 2005), African American race (Lee, Dun, Williams, & Underwood, 2006) and family history, especially among first-degree relatives of patients with bladder cancer or other urologic cancers (Pelucchi, Bosetti, Negri, Malvezzi, & La Vecchia, 2006; Randi et al., 2007). Individuals with a family history of bladder cancer and who smoke significantly increase their risk of bladder cancer by 6.87-fold (Lin et al., 2006).

Cigarette smoking is a major cause of bladder cancer, responsible for approximately 50% of cases in men and 33% in women (Marcus et al., 2000; Zeegers, Kellen, Buntinx, & van den Brandt, 2004; Zeegers, Tan, Dornat, & van Den Brandt, 2000). Aromatic amines found in cigarette smoke are more likely to be responsible for causing bladder cancer than other chemicals found in cigarettes (Vineis & Pirastu, 1997). Another 25% of bladder cancers are attributable to occupational exposure to hazardous chemicals. Chemicals include aromatic amines used in the chemical, dye, rubber, oil, paint, leather, and printing industries (Johansson & Cohen, 1997; Kirkali et al., 2005; Yasunaga et al., 1997). The evidence related to hair dye use or employment as a hairdresser as a potential cause of bladder cancer is inconclusive; however, some individuals with genetic risk who use hair dye and hairdressers who applied hair dye prior to the 1980s may be at higher risk (Rollison, Helzlsouer, & Pinney, 2006; Bolt & Golka, 2007). Radiation therapy used in the management of prostate cancer may increase the risk of developing bladder cancer (Boorjian et al., 2007). The use of cyclophosphamide in the treatment of ovarian cancer may increase a woman's risk of developing bladder cancer months to years after ovarian cancer therapy (Kaldor et al., 1995; Volm, Pfaff, Gnann, & Kreienberg, 2001). Long-term use of phenacetin, an analgesic no longer available in the United States, may increase the risk of bladder cancer (Fortuny et al., 2007). Uncommon in the United States but found in contaminated water in Africa and the Middle East, the parasite and eggs of *Schistosoma haematobium* are a cause of bladder cancer (Bedwani et al., 1998; Blute & Oliva, 2000).

Risk Factors for Cancer of the Penis

Cancer of the penis is a rare malignancy. Human papillomavirus (HPV) infection is responsible for 40%–50% of penile cancer cases (Dillner, Meijer, von Krogh, & Horenblas, 2000). Risk factors include older age, lack of circumcision as a newborn, phimosis, long foreskin, poor hygiene, penile rash, penile tear, smoking, genital warts, ultraviolet radiation exposure, and balanitis xerotica obliterans (BXO) also know as lichen sclerosus (Barnholtz-Sloan, Maldonado, Pow-sang, & Guiliano, 2007; Daling et al., 2005; Harish & Ravi, 1995; Maden et al., 1993; Misra, Chaturvedi, & Misra, 2004; Velazquez et al., 2003). BXO may be a premalignant lesion, and patients with chronic lesions require follow-up and biopsy if circumcision does not remove the problem (Pietrzak, Hadway, Corbishley, & Watkin, 2006). BXO often is associated with penile cancers, and they both may be diagnosed concurrently or sequentially (Pietrzak). BXO may be considered a premalignant lesion in patients without HPV (Velazquez & Cubilla, 2003).

Risk Factors for Renal Cell Cancer

In 2008, approximately 54,390 people in the United States were diagnosed with renal cell cancer (RCC) (Jemal et al., 2008). Risk factors are divided into controllable (environmental) or uncontrollable. Environmental risk factors include cigarette smoking, obesity, diet, and hypertension. Uncontrollable risk factors include family history and the need for dialysis because of renal disease. Some variables that are a mixture of controllable and uncontrollable risk factors include the presence of underlying medical conditions such as diabetes.

Cigarette smoking is responsible for up to 27% of RCC cases in men and 11% of cases in women (Benichou, Chow, McLaughlin, Mandel, & Fraumeni, 1998; Yuan, Castelao, Gago-Dominguez, Yu, & Ross, 1998). As expected, the greater the number of cigarettes smoked per day, the greater a person's risk of developing RCC (Hunt, van der Hel, McMillan, Boffetta, & Brennan, 2005). In addition to active smoking, passive smoking (also known as secondhand smoke) also increases the risk of RCC (Hu, Ugnat, & Canadian Cancer Registries Epidemiology Research Group, 2005).

Obesity with an increasing body mass index of more than 25 kg/m^2 and excess calorie consumption increases the risk of RCC for both men and women and accounts for as much as 27% of cases in men and 29% of cases in women (Bergstrom et al., 2001; Pan, DesMeules, Morrison, Wen, & Canadian

Cancer Registries Epidemiology Research Group, 2006). The mechanisms by which obesity and excess calories promote RCC are unclear but most likely include a complex interaction between a variety of growth factors, insulin resistance, altered hormone levels, and other factors (Calle & Kaaks, 2004).

Hypertension may cause 21% of RCC cases (Benichou et al., 1998). Although the disease process or the drugs used to treat it may be responsible for the increased risk, current studies concluded that the hypertension itself is the most likely etiology perhaps by causing injury to the renal tubule (Lipworth, Tarone, & McLaughlin, 2006; McLaughlin & Lipworth, 2000; Zucchetto et al., 2007). Hypertension also is a risk factor for RCC for a variety of ethnic groups including African Americans and Latinos (Setiawan, Stram, Nomura, Kolonel, & Henderson, 2007).

A family history of having a first-degree relative with RCC increases a person's relative risk of developing RCC (Randi et al., 2007; Zbar et al., 2007). Genetic predispositions for RCC are found in people with tuberous sclerosis complex, von Hippel-Lindau syndrome, hereditary papillary renal carcinoma, hereditary leiomyomatosis and RCC, Birt-Hogg-Dubé syndrome, or hyperparathyroidism-jaw tumor syndrome (Pavlovich & Schmidt, 2004; Rakowski et al., 2006; Sudarshan & Linehan, 2006). These syndromes are responsible for 1%–4% of all RCCs (Pavlovich & Schmidt). A number of the genes responsible for these autosomal dominant familial or genetically associated RCC have been identified (Pavlovich & Schmidt). A significant number of RCC cases are diagnosed in people with the highest genetic risk (Hung et al., 2007).

Patients, especially younger patients, who receive long-term renal dialysis for end-stage renal disease (ESRD) are at risk for RCC, possibly related to virus exposure (Maisonneuve et al., 1999) or from renal cystic disease (Stewart et al., 2003). Approximately 1.3%–1.68% of patients on dialysis develop renal cell cancer. RCC occurs in patients on either peritoneal dialysis or hemodialysis (Kojima et al., 2006; Savaj et al., 2003). In patients who have received a renal transplant for ESRD, cancer may develop in the native kidney or in the transplanted kidney, but the incidence is much higher in the native kidney (Ianhez et al., 2007).

Risk Factors for Testicular Cancer

Testicular cancer (TC) is a rare GU malignancy with an increasing incidence (McGlynn et al., 2003). Cryptorchidism, also known as undescended testicle, is a risk factor, and corrective surgery prior to the onset of puberty reduces the risk of malignancy (Pettersson, Richiardi, Nordenskjold, Kaijser, & Akre, 2007). Should orchiopexy not be performed prior to puberty, the cancer risk is six times higher than when an orchiopexy is performed prior to puberty (Walsh, Dall'Era, Croughan, Carroll, & Turek, 2007). Having a brother with TC increases a man's risk of disease development by nine-fold, and it increases by four-fold when a father has a history of TC (Hemminki & Li, 2004). The presence of the TC precursor, carcinoma in situ, which develops in utero, is an important risk factor (Giwercman, Muller, & Skakkebaek, 1991). Therefore, its identification in at-risk patients is important in risk reduction. Risk factors for CIS may include low parity of the mother, low gestational age, epilepsy, and retained placenta (Aschim, Haugen, Tretli, Daltveit, & Grotmol, 2006); however, more research is needed on these potential risk factors and other risk factors potentially found in the mother, the hormonal milieu, or the fetal development (Bridges & Hussain, 2007; Garner, Turner, Ghadirian, & Krewski, 2005). Race may be a risk factor, as Caucasians have a higher incidence than African Americans. However, the incidence of TC is increasing in African American and Hispanic men (Shah, Devesa, Zhu, & McGlynn, 2007). Age is a risk factor, as most patients present with disease when aged 25–35 (Liu, Wen, Mao, Mery, & Rouleau, 1999).

Summary

Cigarette smoking is a major risk factor for GU malignancies, particularly playing a role in renal cell and bladder cancer. Reducing the smoking incidence would significantly affect the frequency of these two diseases. Additional cancer reductions would occur with reduced exposure to environmental toxins and pollutants in the work setting.

References

Aschim, E.L., Haugen, T.B., Tretli, S., Daltveit, A.K., & Grotmol, T. (2006). Risk factors for testicular cancer—differences between pure non-seminoma and mixed seminoma/non-seminoma? *International Journal of Andrology, 29*(4), 458–467.

Barnholtz-Sloan, J.S., Maldonado, J.L., Pow-sang, J., & Guiliano, A.R. (2007). Incidence trends in primary malignant penile cancer. *Urologic Oncology, 25*(5), 361–367.

Bedwani, R., Renganathan, E., El Kwhsky, F., Braga, C., Abu Seif, H.H., Abul Azm, T., et al. (1998). *Schistosomiasis* and the risk of bladder cancer in Alexandria, Egypt. *British Journal of Cancer, 77*(7), 1186–1189.

Benichou, J., Chow, W.H., McLaughlin, J.K., Mandel, J.S., & Fraumeni, J.F., Jr. (1998). Population attributable risk of renal cell cancer in Minnesota. *American Journal of Epidemiology, 148*(5), 424–430.

Bergstrom, A., Hsieh, C.C., Lindblad, P., Lu, C.M., Cook, N.R., & Wolk, A. (2001). Obesity and renal cell cancer—a quantitative review. *British Journal of Cancer, 85*(7), 984–990.

Blute, R.D., & Oliva, E. (2000). Case 31-2000: A 32-year-old man with a lesion of the urinary bladder. *New England Journal of Medicine, 343*(15), 1105–1111.

Bolt, H.M., & Golka, K. (2007). The debate on carcinogenicity of permanent hair dyes: New insights. *Critical Reviews in Toxicology, 37*(6), 521–536.

Boorjian, S., Cowan, J.E., Konety, B.R., DuChane, J., Tewari, A., Carroll, P.R., et al. (2007). Bladder cancer incidence and risk factors in men with prostate cancer: Results from Cancer of the prostate strategic urologic research endeavor. *Journal of Urology, 177*(3), 883–888.

Borden, L.S., Jr., Clark, P.E., & Hall, M.C. (2005). Bladder cancer. *Current Opinion in Oncology, 17*(3), 275–280.

Bridges, B., & Hussain, A. (2007). Testicular germ cell tumors. *Current Opinion in Oncology, 19*(3), 222–228.

Calle, E.E., & Kaaks, R. (2004). Overweight, obesity, and cancer: Epidemiological evidence and proposed mechanisms. *Nature Reviews Cancer, 4*(8), 579–591.

Daling, J.R., Madeleine, M.M., Johnson, L.G., Schwartz, S.M., Shera, K.A., Wurscher, M.A., et al. (2005). Penile cancer: Importance of circumcision, human papillomavirus, and smoking in in situ and invasive cancer. *International Journal of Cancer, 116*(4), 606–616.

Dillner, J., Meijer, C.J., von Krogh, G., & Horenblas, S. (2000). Epidemiology of human papillomavirus infection. *Scandinavian Journal of Urology and Nephrology, 205*(Suppl.), 194–200.

Fortuny, J., Kogevinas, M., Zens, M.S., Schned, A., Andrew, A.S., Heaney, J., et al. (2007). Analgesic and anti-inflammatory drug use and risk of bladder cancer: A population based case control study. *BMC Urology, 7,* 13.

Garner, M.J., Turner, M.C., Ghadirian, P., & Krewski, D. (2005). Epidemiology of testicular cancer: An overview. *International Journal of Cancer, 116*(3), 331–339.

Giwercman, A., Muller, J., & Skakkebaek, N.E. (1991). Carcinoma in situ of the testis: Possible origin, clinical significance, and diagnostic methods. *Recent Results in Cancer Research, 123,* 21–36.

Harish, K., & Ravi, R. (1995). The role of tobacco in penile carcinoma. *British Journal of Urology, 75*(3), 375–377.

Hemminki, K., & Li, X. (2004). Familial risk in testicular cancer as a clue to heritable and environmental aetiology. *British Journal of Cancer, 90*(9), 1765–1770.

Hu, J., Ugnat, A.M., & Canadian Cancer Registries Epidemiology Research Group. (2005). Active and passive smoking and risk of renal cell carcinoma in Canada. *European Journal of Cancer, 41*(5), 770–778.

Hung, R.J., Moore, L., Boffetta, P., Feng, B.J., Toro, J.R., Rothman, N., et al. (2007). Family history and the risk of kidney cancer: A multicenter case-control study in Central Europe. *Cancer Epidemiology, Biomarkers and Prevention, 16*(6), 1287–1290.

Hunt, J.D., van der Hel, O.L., McMillan, G.P., Boffetta, P., & Brennan, P. (2005). Renal cell carcinoma in relation to cigarette smoking: Meta-analysis of 24 cases. *International Journal of Cancer, 114*(1), 101–108.

Ianhez, L.E., Lucon, M., Nahas, W.C., Sabbaga, E., Saldanha, L.B., Lucon, A.M., et al. (2007). Renal cell carcinoma in renal transplant patients. *Urology, 69*(3), 462–464.

Jemal, A., Siegel, R., Ward, E., Hao, Y., Xu, J., Murray, T., et al. (2008). Cancer statistics, 2008. *CA: A Cancer Journal for Clinicians, 58*(2), 71–96.

Johansson, S.L., & Cohen, S.M. (1997). Epidemiology and etiology of bladder cancer. *Seminars in Surgical Oncology, 13*(5), 291–298.

Kaldor, J.M., Day, N.E., Kittelmann, B., Pettersson, F., Langmark, F., Pedersen, D., et al. (1995). Bladder tumours following chemotherapy and radiotherapy for ovarian cancer: A case control study. *International Journal of Cancer, 63*(1), 1–6.

Kirkali, Z., Chan, T., Manoharan, M., Algaba, F., Busch, C., Cheng, L., et al. (2005). Bladder cancer: Epidemiology, staging and grading, and diagnosis. *Urology, 66*(6, Suppl. 1), 4–34.

Kojima, Y., Takahara, S., Miyake, O., Nonomura, N., Morimoto, A., & Mori, H. (2006). Renal cell carcinoma in dialysis patients: A single center experience. *International Journal of Urology, 13*(8), 1045–1048.

Lee, C.T., Dunn, R.L., Williams, C., & Underwood, W., III. (2006). Racial disparity in bladder cancer: Trends in tumor presentation at diagnosis. *Journal of Urology, 176*(3), 927–934.

Lin, J., Spitz, M.R., Dinney, C.P., Etzel, C.J., Grossman, H.B., & Wu, X. (2006). Bladder cancer risk as modified by family history and smoking. *Cancer, 107*(4), 705–711.

Lipworth, L., Tarone, R.E., & McLaughlin, J.K. (2006). The epidemiology of renal cell cancer. *Journal of Urology, 176*(6, Pt. 1), 2353–2358.

Liu, S., Wen, S.W., Mao, Y., Mery, L., & Rouleau, J. (1999). Birth cohort effects underlying the increasing testicular cancer incidence in Canada. *Canadian Journal of Public Health, 90*(3), 176–180.

Maden, C., Sherman, K.J., Beckmann, A.M., Hislop, T.G., Teh, C.Z., Ashley, R.L., et al. (1993). History of circumcision, medical conditions, and sexual activity and risk of penile cancer. *Journal of the National Cancer Institute, 85*(1), 19–24.

Maisonneuve, P., Agodoa, L., Gellert, R., Stewart, J.H., Buccianti, G., Lowenfels, A.B., et al. (1999). Cancer in patients on dialysis for end-stage renal disease: An international collaborative study. *Lancet, 354*(9173), 93–99.

Marcus, P.M., Hayes, R.B., Vineis, P., Carcia-Closas, M., Caporaso, N.E., Autrup, H., et al. (2000). Cigarette smoking, N-acetyltransferase 2 acetylation status, and bladder cancer risk: A case-series meta-analysis of a gene-environment interaction. *Cancer Epidemiology, Biomarkers and Prevention, 9*(5), 461–467.

McGlynn, K.A., Devesa, S.S., Sigurdson, A.J., Brown, L.M., Tsao, L., & Tarone, R.E. (2003). Trends in the incidence of testicular germ cell tumors in the United States. *Cancer, 97*(1), 63–70.

McLaughlin, J.K., & Lipworth, L. (2000). Epidemiologic aspects of renal cell cancer. *Seminars in Oncology, 27*(2), 115–123.

Misra, S., Chaturvedi, A., & Misra, N.C. (2004). Penile carcinoma: A challenge for the developing world. *Lancet Oncology, 5*(4), 240–247.

Pan, S.Y., DesMeules, M., Morrison, H., Wen, S.W., & Canadian Cancer Registries Epidemiology Research Group. (2006). Obesity, high energy intake, lack of physical activity, and the risk of kidney cancer. *Cancer Epidemiology, Biomarkers and Prevention, 15*(12), 2453–2460.

Pavlovich, C.P., & Schmidt, L.S. (2004). Searching for the hereditary causes of renal-cell carcinoma. *Nature Reviews Cancer, 4*(5), 381–393.

Pelucchi, C., Bosetti, C., Negri, E., Malvezzi, M., & La Vecchia, C. (2006). Mechanisms of disease: The epidemiology of bladder cancer. *Nature Clinical Practice Urology, 3*(6), 327–340.

Pettersson, A., Richiardi, L., Nordenskjold, A., Kaijser, M., & Akre, O. (2007). Age at surgery for undescended testis and risk of testicular cancer. *New England Journal of Medicine, 356*(18), 1835–1841.

Pietrzak, P., Hadway, P., Corbishley, C.M., & Watkin, N.A. (2006). Is the association between balanitis xerotica obliterans and penile carcinoma underestimated? *BJU International, 98*(1), 74–76.

Rakowski, S.K., Winterkorn, E.B., Paul, E., Steele, D.J., Halpern, E.F., & Thiele, E.A. (2006). Renal manifestations of tuberous sclerosis complex: Incidence, prognosis, and predictive factors. *Kidney International, 70*(10), 1777–1782.

Randi, G., Pelucchi, C., Negri, E., Talamini, R., Galeone, C., Franceschi, S., et al. (2007). Family history of urogenital cancers in patients with bladder, renal cell and prostate cancers. *International Journal of Cancer, 121*(12), 2748–2752.

Rollison, D.E., Helzlsouer, K.J., & Pinney, S.M. (2006). Personal hair dye use and cancer: A systematic literature review and evaluation of exposure assessment in studies published since 1992. *Journal of Toxicology Environmental Health, Part B: Critical Reviews, 9*(5), 413–439.

Savaj, S., Liakopoulos, V., Ghareeb, S., Musso, C., Sahu, K., Bargman, J.M., et al. (2003). Renal cell carcinoma in peritoneal dialysis patients. *International Urology and Nephrology, 35*(2), 263–265.

Setiawan, V.W., Stram, D.O., Nomura, A.M., Kolonel, L.N., & Henderson, B.E. (2007). *American Journal of Epidemiology, 166*(8), 932–940.

Shah, M.N., Devesa, S.S., Zhu, K., & McGlynn, K.A. (2007). Trends in testicular germ cell tumours by ethnic group in the United States. *International Journal of Andrology, 30*(4), 206–214.

Stewart, J.H., Buccianti, G., Agodoa, L., Gellert, R., McCredie, M.R., Lowenfels, A.B., et al. (2003). Cancers of the kidney and urinary tract in patients on dialysis for end-stage renal disease: Analysis of data from the United States, Europe, and Australia and New Zealand. *Journal of the American Society of Nephrology, 14*(1), 197–207.

Sudarshan, S., & Linehan, W.M. (2006). Genetic basis of cancer of the kidney. *Seminars in Oncology, 33*(5), 544–551.

Velazquez, E.F., Bock, A., Soskin, A., Codas, R., Arbo, M., & Cubilla, A.L. (2003). Preputial variability and preferential association of long phimotic foreskins with penile cancer. *American Journal of Surgical Pathology, 27*(7), 994–998.

Velazquez, E.F., & Cubilla, A.L. (2003). Lichen sclerosus in 68 patients with squamous cell carcinoma of the penis: Frequent atypias and correlation with special carcinoma variants suggests a precancerous role. *American Journal of Surgical Pathology, 27*(11), 1448–1453.

Vineis, P., & Pirastu, R. (1997). Aromatic amines and cancer. *Cancer Causes and Control, 8*(3), 346–355.

Volm, T., Pfaff, P., Gnann, R., & Kreienberg, R. (2001). Bladder carcinoma associated with cyclophosphamide therapy for ovarian cancer occurring with a latency of 20 years. *Gynecologic Oncology, 82*(1), 197–199.

Walsh, T.J., Dall'Era, M.A., Croughan, M.S., Carroll, P.R., & Turek, P.J. (2007). Prepubertal orchiopexy for Cryptorchidism may be associated with lower risk of testicular cancer. *Journal of Urology, 178*(4, Pt. 1), 1440–1446.

Yasunaga, Y., Nakanishi, H., Naka, N., Miki, T., Tsujimura, T., Itatani, H., et al. (1997). Alterations of the *p53* gene in occupational bladder cancer in workers exposed to aromatic amines. *Laboratory Investigations, 77*(6), 677–684.

Yuan, J.M., Castelao, J.E., Gago-Dominguez, M., Yu, M.C., & Ross, R.K. (1998). Tobacco use in relation to renal cell carcinoma. *Cancer Epidemiology, Biomarkers and Prevention, 7*(5), 429–433.

Zbar, B., Glenn, G., Merino, M., Middelton, L., Peterson, J., Toro, J., et al. (2007). Familial renal carcinoma: Clinical evaluation, clinical subtypes and risk of renal carcinoma development. *Journal of Urology, 177*(2), 461–465.

Zeegers, M.P., Kellen, E., Buntinx, F., & van den Brandt, P.A. (2004). The association between smoking, beverage consumption, diet and bladder cancer: A systematic literature review. *World Journal of Urology, 21*(6), 392–401.

Zeegers, M.P.A. Tan, F.E.S., Dorant, E., & van den Brandt, P.A. (2000). The impact of characteristics of cigarette smoking on urinary tract cancer risk: A meta-analysis of epidemiologic studies. *Cancer, 89*(3), 630–639.

Zucchetto, A., Dal Maso, L., Tavani, A., Montella, M., Ramazzotti, V., Talamini, R., et al. (2007). History of treated hypertension and diabetes mellitus and risk of renal cell cancer. *Annals of Oncology, 18*(3), 596–600.

CHAPTER 2

Anatomy and Physiology of the Genitourinary System

Maureen E. O'Rourke RN, PhD

Introduction

In 2008, an estimated 134,830 tumors arising from the genitourinary (GU) system (excluding the prostate) were diagnosed (American Cancer Society, 2008). Nurses need knowledge of the normal anatomy and physiology of the GU system to guide patient assessment and differentiation from pathophysiologic changes. This knowledge also is critical for accurate patient and family education. Figure 2-1 illustrates an overview of the anatomy of the GU system.

The Kidneys

Anatomy

The kidneys are bean-shaped structures, approximately the size of a clenched fist. They are reddish-brown in color and measure approximately 10 cm in length by 5 cm in width (Moore, Dalley, & Agur, 2006). Each weighs approximately 150 grams in the adult (Guyton & Hall, 1997). The kidneys are located one each on the right and left side of the retroperitoneal cavity and extend from the L1–L4 region in the erect position. The right kidney lies slightly lower than the left because of the size of the right lobe of the liver. The kidneys move slightly with respiration because of their close relationship with the diaphragm. The diaphragm serves as a barrier between the kidneys, the pleural cavity, and the 12 pairs of ribs (Moore et al.). Both kidneys are embedded in perirenal fat and are cushioned by a protective layer called the renal or Gerota's fascia. This fascia serves to anchor the kidneys to surrounding structures, thereby preventing injury from jarring or trauma to the body. The fascia also acts as a barrier for infection that may arise from the kidneys and spread to other parts of the body (Kelley & Petersen, 2007). Additionally, the kidneys are each encased in a dense fibrous protective covering called the renal capsule. See Figure 2-2 for a coronal midsection view of a kidney.

Anatomically, the kidneys are divided into five segments in accordance with their vascular supply: apical, upper anterior, middle inferior, inferior, and posterior. These divisions assist in the planning of surgical intervention (Kelley & Petersen, 2007).

Each kidney has a distinct indentation, the hilus, on the medial border, where the ureter, nerves, and renal blood ves-

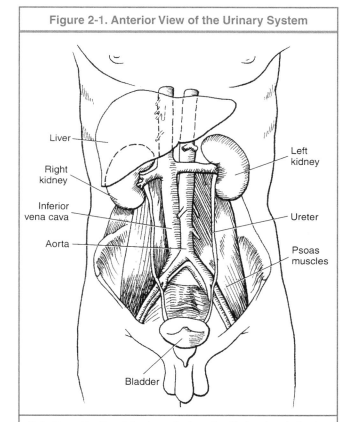

Figure 2-1. Anterior View of the Urinary System

Note. From *Sectional Anatomy for Imaging Professionals* (2nd ed., p. 382), by L.L. Kelley and C.M. Petersen, 2007, St. Louis, MO: Elsevier Mosby. Copyright 2007 by Elsevier Mosby. Reprinted with permission.

Figure 2-2. Coronal Midsection View of the Kidney

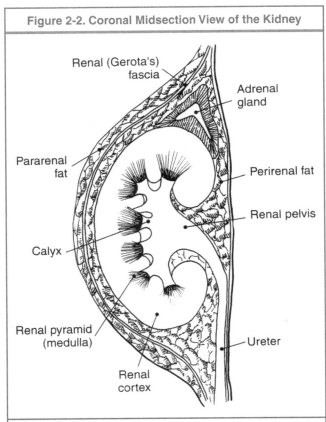

- Renal (Gerota's) fascia
- Adrenal gland
- Pararenal fat
- Perirenal fat
- Renal pelvis
- Calyx
- Renal pyramid (medulla)
- Ureter
- Renal cortex

Note. From *Sectional Anatomy for Imaging Professionals* (2nd ed., p. 383), by L.L. Kelley and C.M. Petersen, 2007, St. Louis, MO: Elsevier Mosby. Copyright 2007 by Elsevier Mosby. Reprinted with permission.

Blood supply to the kidneys encompasses 21% of the total cardiac output, approximately 1,200 ml/minute (Guyton & Hall, 1997). At the location of the hilum, the renal artery enters the kidney along with the renal vein, then braches off into the interlobar, arcuate, and interlobular, or radial, arteries. Further branching of this arterial tree leads to the afferent arterioles, which in turn lead to the glomerular capillary tufts within the glomeruli (Guyton & Hall). At the distal ends of the capillaries of each glomerulus, the capillaries coalesce forming the efferent arteriole. This leads to a second capillary network called the peritubular capillaries that surround the renal tubules (Guyton & Hall). See Figure 2-3 for a view of the major blood vessels that supply the kidney and the microcirculation supply to the nephron.

Figure 2-3. Section of Kidney Showing Major Blood Vessels That Supply Blood Flow to the Kidney, and Schematic of the Microcirculation of Each Nephron

- Interlobar arteries
- Arcuate arteries
- Renal artery
- Segmental arteries
- Interlobular arterioles
- Efferent arteriole
- Glomerulus
- Proximal tubule
- Juxtaglomerular apparatus
- Afferent arteriole
- Cortical collecting tubule
- Distal tubule
- Bowman's capsule
- Arcuate artery
- Loop of Henle
- Arcuate vein
- Peritubular capillaries
- Collecting duct

Note. From *Human Physiology and Mechanisms of Disease* (6th ed., p. 213), by A.C. Guyton and J.E. Hall, 1997, Philadelphia: Saunders. Copyright 1997 by Saunders. Reprinted with permission.

sels enter and exit the organ. Both kidneys are composed of an outer cortex and an inner medulla. The cortex comprises the outer one-third of renal tissue and contains the basic functional units called nephrons. Each kidney has an estimated one to two million nephrons. The medulla is the area of the kidney where filtration and the concentration of waste take place. The cortex consists primarily of connective tissue and projects outward into a region in the medullary area as renal columns. Renal corpuscles, which are tufts of capillaries, and the glomerulus are surrounded by the glomerular capsule and contained in the cortex. Each nephron is composed of the glomerulus and convoluted tubules. These collecting tubules form the basis of the urinary filtration system (Chung & Chung, 2008; Kelley & Peterson, 2007).

The renal medulla is the inner portion of the kidney. This portion contains 8–12 segments called renal pyramids, which contain both the loops of Henle and the collecting tubules of the nephrons. Arising from the apices of the renal pyramids are the 7–14 minor calyces, which ultimately merge into the 2 or 3 major calyces and join to empty into the renal pelvis. The renal pelvis is the largest dilated segment of the collecting system and leads directly into the ureter (Chung & Chung, 2008; Kelley & Peterson, 2007).

Venous drainage from the kidneys is through the inter-lobular veins, which carry blood to the arcuate veins. Blood next travels from the arcuate veins to the interlobar veins, which join to form the renal vein at the location of the hilum. The renal veins empty into the inferior vena cava (Kelley & Petersen, 2007).

Nerves to the kidneys are of both sympathetic and para-sympathetic origin and arise from the renal nerve plexus. The renal nerve plexus is supplied by the abdominopelvic and splanchnic nerves (Moore et al., 2006).

Physiology

The functions of the kidneys are numerous and include the regulation of fluid and electrolytes as well as osmolality, regulation of acid-base balance, metabolic waste excretion, arterial pressure regulation, and hormonal secretion.

Filtration

The formation of urine begins with glomerular filtration. Efficient filtration is dependent upon rapid renal blood flow at a consistent pressure rate. The porous glomerular capillaries lie between the afferent and efferent arterioles and function to filter large quantities of both water and solutes from the plasma. The glomerulus functions as a sieve and filters while preventing the loss of essential components such as red blood cells (RBCs) and plasma proteins. This selective filtration is determined by molecular size, electrical charge, protein binding, configuration, and rigidity. Smaller molecules, such as water and ions including sodium, potassium, chloride, phosphorus, magnesium, and calcium are filtered without restriction. Larger molecules such as plasma proteins and albumin are not allowed to pass through the filtration system if it is functioning normally. The filtration barrier has a nega-tive charge; hence, the movement of less negatively charged molecules is restricted to a greater degree than more positively charged or neutral particles. Ellipse-shaped molecules filter more easily than round molecules. Drugs and ions that are bound to proteins are not filtered through the glomerulus. Thus, normal glomerular filtrate is protein free but contains crystalloids such as sodium, potassium, chloride, creatinine, urea, uric acid, and magnesium in approximately the same concentration as the plasma (Guyton & Hall, 1997; Holechek, 1992).

A potentially useful lay analogy of the process is as fol-lows. Think of the filtration process as though you were cleaning out your desk drawer. The glomerulus dumps all of the contents of your dirty desk drawer onto the desktop. The large items, such as the dividers in the drawer, remain and are not discarded. Small items such as paperclips and rubber bands fall out. By processes of active and passive transport, the proximal and distal tubules are able to selectively put back into the desk drawer exactly what you need, such as paperclips and thumbtacks—nothing more and nothing less.

Some substances are replaced into the blood purposely while others are purposely filtered out. If the glomerulus is dam-aged and becomes too leaky, large items, which should "stay in the desk drawer," are allowed to fall or leak out, resulting in proteinuria, hematuria, and similar conditions.

Renal Blood Flow

Renal blood flow is controlled by both intrinsic and extrin-sic factors. Intrinsic factors include

- An autoregulatory mechanism: Despite mean arterial pres-sure (MAP) changes within a range of 80–180 mm Hg, an intra-renal system maintains consistent renal blood flow. However, constant renal blood flow cannot be maintained if the MAP is outside of this range. The autoregulatory function maintains renal blood flow as a constant despite the influence of stressors such as exercise, emotional up-sets, and postural changes, although these stressors can cause systemic blood pressure changes. This mechanism is attributed to baroreceptors (also called stretch recep-tors) in the afferent arterioles. With increases in the MAP, baroreceptors respond to the stretching of the vascular wall and cause afferent arteriolar constriction, which prevents the transmission of the elevated arterial pressure to the glomerulus. This, in turn, maintains normal glomerular filtration. Alternatively, if the MAP falls below the desired range, arteriolar dilation occurs to maintain pressure and normal glomerular filtration. In the absence of autoregula-tion, relatively small incremental changes in systemic blood pressure would increase or decrease glomerular filtration rates (GFR) and could greatly affect urine output (Guyton & Hall, 1997; Holechek, 1992).

- Renin-angiotensin mechanism: The kidneys produce a proteolytic enzyme called renin in response to any change in extracellular fluid volume, which may affect MAP and systemic blood pressure. Renin facilitates the splitting of angiotensin I from angiotensinogen. Angiotensin II is split off from angiotensin I. Angiotensin II, a potent vasoconstric-tor, stimulates the release of aldosterone from the adrenal cortex (Holechek, 1992; Sharp, 2006).

- Eicosanoids and kinins: The kidneys produce these vaso-active substances, which include chemicals such as some prostaglandins, leukotrienes, and thromboxane. Leuko-trienes and thromboxane are vasoconstrictive; however, their role in maintaining renal blood flow and GFR is unclear (Holechek, 1992). Prostaglandins and bradykinin are contributing factors in regulating renal blood flow, with a modest vasodilator effect. They may oppose some of the effects of renal vasoconstrictive agents on the afferent ar-terioles and may prevent excessive reduction in renal blood flow and GFR (Guyton & Hall, 1997).

Extrinsic factors that regulate renal blood flow include the sympathetic nervous system, antidiuretic hormone, angio-tensin II, dopamine, and histamine. A number of additional hormonal factors also influence renal hemodynamics, including the endothelium-derived factor, endothelin, and atrial natriuretic peptide (Holechek, 1992).

- Sympathetic nervous system (SNS): All blood vessels of the kidneys receive rich innervation from the SNS. The SNS is able to detect systemic volume changes through cardiac and arterial baroreceptors. Activation of the SNS causes constriction of the renal arterioles, decreasing GFR and renal blood flow. This function of the SNS is most important during major and acute hypovolemic disturbances lasting minutes to hours, such as severe hemorrhage or brain ischemia (Guyton & Hall, 1997).
- Antidiuretic hormone (ADH): Also called vasopressin, ADH is produced in the posterior pituitary gland and is released in hypovolemic states. ADH "increases permeability of the nephron membrane to water, allowing for water reabsorption" (Davies, 2006, p. 638) and increases circulatory volume and renal perfusion, thus maintaining MAP. Production of ADH diminishes as serum osmolality and extracellular volume normalize (Holechek, 1992).
- Dopamine: Within the renal blood vessels, dopamine receptors respond to endogenous low-dose dopamine, increasing renal blood flow and GFR (Holechek, 1992).
- Histamine: This compound increases GFR and renal blood flow by dilation of the efferent and afferent arterioles. This function is important in cases of allergic reactions.
- Angiotensin II: Aside from being formed within the kidney, angiotensin II is a circulating hormone, which preferentially constricts efferent arterioles to maintain GFR in situations when arterial pressure decreases or volume is depleted (Guyton & Hall, 1997).
- Atrial natriuretic peptide (ANP): ANP is secreted by the right atrium in response to increased right atrial pressure and dilation. It induces vasoconstriction of the afferent arterioles and vasodilation of the afferent arterioles, increasing GFR. ANP blocks ADH release and increases sodium and water loss. Ultimately, it results in reduced peripheral and renal vasoconstriction and decreased circulatory volume (Holechek, 1992).

Maintenance of Fluid and Electrolyte Balance

- Sodium and potassium regulation: The kidney is essential in maintaining the normal potassium balance within the body. Potassium (K) is the most abundant positively charged ion or cation and is present predominantly in the intracellular fluid (ICF). Normally, the delicate balance of ICF versus extracellular fluid (ECF) potassium concentration is maintained by the sodium-potassium adenosine triphosphatase pump located within cell membranes. The pump actively transports sodium (Na) out of the cell and K into the cell. Additionally, some transport takes place via passive movement. Cells are much more permeable to K than Na, and consequently, K continually diffuses along a concentration gradient from the ICF to the ECF. Sodium diffuses back into cells at a much slower rate, leaving cells

with a net positive charge loss so that the interior of cells has a negative electrical potential compared to the ECF (Ludlow, 1993).

- In response to the amount of K ingested, the kidney is able to regulate the excretory rate of it. More than 90% of K intake is excreted each day. K is filtered freely through the glomeruli maintaining a plasma concentration that generally is equal to the concentration, which enters the proximal tubule. Additionally, increases in K plasma concentration stimulate aldosterone secretion from the adrenal cortex, which further enhances K secretion into the luminal fluid. Nephron segments will reabsorb or excrete K depending on the balance of K within the body. Substantial K reabsorption takes place along the proximal tubule and the ascending loop of Henle. However, the concentration of K entering the distal convoluted tubule is lower than the plasma concentration (Ludlow, 1993).
- The rate of flow in the collecting tubules also affects serum K concentration. With increased rate of luminal flow, there is less time for K to be secreted into the lumen of the tubules. With decreased luminal flow rates, mean K concentrations within the lumen are higher because a longer time is available for K to enter the lumen. In the presence of loop or thiazide diuretics, NaCl and water reabsorption are inhibited with a subsequent increase in luminal flow rates. This leads to increased K secretion and excretion and is the mechanism by which diuretics cause potassium depletion (Ludlow, 1993).
- The internal regulation of K also is affected by the body's acid-base balance. In the case of acidosis, K moves into the ECF to maintain neutrality. This results in a rise in plasma K concentration and leads to a decreased amount of K available to enter the luminal fluid. In the case of alkalosis, the reverse is true. Plasma K concentration falls, and ICF K concentration increases. During metabolic alkalosis, K secretion into the luminal fluid increases (Ludlow, 1993).
- Active reabsorption of Na takes place within the proximal tubule. Water and chloride reabsorption occur passively within this location. Chloride is actively reabsorbed in the thick ascending limb of the loop of Henle (Yucha, 1993a).
- Regulation of phosphate, magnesium, and calcium: The maintenance of phosphate, magnesium, and calcium also are a part of renal control. Renal excretion is the primary method of phosphate regulation by the body. Ninety percent of plasma phosphate is filtered through the glomerulus and reabsorbed by the proximal tubule. Urinary excretion is affected by both dietary intake and parathyroid hormone levels (Yucha, 1993b).
- Magnesium homeostasis is maintained though renal reabsorption and excretion. The major site for magnesium reabsorption is the thick ascending loop of Henle. Excretion varies with dietary changes, changes in ECF

volume, calcium levels, and thiazide diuretics. With high dietary intake, magnesium reabsorption in the proximal tubule and loop of Henle decreases drastically. Conversely, magnesium conservation takes place when low levels cause the enhanced reabsorption, which takes place within the thick ascending limb of the loop of Henle (Yucha, 1993b).

Erythropoietin Production

The kidneys regulate RBC production within the bone marrow though the production and release of erythropoietin. The basic regulator of RBC production is tissue oxygenation. Any decrease in tissue oxygenation such as low hemoglobin levels, diminished blood flow, or low blood volume serves as a trigger for increased RBC production. Erythropoietin is a circulating glycoprotein that is classified as a hormone, which regulates RBC production. Although it is uncertain precisely where in the kidney erythropoietin is made physiologically, it is believed that this takes place in the juxtamedullary region (Donnelly, 2003).

The Ureters

Anatomy

Ureters are muscular tubules that extend from the renal pelvis of each kidney into the urinary bladder. The ureters, one on each side, are located in the retroperitoneum and descend along the psoas muscle. The ureters receive blood along their course from the aorta and the renal, gonadal, common and internal iliac, umbilical, superior and inferior vesical, and middle rectal arteries. Neurologically, the ureters are innervated by the sympathetic lumbar and parasympathetic splanchnic nerves (Chung & Chung, 2008).

Physiology

The ureters function simply as narrow muscular transport tubules for carrying urine from the kidney to the bladder.

The Bladder and Urethra

Anatomy

The urinary bladder is an inverted pyramid-shaped muscular organ resting on the pelvic floor, situated within the perineum, and lying posterior to the symphysis pubis. In females, it sits slightly lower than in males. In its empty state, four surfaces can be defined. The superior surface of bladder's body, or the apex, is covered by peritoneum with loops of both the ileum and sigmoid colon resting upon it. The posterior surface, or fundus, is the base of the bladder. In females, the

fundus is related to the anterior vaginal wall, and in males to the rectal wall. The two inferolateral surfaces are in contact with the fascia, which covers the levator ani muscles. Where the two inferolateral surfaces meet with the posterior surface is the neck of the bladder, and this continues into the urethra. The bladder neck contains the internal urethral sphincter. This is responsible for involuntary control over the release of urine from the bladder itself. The walls of the bladder mainly are composed of smooth detrusor muscle. The bladder is anchored to the pelvis by peritoneal ligaments, specifically, the median umbilical ligament and two lateral umbilical ligaments. In females, the pubovesical ligament holds the bladder neck in place. The puboprostatic ligament performs this function in males (Chung & Chung, 2008; Kelley & Peterson, 2007).

The urinary bladder receives its primary blood supply from the superior and inferior vesical arteries, and in females from the vaginal artery. The prostatic or vesical plexus, emptying into the internal iliac vein, drains venous blood. Both the obturator and inferior gluteal arteries supply small branches to the bladder (Moore et al., 2006).

Neural innervation to the bladder is via the vesical and prostatic plexuses, which are extensions of the hypogastric plexuses. Parasympathetic nerves originating in the spinal cord area of S2–S4 cause the bladder muscle to contract and relax the internal sphincter resulting in bladder emptying (Chung & Chung, 2008). These parasympathetic fibers provide motor impulses to the detrussor muscle and inhibitory impulses to the internal urethral sphincter of the male bladder. When stretching from urine in the bladder stimulates visceral afferent fibers, the bladder reflexively contracts, the urethral sphincter relaxes, and urine is released from the bladder into the urethra. This reflex can be suppressed with training. Sympathetic innervation stimulates ejaculation while simultaneously closing the internal urethral sphincter by contraction, thereby avoiding reflux of semen into the bladder (retrograde ejaculation) (Moore et al., 2006).

The bladder floor contains three openings, two of which are created by the entering ureters. The third opening is created by the urethra exiting the area. These three openings form a triangular-shaped region known as the trigone (Kelley & Peterson, 2007).

In both males and females, the urethra passes directly through the urogenital diaphragm, which contains the urethral sphincter muscle. This is responsible for voluntary closure of the bladder to retain urine. The female urethra is shorter than the male (3–4 cm versus 18–20 cm). Additionally, the female urethra is more easily distended, allowing easier passage of cystoscopes and urinary catheters. In the female, the urethra descends both inferiorly and anteriorly and is embedded in the anterior vaginal wall. The external urethral opening in females is located between the clitoris and vaginal opening. The location, shorter length, and distensible nature of the female urethra make women more prone to urinary tract infections (Moore et al., 2006). The longer male urethra extends from the inferior portion of the bladder to the penile tip and is divided anatomically into three regions: the prostatic urethra, the membranous urethra, and the penile urethra. The prostatic urethra passes through the middle of the prostate gland. Hence, it can become compressed from prostatic hypertrophy or tumor growth. The most narrow and shortest portion of the male urethra is the membranous portion. The longest segment is the penile urethra, extending from the external urethral sphincter to the tip of the penis (Kelley & Peterson, 2007).

Located posterior to the membranous urethra are the two bulbourethral, or Cowper's, glands. Their function is to secrete an alkaline fluid, which is a component of seminal fluid, into the membranous urethra (Kelley & Petersen, 2007).

Physiology

The functions of the bladder and the urethra are simple when compared to the complexity of renal physiology. The urethra functions as a narrow, muscular tube exporting urine from the bladder. In males, the urethra also functions to carry seminal fluid consisting of sperm and glandular secretions. The ejaculatory ducts are minute slit-like openings that communicate directly with the prostatic urethra. At this point, the reproductive and urinary tracts merge in males (Moore et al., 2006).

The bladder functions mainly as a collection and storage vesical for urine. Urination, or micturition, is initiated by stimulation of the baroreceptors in the detrusor muscle of the bladder wall via increasing urinary volume. Afferent impulses arise from the baroreceptors and enter the spinal column at the level of S2–S4 by way of the pelvic splanchnic nerves. Abdominal muscle contraction increases intra-abdominal and pelvic pressure assisting in emptying the bladder. Sympathetic fibers relax the bladder muscular wall and cause the internal sphincter to contract. Parasympathetic neural fibers cause contraction of the detrusor muscle and relax the internal sphincter enhancing the urge to void. Somatic fibers of the pudendal nerve cause a voluntary relaxation of the external urethral sphincter, allowing the bladder to empty. At the end of micturition, the external urethral sphincter contracts, stopping urine flow. In males, the bulbospongiosus muscles assist in expelling the final drops of urine from the urethra (Chung & Chung, 2008).

The Penis

Anatomy

The penis is the male external reproductive organ and is composed of three main parts: the glans, the root, and the body. See Figure 2-4 for a coronal view of the male reproductive anatomy and Figure 2-5 for the anatomy of the penis. The penis root is attached to the pubic arch via the suspensory ligaments, while the body is free of ligamental attachment. The root is composed of three cylindrical bodies of erectile tissue: the pair of corpora cavernosa and the corpus spongiosum. Each cavernosa is encapsulated by an outer fibrous covering called the tunica albuginea. Superficial to this is the deep fascia of the penis, also called Buck's fascia (Moore et al., 2006). The corpora cavernosa are located dorsally, whereas the corpus spongiosum is located within the undersurface of the penis. Networks of collagen fibers and spaces that become enlarged when filled with blood during an erection are within the corpora cavernosa. The corpora cavernosa are fused; however, posteriorly they are separated, generally incompletely, by the septum penis (Moore et al.). The area where they are not fused is referred to as the crura of the penis.

The corpus spongiosum contains the spongy urethra and dense venous plexuses, which are necessary for erectile function. The corpus spongiosum forms the bulb of the penis. This is located between the two crura (Moore et al., 2006). The bulbospongiosus muscles are located one on each side of the midline of the penis, covering the bulb and posterior portion of the corpus spongiosum.

The root of the penis is attached to the pubic arch. The body of the penis is suspended from the pubic symphysis and is free or pendulous. The body contains no muscle tissue and consists of thin skin, connective tissue, lymphatic channels, blood vessels, fascia, the corpora cavernosa, and the corpus spongiosum. At its distal end, the corpus spongiosum expands and forms the cone-shaped glans penis, also referred to as the head of the penis. The skin of the penis is more darkly pigmented than other body skin in general. At the neck of the glans is a double layer of skin, which comprises the prepuce, or foreskin. In uncircumcised males, this covers the glans to some extent (Moore et al., 2006).

Blood is supplied to the penis mainly by branches of the internal pudendal arteries. Venous drainage is via the superficial and deep dorsal veins of the penis, along with the internal pudendal vein (Moore et al., 2006).

The penis is innervated by S2–S4 spinal cord segments, which pass through the pelvic splanchnic and pudendal nerves. The dorsal nerve of the penis provides the primary sensory and sympathetic innervation. The glans penis has a rich supply of sensory nerve endings (Moore et al., 2006).

Physiology

Erection

Erection of the penis occurs as a gradual buildup in response to a variety of stimuli, including pleasurable sights, sounds, smell, and tactile sensation. Sensory stimuli result in stimulation of the afferent fibers of the central nervous system. Efferent impulses pass down the spinal cord to parasympathetic fibers in the sacral segments. The parasympathetic fibers

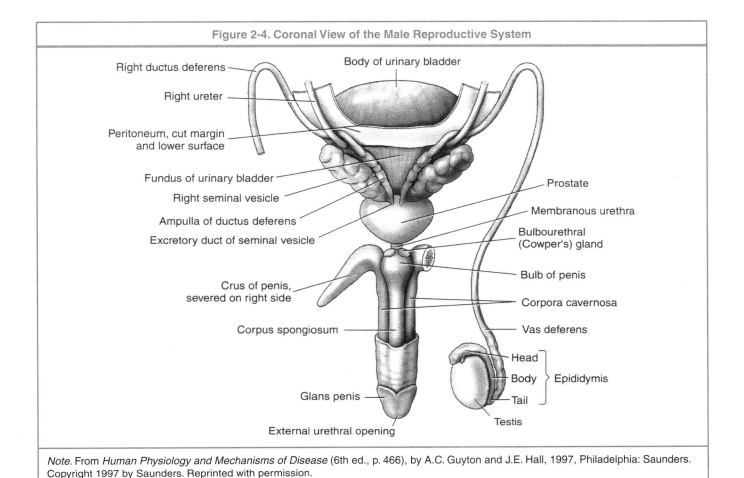

Figure 2-4. Coronal View of the Male Reproductive System

Right ductus deferens

Right ureter

Peritoneum, cut margin and lower surface

Fundus of urinary bladder

Right seminal vesicle

Ampulla of ductus deferens

Excretory duct of seminal vesicle

Crus of penis, severed on right side

Corpus spongiosum

Glans penis

External urethral opening

Body of urinary bladder

Prostate

Membranous urethra

Bulbourethral (Cowper's) gland

Bulb of penis

Corpora cavernosa

Vas deferens

Head
Body ⟩ Epididymis
Tail

Testis

Note. From *Human Physiology and Mechanisms of Disease* (6th ed., p. 466), by A.C. Guyton and J.E. Hall, 1997, Philadelphia: Saunders. Copyright 1997 by Saunders. Reprinted with permission.

synapse on postganglionic neurons, which join the internal pudendal arteries. These arteries enter the erectile tissue at the root of the penis, causing vasodilation and a massive increase in blood flow in the spaces of the erectile tissue. Both the corpus cavernosa and spongiosum engorge with blood and expand. As this occurs, the venous outflow is blocked, maintaining the erection. The penis increases in both length and diameter during this time. When the climax of sexual activity is reached, ejaculation either takes place or is inhibited. At this point, the arteries undergo constriction and the penis returns to its resting flaccid state (Snell, 2000).

Ejaculation

During the excitement phase of sexual activity, the bulbourethral glands provide lubrication to the external urinary meatus of the glans penis. Friction along the glans combined with other afferent nervous system impulses, results in sympathetic fiber discharge to the smooth muscles of the duct of the epididymis, vas deferens, prostate, and seminal vesicles. As the smooth muscles contract, sperm and secretions from the seminal vesicles and prostate are discharged into the prostatic urethra. This fluid joins with fluid secreted by the bul-

bourethral and penile urethral glands and ultimately is ejected when the bulbospongiosus muscles contract, compressing the urethra. The bladder sphincter contracts simultaneously, preventing a reflux of sperm and seminal fluid (semen) into the bladder (Snell, 2000).

Scrotum

Anatomy

The scrotum is a fibromuscular pouch that serves to enclose the testes, epididymis, and lower portions of the spermatic cord. Three layers of fascia and a layer of connective tissue embedded with smooth muscle fibers comprise the scrotum. The connective and muscle tissue layer is referred to as the dartos tunica. This forms an internal septum dividing the scrotum into right and left compartments, with each containing a testis (Kelley & Petersen, 2007). The outer appearance is wrinkled because of the response of the dartos tunica, which constricts and pulls the testis close to the body when exposed to cooler temperatures.

Figure 2-5. Anatomy of the Penis

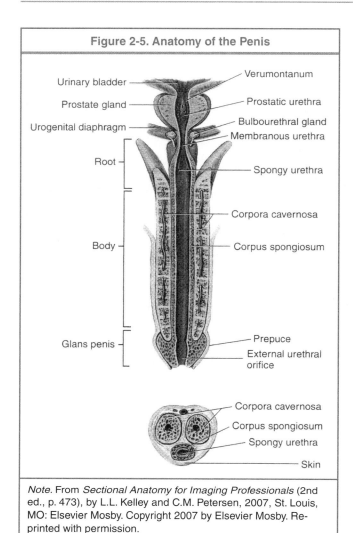

Note. From *Sectional Anatomy for Imaging Professionals* (2nd ed., p. 473), by L.L. Kelley and C.M. Petersen, 2007, St. Louis, MO: Elsevier Mosby. Copyright 2007 by Elsevier Mosby. Reprinted with permission.

Arterial supply to the scrotum is via the anterior scrotal arteries, pudendal arteries, and posterior scrotal arteries. The cremesteric arteries also contribute to arterial blood supply. Venous drainage of the scrotum is through the scrotal veins, which drain into the pudendal veins (Moore et al., 2006).

Innervation to the anterior portion of the scrotum is supplied by the lumbar plexus and anterior and posterior scrotal nerves. Sympathetic fibers from these nerves assist in thermoregulation of the scrotum by stimulating contraction of the dartos smooth muscle or stimulating scrotal sweat glands (Moore et al., 2006).

Physiology

The main function of the scrotum is to serve as a protective sac surrounding the testes. The scrotum is responsible for thermoregulation of the testes, an invaluable function for survival of sperm. This is accomplished by allowing the testes to be suspended outside of the peritoneum where the environment is cooler.

Testes

Anatomy

The testes are paired, firm, ovoid male gonadal glands that produce sperm cells and male hormones, primarily testosterone. The testes develop retroperitoneally and descend into the scrotal sacs (Chung & Chung, 2008). See Figure 2-6 for a lateral view of the male reproductive system and Figure 2-7 for a view of the testicles. Each testis is suspended in a scrotal sac. The left testis generally hangs slightly lower than the right. Each testis is covered by a fibrous outer surface called the tunica albuginea. This thickens into the mediastinum of the testes, and from this internal ridge, fibrous septa extend inward. Contained in the testes are long, tightly coiled seminiferous tubules within which sperm are produced. A network of tubules is formed as up to 800 seminiferous tubules join the straight tubules leading to the rete testis (Kelley & Petersen, 2007). The rete testis is a network of canals lying within the mediastinum of each testis (Moore & Dalley, 2006).

Each testis is covered by the tunica vaginalis, except in the area where the testis attaches to the spermatic cord and epididymis. Tiny slits called the sinus of the epididymis are

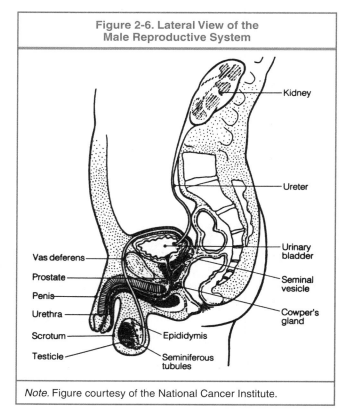

Figure 2-6. Lateral View of the Male Reproductive System

Note. Figure courtesy of the National Cancer Institute.

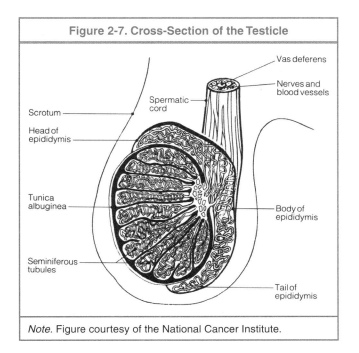

Figure 2-7. Cross-Section of the Testicle

Note. Figure courtesy of the National Cancer Institute.

within the tunica vaginalis. The testes are able to move freely within the scrotal sac because of the presence of a small amount of fluid between the layers of the tunica vaginalis (Moore et al., 2006).

Blood flow to the testes is supplied by the testicular arteries, which arise from the anterior abdominal aorta. Venous drainage from the testes and epididymis is via the pampiniform venous plexus. The veins of this network converge to form the right and left testicular veins. These veins are also part of the thermoregulatory system, which protects the testes (Moore et al., 2006). The right testicular vein drains into the inferior vena cava, while the left testicular vein drains directly into the high pressure left renal vein.

The autonomic testicular plexus of nerves arises from the testicular artery and contains vagal parasympathetic and visceral afferent fibers, as well as sympathetic fibers from the T7 region of the spinal cord (Moore et al., 2006).

Physiology

The testes perform two main functions: the production of sperm and the production of male sex hormones. Although the testes secrete several male hormones (collectively called androgens), the most abundant and significant is testosterone. Testosterone is formed by the interstitial cells of Leydig within the seminiferous tubules under the influence of luteinizing hormone (LH) secreted by the anterior pituitary gland. Testosterone is responsible for the masculine characteristics of the body, including hair and muscle distribution, muscle development, thickening of the bone matrix, the development of a bass voice, and skin thickness. Testosterone in

fetal development is responsible for the growth of the penis, scrotum, prostate, seminal vesicles, and genital ducts and suppression of the development of female genital organs (Guyton & Hall, 1997).

The conversion of spermatogonia into spermatocytes occurs within the seminiferous tubules. This process is stimulated by the release of follicle-stimulating hormone (FSH) from the anterior pituitary gland, coupled with testosterone secretion by the interstitial cells. Spermatogenesis is dependent upon both functioning interstitial cells and a functioning anterior pituitary gland, as both LH and FSH are necessary for this process to occur (Guyton & Hall, 1997).

Epididymis and Vas Deferens

Anatomy

The epididymis is a firm structure, which lies posterior to the testis. On its medial side is the vas deferens. The epididymis is composed of a head, a body, and a tail. The groove separating the testis and the epididymis is called the sinus of the epididymis. The epididymis is essentially a coiled tube, nearly 20 feet or 6 meters long. The vas deferens is the tube that emerges from the tail of the epididymis, connecting it to the spermatic cord (Snell, 2000)

Physiology

The main function of the epididymis is to provide a storage space for the maturation of spermatozoa. Fluid absorption takes place within the epididymis, as well as the addition of substances to the seminal fluid, which nourishes the sperm as they mature (Snell, 2000).

Summary

A thorough understanding of normal anatomy and physiology of the GU system forms the basis for interpretation of changes associated with primary malignancies and metastatic disease. This information is critical for nursing assessment, the planning and implementation of nursing interventions, and patient education.

The author acknowledges Kenneth S. O'Rourke, MD, for his thoughtful review and many helpful suggestions.

References

American Cancer Society. (2008). *Cancer facts and figures 2008.* Atlanta, GA: Author.

Chung, K.W., & Chung, H.M. (2008). *Gross anatomy* (6th ed.). Philadelphia: Lippincott Williams & Wilkins.

Davies, M.J. (2006). Acute renal failure. In D. Camp-Sorrell & R. Hawkins (Eds.), *Clinical manual for the advanced practice nurse* (2nd ed., pp. 637–638). Pittsburgh, PA: Oncology Nursing Society.

Donnelly, S. (2003). Why is erythropoietin made in the kidney? The kidney functions as a "critmeter" to regulate the hematocrit. *Advances in Experimental Medicine and Biology, 543,* 73–87.

Guyton, A.C., & Hall, J.E. (1997). *Human physiology and mechanisms of disease* (6th ed.). Philadelphia: Saunders.

Holechek, M.J. (1992). Glomerular filtration and renal hemodynamics. *ANNA Journal, 19*(3), 237–248.

Kelley, L.L., & Petersen, C.M. (2007). *Sectional anatomy for imaging professionals* (2nd ed.). St. Louis, MO: Elsevier Mosby.

Ludlow, M. (1993). Renal handling of potassium. *ANNA Journal, 20*(1), 52–58.

Moore, K.L., Dalley, A.F., & Agur, A.M.R. (2006). *Clinically oriented anatomy* (5th ed.). Philadelphia: Lippincott Williams & Wilkins.

Sharp, K. (2006). Hypertension. In D. Camp-Sorrell & R.A. Hawkins (Eds.), *Clinical manual for the advanced practice nurse* (2nd ed., pp. 329–347). Pittsburgh, PA: Oncology Nursing Society.

Snell. R.S. (2000). *Clinical anatomy for medical students* (6th ed.). Philadelphia: Lippincott Williams & Wilkins.

Yucha, C.B. (1993a). Renal control of calcium. *ANNA Journal, 20*(4), 440–445.

Yucha, C.B. (1993b). Renal control of phosphorus and magnesium. *ANNA Journal, 20*(4), 447–451.

CHAPTER 3

Pathophysiology

Maryann Carousso, MSN, RN, AOCNP®, Anne Marie Flaherty, RN, MS, AOCNS®, and Jeanne Held-Warmkessel, MSN, RN, AOCN®, ACNS-BC

Introduction

Nurses require an understanding of the pathophysiology, carcinogenesis, signs, and symptoms of the disease process in order to discuss staging, grading, and diagnostic tests used in genitourinary (GU) cancer diagnosis and patient management. The purpose of this chapter is to discuss these issues in order to form a basis of understanding of the treatment of bladder, penile, renal, and testicular cancers.

Bladder Cancer

Introduction

Bladder cancer is the fourth most common cancer and the eighth most common cause of cancer-related deaths. The incidence and death rates for bladder cancer are approximately 75% lower in women than in men (Jemal et al., 2008). This disease has far-reaching implications for both genders regarding altered sexuality, body image, quality of life, and role function. This section will review the pathophysiology of bladder cancer with the goal of educating nurses with the knowledge required to care for patients with bladder cancer, as well as information that nurses should share with patients so that they can make informed choices.

Cancer Cell of Origin

Bladder cancer originates in the epithelial cells of the urothelial lining of the GU tract that extends from the renal pelvis to the proximal urethra (Hoglund, 2007; Kakizoe, 2006). It is frequently multifocal and heterogeneous in nature, and patients may present with multiple concurrent tumors throughout the urothelial lining of the GU tract (Cheng et al., 2000; Kakizoe; Koss, Tiamson, & Robbins, 1974).

Risk Factors

Bladder cancer risk factors include cigarette smoking, infection with the organism *Schistosoma haematobium*, older age, exposure to arylamines, and occupations such as working in chemical plants (Borden, Clark, & Hall, 2005). In comparison with nonsmokers, a smoker's risk of developing bladder cancer is three times greater (Zeegers, Tan, Dorant, & van den Brandt, 2000). Aromatic amines are the chemicals that have been identified in cigarette smoke as the carcinogens causing bladder cancer (Vineis & Pirastu, 1997). After smoking, the next most common cause of bladder cancer is exposure to chemicals (Botteman, Pashos, Redaelli, Laskin, & Hauser, 2003). See Chapter 4 for more information about risk factors.

Types of Bladder Cancers

Approximately 90%–93% of bladder cancers in the United States are transitional cell carcinomas (TCC) of urothelial histology (O'Donnell, 2007; Ross, Yu, & Yuan, 2006). Although the most common type is squamous cell carcinoma (SCC) in other parts of the world, this histology is rare in the United States (Gilligan & Dreicer, 2007). The remaining 7%–10% of bladder cancers are cell types such as small cell or neuroendocrine, adenocarcinoma, glandular, or undifferentiated (Cheng et al., 2004; O'Donnell; Ross et al.). Sarcomas are rare and include leiomyosarcomas, rhabdomyosarcomas, angiosarcomas, and malignant fibrous histiocytomas (Lott, Lopez-Beltran, Montironi, MacLennan, & Cheng, 2007).

Staging

In the United States, bladder cancer is staged using the American Joint Committee on Cancer (AJCC) guidelines. In other parts of the world, the World Health Organization (WHO) system, originally published in 2004, is the most commonly used staging system (Kirkali et al., 2005). The AJCC system is based on the tumor, node, and metastasis (TNM) system of disease description (Greene, Compton, Fritz, Shah, & Winchester, 2006). Bladder cancer is staged based on how deep the tumor invades the bladder through the epithelium, subepithelial connective tissue, the muscle (called the muscularis), and the perivesical fat (Greene et al., 2006). Based on the most recent version of the TNM system (Greene et al., 2006), Ta tumors are noninvasive and confined to the mucosa. Carcinoma in situ tumors are staged as Tis. T1 tumors involve the subepithelial layer. T2 tumors invade the muscle. T2, T3, and T4 tumors are divided into "a" and "b" based on their depth of invasion. For example, T2a tumors involve the superficial muscle layer, whereas T2b tumors have grown into the outer part of the muscle layer. T3 tumors have grown through and outside the bladder wall into the perivesical tissues. T3a tumors have microscopic involvement, and T3b tumors have macroscopic invasion. T4 tumors have invaded the neighboring organs such as the prostate or uterus. T4a tumors involve the prostate, uterus, or vagina, and T4b tumors involve the pelvic wall or abdominal wall (Greene et al., 2006).

Nodal metastases are divided into N0–N3. With N0 disease, no metastases are present in the lymph nodes. With N1 disease, there is metastasis in one lymph node and the node's size is smaller than 2 cm at the greatest dimension. N2 disease is in one lymph node that is 2–5 cm in diameter at the greatest dimension or in multiple nodes; all smaller than 5 cm. N3 lymph node metastases are greater than 5 cm (Greene et al., 2006). Distant metastases are either absent (M0) or present (M1).

Using the TNM system, bladder cancer is staged as follows (Greene et al., 2006).
• Stage I is T1N0M0.
• Stage II is T2a–T2bN0M0.
• Stage III is T3a–T4aN0M0.
• Stage IV is T4b or any T size with N1–3 and M0–1.

Specific tests used to determine the extent of disease in patients with invasive bladder cancer will be discussed later in this section.

Tumor Grading

Tumor grades are used to predict the behavior of the tumor, with higher-grade tumors behaving in an aggressive manner (rapidly progressing) and lower-grade tumors behaving in a less aggressive (slowly progressing) manner (Kirkali et al., 2005). Bladder cancer may be low grade (G1), moderate-to-high grade (G2), or high grade (G3) (O'Donnell, 2007). Both noninvasive and invasive tumors should be graded only as low-grade or high-grade. Some pathologists still use the G2 classification; therefore, G2 should be considered high-grade (Epstein, Amin, Reuter, & Mostofi, 1998; Shipley et al., 2005). TCC exists in two types of clinically distinct forms, superficial or invasive. The majority of TCCs are papillary (or superficial). These tumors do not progress beyond the mucosal (Ta) or submucosal tissue (T1) layers and tend to

not infiltrate into deeper tissues, although some may behave in an aggressive manner. Ta tumors may be classified by the new term, *papillary urothelial neoplasm of low malignant potential* (Jones & Cheng, 2006). Tumors that invade the mucosal layer are common and tend to be low grade, but may also occur as high-grade tumors (Sylvester et al., 2005). High-grade tumors may progress to be life-threatening (Herr, 2000). Tumors that invade the submucosal layer tend to be higher grade. Some researchers do not consider these to be superficial tumors, as the tumors exhibit malignant behavior and are potentially fatal (Soloway, Lee, Steinberg, Ghandi, & Jewett, 2007). Superficial tumors may be exophytic, unifocal, and multifocal, and they often recur (Donat, 2003). Recurrence may manifest as superficial disease or the development of invasive bladder cancer. Carcinoma in situ is the third type of superficial bladder cancer and is a high-grade dysplasia or lesion. It is a cancer precursor (Kirkali et al.; O'Donnell) and is considered malignant (Sylvester et al.). The presence of carcinoma in situ increases the risk of invasive disease (Hudson & Herr, 1995), as higher-grade tumors are more likely to behave in an aggressive manner (Jordan, Weingarten, & Murphy, 1987). The second type of TCC is invasive through the mucosal and submucosal layers and into the muscle layer of the bladder (T2 or greater) and behaves in an aggressive manner (O'Donnell; Ross et al., 2006).

Carcinogenesis

Bladder cancer progresses through a process of development associated with chromosomal changes. Droller (2005) hypothesized that bladder cancer transitions from normal tissue to papillary tumors that are low grade. This is attributed to abnormalities and alterations in chromosome 9 that are linked to the development of bladder cancer. Deletions of chromosome 9 are most likely the earliest changes associated with bladder cancer (van Oers et al., 2006). Changes in chromosome 9 are also associated with flat urothelial hyperplastic lesions, which could be the first step in the bladder cancer process (van Oers et al.). Lindgren et al. (2006) have shown that chromosome 9 may be associated with tumor development and not tumor initiation. Loss of heterozygosity of chromosome 9q may be associated with the loss of a tumor suppressor gene (possibly *TSC1*) that allows for the development of invasive bladder cancer (Hirao et al., 2005). Lower grade tumors are associated with alterations in fibroblast growth factor 3 receptor, a type of tyrosine kinase receptor that regulates cell growth, differentiation, and angiogenesis in greater frequency than in high-grade tumors (Lindgren et al.).

Chromosome 17 alterations are associated with tumor invasion and high-grade tumors (Droller, 2005). Changes in chromosome 17, along with changes in chromosomes 3 and 7, are associated with T3–T4 tumors (Gallucci et al., 2005). In addition, the *p63* gene on chromosome 3 plays an early role in cancer development (Comperat et al., 2007). The normal role of *p63* is to promote urothelial differentiation (Zigeuner et al., 2004). Multiple other chromosomal changes have been identified in patients with bladder cancer, including chromosome gains, losses, deletions, and amplifications (Mhawech-Fauceglia, Cheney, & Schwaller, 2006). Several carcinogenesis pathways have been discovered that incorporate the identified genetic alterations. However, more research is needed to identify the roles that tumor suppressor genes, oncogenes, and other chromosomal alterations play in the development of bladder cancer.

Signs and Symptoms

Frequently associated with urinary tract infections (UTIs), menstruation, or other "benign" GU problems, hematuria is the most common symptom of bladder cancer. Because of its intermittent nature, patients often ignore hematuria. The hematuria is most often painless and visible (gross hematuria) throughout the voiding process from the beginning to the end of micturition (Heney, 2006). Microscopic hematuria occurs less frequently. If pain is present with the hematuria, it may be associated with inflammation from calculi or infection (Heney), and a search for these etiologies should be pursued. As most bladder tumors produce symptoms leading to diagnosis, bladder cancer is rarely found on autopsy (Wijkstrom et al., 2000). Patients may complain of frequency, urgency, burning, or dysuria (Droller, 2005; Heney).

Sites of Metastatic Disease

Bladder cancer metastasizes via the lymphatic and hematologic systems. Common sites of disease spread include the lymph nodes in the pelvis, the pelvis and its viscera, the retroperitoneum, skeleton, liver, lung, peritoneum, kidney, adrenal glands, pleura, and intestine (Hassan, Cookson, Smith, & Chang, 2006; Wallmeroth et al., 1999).

The disease may grow and invade the local structures, producing symptoms related to invasion of the prostate, uterus, or vagina, such as erectile problems, difficulty voiding, or bleeding. Bladder outlet obstruction may develop from prostatic involvement resulting in obstructive symptoms. Occasionally, patients may experience acute severe pain or irritative symptoms (Heney, 2006). Metastatic disease to bone may produce symptoms such as pain. Liver metastases may produce jaundice, whereas lung metastases may produce a cough, shortness of breath, or dyspnea. Lymph node metastases may compress soft tissues such as the ureters and cause hydronephrosis, flank pain, and lower extremity edema. Renal impairment or failure may develop. A mass may be palpable in the pelvis (Kirkali et al., 2005). Anorexia, weight loss, and bowel obstruction may occur with advanced disease; however, brain metastases are rare. Approximately half of patients with disease that involves the muscle layer of the bladder have occult metastases at the time of diagnosis (Slack & Prout, 1980).

Diagnostic Studies

Bladder cancer is diagnosed with laboratory studies, urine cytology, urinary marker tests, intravenous pyelography (IVP), ultrasonography (ultrasound), or cystoscopy. Of these, cystoscopy is the gold standard. Explanations of these diagnostic studies follow.

Laboratory Studies

All patients should be evaluated with a routine urinalysis, urine culture and sensitivity, and complete blood count. In patients with invasive bladder cancer, alkaline phosphatase, creatinine clearance, and a comprehensive metabolic panel that includes liver function tests and electrolytes should be completed. Patients being considered for surgery require coagulation studies.

Urine Cytology

In the presence of hematuria that is not the result of a gynecologic problem or menses, the patient should be evaluated for other causes of hematuria, such as a UTI, calculi, or a prostate disorder in males. A urinalysis and culture and sensitivity should be performed. In the absence of any other etiology, the patient should undergo urine cytologic evaluation. This is done using a voided urine specimen and subjecting the specimen to cytology and flow cytometry. Urine cytology is a reliable method of identifying the presence of abnormal cells with greater than 90% specificity and 40%–60% sensitivity (Shipley et al., 2005). Daily specimens examined over three days will likely produce a diagnosis (Geisse & Tweeddale, 1978). The specimens need to be obtained after the first voided specimen of the day, either midmorning or at random (Young & McKee, 2006). Overnight specimens may contain cells not useful for evaluation because of cell deterioration (Young & McKee). Although these tests are useful, no currently available urine test can take the place of invasive bladder evaluations with cystoscopy (Planz et al., 2005), which is presented in detail later in this section.

Urinary Marker Tests

Cytology is very useful in the detection of high-grade bladder cancer but is not as effective for low-grade disease detection (Amiel, Shu, & Lerner, 2004). This has led to the search for urine tests that can be used to detect or assist with the detection of other types of bladder cancer. Urinary marker tests may be used in conjunction with cystoscopy to improve cancer detection (O'Donnell, 2007). Available tests measure tumor membrane antigens, nuclear matrix proteins (NMP22), bladder tumor-associated antigens, or chromosomal abnormalities in cells in either a voided specimen or a specimen obtained by bladder barbotage (injection, removal, and reinjection or flushing of saline into bladder via an instrument placed in the urethra) (Droller, 2005; Gibanel et al., 2002; Grossman et al., 2005; O'Donnell; Varella-Garcia, Akduman, Sunpaweravong, Di Maria, & Crawford, 2004). Urinary marker tests are more sensitive than cytology but lack its specificity (Bassi et al., 2005).

Intravenous Pyelography

IVP involves the use of systemically injected dye followed by a pelvic radiograph to evaluate the bladder and urethra, as well as the upper parts of the renal system, such as the kidneys and ureters. The use of dye is contraindicated in patients with a dye or shellfish allergy. IVP is useful in identifying upper renal system causes of hematuria such as renal calculi (Guimaraes & Harisinghani, 2006). However, IVP rarely identifies upper urinary tract cancers (Goessl, Knispel, Miller, & Klan, 1997) and therefore is not a necessary part of the initial workup for many patients (Kirkali et al., 2005). IVP is useful in patients with high-risk superficial bladder cancer, as it is helpful in finding synchronous tumors in the upper urinary tract (Bajaj, Sokhi, & Rajesh, 2007).

Ultrasonography

The exact role of ultrasound in the diagnosis of bladder cancer is undetermined (Guimaraes & Harisinghani, 2006). The test offers the advantages of being noninvasive and inexpensive, requiring no preparation, and not using contrast dye. In the evaluation of 1,007 patients with hematuria, ultrasound had 63% sensitivity and 99% specificity (Datta, Allen, Evans, Vaughton, & Lucas, 2002). However, ultrasound does not show the ureters well unless pathology is present such as hydronephrosis (Guimaraes & Harisinghani).

Cystoscopy

Cystoscopy is the gold standard in evaluation of the bladder for cancer. It is required to evaluate the etiology of hematuria not explained by another disease process or diagnostic test. Cystoscopy evaluates the urethra and the lining of the bladder using a lighted instrument inserted via the urethra. The size, number, appearance, architecture, and other features of bladder tumors are seen during cystoscopy. Abnormal areas, their adjacent areas, and the area where the urethra traverses the prostate and the bladder neck are biopsied and sent for pathologic evaluation (Droller, 2005). Random biopsies of the bladder urothelial lining are done only when visible lesions are not present and when other diagnostic tests do not reveal a cause of bleeding (Droller). Otherwise, only biopsies of visible lesions are performed. A biopsy of the muscle layer below the visible tumor is required to ensure that muscle-invasive disease is not missed, as this could potentially result in under-staging a patient's disease (Droller; Brauers, Buettner, & Jakse, 2001).

Fluorescence Cystoscopy

The investigational procedure of fluorescence cystoscopy involves instillation of a photoactive chemical, hexaminolevulinate, into the bladder during cystoscopy, and then examining the bladder with blue light instead of the white light used in routine cystoscopy (Grossman et al., 2007). Clinical trials are under way to determine if this approach is an improvement over standard cystoscopy.

Retrograde Pyelography

Performed during the cystoscopy, retrograde pyelography involves the placement of small catheters inserted into the upper urinary tract via the cystoscope, which are used to inject dye to detect upper urinary tract tumors. Radiographs are then taken to visualize the upper sections of the urinary tract.

Evaluation Under Anesthesia

With the patient under anesthesia, the physician performs a bimanual evaluation of the bladder prior to and after resection of the bladder tumor. The presence of a palpable tumor prior to transurethral resection indicates that a large tumor is present and may have spread to nearby organs and tissues. If the tumor is still palpable after removal, it indicates a poor prognosis (Droller, 2005).

Staging Tests

Chest Radiograph

A chest x-ray should be done as part of the workup of the patient with invasive bladder cancer to examine the chest and lungs for metastasis and other pathology (e.g., cardiomyopathy, chronic obstructive pulmonary disease) that could contribute to the decision-making process related to treatment.

Computed Tomography

Computed tomography (CT) scan of the abdomen and pelvis are performed as part of the hematuria workup and cancer staging. It should be performed prior to the removal of the tumor for the most accurate determination of diagnosis and extent of disease (Zhang, Gerst, Lefkowitz, & Bach, 2007). CT scan is considered the test of choice for evaluation of hematuria, high-grade bladder cancer, muscle-invading bladder cancer, and metastatic disease. In combination with urography, the administration of IV dye or CT urography (CTU) shows details related to multiple GU pathologies, lymph node metastases, and local versus regional tumor invasion (Albani, Ciaschini, Streem, Herts, & Angermeier, 2007; Zhang et al.). CTU is considered the best diagnostic study for patients who are able to receive IV contrast. Its ability to clearly project the upper parts of the GU tract is better than other imaging tests (Zhang et al.); however, it is limited by less sensitivity to lower GU tract lesions (Albani et al.).

Magnetic Resonance Imaging

Magnetic resonance imaging (MRI) offers the patient improved evaluation of the lower GU tract and bladder tumor staging over CTU because of the addition of gadolinium-enhanced dynamic technique imaging (Tanimoto et al., 1992).

In a study of 35 patients with bladder cancer who were staged using both CT and MRI, CT was 55% accurate, and MRI was 75% accurate. However, the difference in accuracy was not statistically significant (Kim et al., 1994). In advanced disease, both CT and MRI are accurate (Kim et al.). A more recent study demonstrated that MRI is able to differentiate superficial tumors from invasive tumors and tumors confined to the bladder from those that have spread beyond the bladder (Tekes et al., 2005).

Nursing History and Assessment

A thorough nursing history is essential in providing comprehensive care to the patient with bladder cancer. The past medical history should include information about the use of antineoplastic agents to treat other cancers or immune system dysfunction. Nurses should specifically ask about cyclophosphamide exposure, as its use may increase the risk of bladder cancer. The history also needs to include information about (Heney, 2006; Pashos, Botteman, Laskin, & Redaelli, 2002)

- The use of a chronically indwelling urinary bladder catheter
- Smoking history
- Occupation
- Any potential exposure to carcinogens
- Menstruation and pain with menses in female patients
- The appearance of blood in the urine. Determine what medications the patient takes or has received that may cause the urine to be discolored red, or foods that have been consumed, such as fresh beets, that color the urine red.
- Medications for pain and the type, length, and frequency of usage
- The patient's urologic history and micturition history, as well as signs and symptoms. Some patients have discomfort over the bladder in the suprapubic area.
- Changes in bladder function
- The presence of irritative voiding symptoms such as frequency, urgency, burning, or dysuria (Heney, 2006)
- If the entire stream of urine is red or if just the beginning or end. If blood is present at the beginning only, it is associated often with blood from the bladder neck or trigone. If blood is present at the end of the stream, it may be related to prostatic disease (Heney, 2006). Hematuria is associated with a variety of physical activities such as running, biking, and sports; therefore, ask about exercise and physical activity (Fassett, 1984; Jones & Newhouse, 1997; Leibovitch & Mor, 2005).
- Pain—its location, duration, onset, and precipitating factors
- Recent weight loss or appetite loss, cough, changes in bowel habits, and other signs of metastatic disease

Weigh the patient and take vital signs as baseline assessments. While a routine head-to-toe physical assessment is performed, the nurse should focus the assessment on the GU tract, abdomen, and pelvis. The bladder and pelvic area should be palpated. However, it is rare that a mass is felt unless the disease is advanced. Occasionally, a suprapubic mass may be felt, so this area requires special attention. The inguinal area should be evaluated for palpable lymph nodes. A digital rectal examination should be performed to palpate the prostate and bladder areas in men. In women, the vaginal area also should be palpated (Heney, 2006). Sites of pain should be examined, palpated, and assessed. Last, nurses should examine the lower extremities for edema and, if present, grade severity.

Penile Cancer

Introduction

Penile cancer is a compilation of carcinomas in situ and invasive carcinoma. Carcinomas in situ of the penis include Bowen disease, erythroplasia of Queyrat, and Bowenoid papulosis—all of which, if untreated, can progress to an invasive carcinoma (Micali, Schwartz, & Nasca, 2006). SCC accounts for 95% of invasive carcinomas of the penis (Micali, Nasca, Innocenzi, & Schwartz, 2006).

Types of Penile Cancer

The clinical presentation and histopathologic characteristics of the four most common premalignant lesions of the penis are described in Table 3-1. Whether Bowenoid papulosis is truly part of this group or is a separate disease is controversial. Erythroplasia of Queyrat and Bowen disease are penile intraepithelial neoplasias. Bowenoid papulosis is considered a type of cutaneous dysplasia that may not become an in situ carcinoma, and therefore has a much better prognosis (Ammin, Tamboli, & Cubilla, 2003).

Balanitis xerotica obliterans (BXO), also called lichen sclerosus (LS), is not a malignancy. Rather, it is a premalignant condition that causes cellular and structural changes that make the development of an invasive tumor more likely. BXO and LS cause phimosis, which is a constricted prepuce, or top of the foreskin, resulting in nonretractile foreskin (Andriole, 2008). Phimosis can lead to chronic inflammation of the glans and foreskin and is associated with penile cancer. In one study, 35% of patients with penile cancer had phimosis compared to 7.5% in the control group of uncircumcised men (Daling et al., 2005; Reddy, Devendranath, & Pratap, 1984). Tseng, Morgenstern, Mack, and Peters (2001) found that phimosis was the strongest predictor of invasive penile cancer when analyzing 100 cases of patients with penile cancer compared to 100 control participants.

The invasive types of tumors are listed in Table 3-2 with their characteristics and incidence. Penile horn, in and of itself, is not a malignant condition, but it can evolve into a malignancy or form as a result of invasive cancer (Andriole,

Table 3-1. Premalignant Lesions Associated With Penile Cancer

Premalignant Lesions	Clinical Presentation	Histopathology
Erythroplasia of Queyrat (Penile intraepithelial neoplasm) 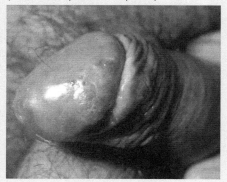	Bright red velvety plaque on the glans or foreskin. Common in older adult, uncircumcised white men. Malignant transformation more common.	Epithelial hypoplasia, disorderly, dysplastic cells that display nuclear atypia and replace mature keratinocytes. Large number of plasma cells.
Bowen disease (Penile intraepithelial neoplasm)	Solitary, dull red plaque on the shaft with areas of crusting and drainage. Rarely found in older adult white men. Approximately 5% transform to squamous cell carcinoma (SCC).	Similar to erythroplasia of Queyrat except less epithelial hypoplasia and more multinucleated cells.
Bowenoid papulosis 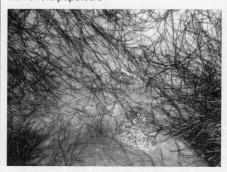	Warty, red or purplish, elevated papules on the shaft of very sexually active young men. Considered a syndrome associated with human papillomavirus (HPV). Low malignant transformation potential and may be associated with immunosuppression.	Epidermal thickening, atypical basaloid keratinocytes with large, hyperchromatic, pleomorphic nuclei, atypical mitotic figures, individual cell necrosis, and dyskeratosis in a benign environment.
Balanitis xerotica obliterans or lichen sclerosus 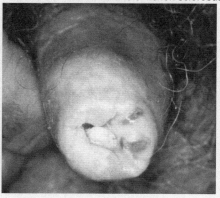	Well-defined, marginated white patch on the glans penis or prepuce and may involve urethral meatus. Symptoms include pain, difficulty urinating caused by meatal stricture, and painful erection. The condition may be associated with HPV. Although this condition is considered benign, it has been associated with development of SCC.	Thinning and hyperkeratosis of epithelium, basal cell layer showing degeneration, band-like infiltrate of lymphocytes and plasma cells in the dermis, hyalinization of collagen in the upper dermis.

Note. Based on information from Andriole, 2008; Micali, Nasca, et al., 2006; Micali, Schwartz, et al., 2006; Pietrzak et al., 2006; Stancik & Holtl, 2003.

Photos courtesy of eMedicine.com, available at http://www.emedicine.com/derm/topic919.htm. Reprinted with permission.

Table 3-2. Invasive Penile Cancer

Location	Description	Comments
Penile horn 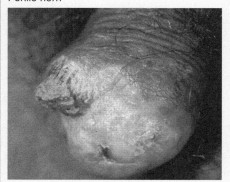	Not considered malignant, but it may be associated with benign or invasive carcinomas. Most often seen in older men who were circumcised as adults with a long-standing history of chronic inflammation on the glans. Appears as a hard and conical keratotic outgrowth, yellow/white with a bulging erythematous base.	30% may reveal a squamous cell carcinoma (SCC). Most malignant penile horns are low grade and rarely metastasize.
Verrucous carcinoma, Buschke-Lowenstein tumor, giant condyloma acuminatum 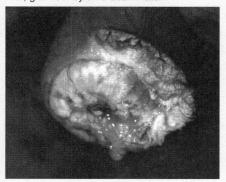	These three lesions may be different or one and the same. All present as a large fungating mass, which is aggressive and invasive to local tissue and structures. Rarely metastasizes unless it evolves into SCC when associated with x-ray exposure or human papillomavirus (6, 11, 16, and 18). May be considered a well-differentiated SCC of low-grade potential.	These account for 5%–24% of squamous cell penile cancer.
Squamous Cell Carcinoma 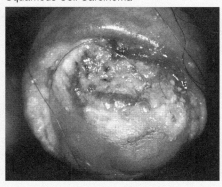	50% are well differentiated. 30% are moderately differentiated. 20% are poorly differentiated. Lesions contain heavy keratinization, epithelial pearl formation, increased mitotic activity, and hyperchromic enlarged nuclei.	SCC accounts for 95% of penile cancers.
Other non–squamous cell penile cancers: melanoma, basal cell carcinoma, sarcoma, lymphoma	Have characteristics of the primary histology type of the tumor.	These comprise the remaining 5% of penile cancers.

Note. Based on information from Andriole, 2008; Micali, Nasca, et al., 2006; Micali, Schwartz, et al., 2006; Pietrzak et al., 2006; Stancik & Holtl, 2003.

Photos courtesy of eMedicine.com, available at http://www.emedicine.com/derm/topic919.htm. Reprinted with permission.

2008; Cruz Guerra et al., 2005). Verrucous carcinoma is a well-differentiated type of anogenital SCC and therefore has a more slowly progressing disease with a better prognosis. It is associated with human papillomaviruses (HPVs), with the most common types being HPV 16 and 18 (Andriole; Brosman, 2008).

SCC can be subdivided according to histologic features, and Table 3-3 lists these with their specific features. The usual variant comprises 60% of all cases and has intermediate aggressive characteristics. Basaloid is the most aggressive penile carcinoma and is associated with HPV. The exact relationship of HPV to penile cancer has not been established, but some researchers suggest that two separate types of penile cancer exist: one associated with HPV and sexual transmission in younger men, and the other nonviral with an unknown cause that occurs in older men (Micali, Nasca, et al., 2006; Nasca, Innocenzi, & Micali, 1999; Rubin et al., 2001).

Carcinogenesis

HPV has been associated with specific types of penile cancer and may initiate the disease through its oncogenes. Kayes, Ahmed, Arya, and Minhas (2007) reviewed 49 publications

Table 3-3. Histologic Subtypes of Squamous Cell Carcinoma

Subtype	Characteristics
Usual variant	Most common (60%) subtype, intermediate risk for metastatic spread; intermediate prognosis
Verruciform variant	Massive hyperplasia is typical; accounts for 3% of cases
Pseudohyperplastic	Occurs in older patients with lichen sclerosus with low risk of metastasis
Basaloid variant	Associated with human papillomavirus, has poor prognosis and more aggressive features, is high-grade; vascular invasion. Occurs in 10% of cases.
Sarcomatoid variant	Histologically resembles sarcoma; accounts for 4% of cases
Adenosquamous Variant	Has presentation of both glandular (adeno) arrangement of cells and squamous cells; accounts for 1% of cases
Mixed variant	May contain any of a combination of the above subtypes

Note. Based on information from Cubilla, Piris, et al., 2001; Cubilla, Reuter, et al., 2001; Micali, Schwartz, et al., 2006; Micali, Nasca, et al., 2006.

reporting molecular and genetic changes in HPV-dependent and HPV-independent penile carcinomas. These oncogenic proteins have a role in controlling cellular differentiation, proliferation, and apoptosis (Walboomers et al., 1999). More recently, Bleeker et al. (2009) updated this information and created a schematic overview of early and late molecular events. This schematic is presented in Figure 3-1 and illustrates HPV-mediated and HPV-independent molecular changes.

HPV-mediated carcinogenesis arises from effects of the virus initiating genetic alterations to transform the infected cell into a malignant one. HPV does this by exerting an oncogenic effect through the expression of oncoproteins E6 and E7. These oncoproteins then inactivate *TP53* and *RB* tumor suppressor genes. Specifically, E7 inactivates *RB*, which then leads to overexpression of p16, and E6 inactivates *p53*, which causes dysregulation of the cell cycle (Bleeker et al., 2009).

HPV-independent carcinogenesis affects the same pathways but through different mechanisms. The p16 pathway is disrupted by either p16 promoter methylation or overexpression of the *BMI-1* gene, which also can disrupt the p14 pathway. Somatic mutations of *TP53*, overexpression of *MDM2*, and mutation of p14 have been identified in penile carcinogenesis (Bleeker et al., 2009).

Common and late molecular events involve alterations in *ras*, *myc*, E-cadherin, matrix metalloproteinases (MMPs), cyclooxygenase (COX), and prostaglandin synthesis. Ki-67 is a nuclear protein positively expressed in some penile cancers and reflects the growth fraction within tumors (Kayes et al., 2007). Cyclin D1 is a cell cycle activator, and its overexpression may be used as a prognostic factor of poor outcome in penile carcinoma (Papadopoulos et al., 2007). The COX pathway and prostaglandin production are involved with tumor invasion as well as carcinogenesis. COX-2 and prostaglandin E synthase-1 were found to be upregulated in a small sample of both invasive and dysplastic penile lesions (Golijanin et al., 2004). MMPs and E-cadherin are involved with invasion and metastasis; low levels of E-cadherin suggest a high risk of lymph node involvement, and high MMP-9 levels suggest a high risk for disease recurrence (Campos, Lopes, Guimares, Carvalho, & Soares, 2006). Serine protease inhibitors that are the product of two genes, *SERPINB* and *SERPINB4*, also have been implicated in penile carcinogenesis and have been studied as possible tumor markers and predictors of lymph node metastases. Currently, SCC antigen derived from the serpin family is not a sensitive marker of tumor burden, but it does have prognostic value for disease-free survival in patients who had surgery for penile cancer (Zhu et al., 2008).

Clinical Signs and Symptoms

Primary penile SCC can occur on any part of the penis, but the most common sites are the glans (34%) and the prepuce

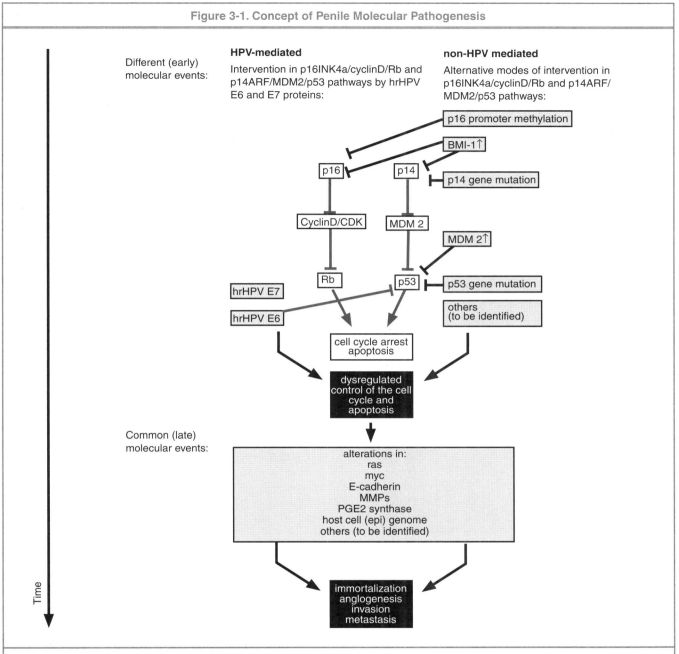

Figure 3-1. Concept of Penile Molecular Pathogenesis

Note. From "Penile Cancer: Epidemiology, Pathogenesis, and Prevention," by M. Bleeker, D. Heideman, P. Snijders, S. Horenblas, J. Dillner, and C. Meijer, 2009, *World Journal of Urology, 27*(2), p. 146. Copyright 2009 by Springer. Reprinted with permission.

(15%), whereas the least common is the shaft (less than 2%) (Barnholtz-Sloan, Maldonado, Pow-sang, & Guiliano, 2007). The appearance of the lesion at the time of presentation can vary greatly, and many men delay seeking medical intervention. The average time from when a man recognizes a problem to when he seeks medical care is 10 months, with 50% of men having had the lesion for more than one year (Pettaway, Lynch, & Davis, 2007; Sufrin & Huben, 1991).

Penile cancer usually presents as itching and burning with a lesion that can be either papillary or flat. The papillary lesion appears as a well-defined outgrowth, whereas a flat lesion appears red with superficial erosion and deep tissue invasion (Burgers, Bodalament, & Drago, 1992). Sufrin and Huben (1991) published a review of more than 4,000 penile cancer cases and found that 47% presented with a papillary lesion, 35% had a sore or flat lesion, and 17% had an inflammatory-type of lesion. More than half of the lesions were greater than 2 cm in size at presentation, and 14% invaded the shaft of the penis (Burgers et al.).

Buck's fascia in the penis creates a barrier that prevents local extension and protects the corporal bodies from invasion. Should the penile lesion progress beyond Buck's fascia and the tunica albuginea, extensive tissue destruction and vascular invasion occur involving the urethra with either fistula formation or obstruction. Secondary infection may be present, and pain is less severe than would be expected with such massive tissue invasion (Andriole, 2008).

Sites of Metastases

Penile carcinoma invades via a horizontal and a vertical approach. Horizontal spreading to adjacent epithelium can involve the glans, coronal sulcus, and foreskin of the penis, as well as the urethral mucosa. Vertical spreading can lead to invasion of the various internal structures of the penis including the fascia, tunica albuginea, and corpora cavernosa (Micali, Nasca, et al., 2006). Because of the pathway of lymphatic drainage from the penis, penile cancer spreads initially to the ipsilateral superficial inguinal lymph nodes, followed by the deep inguinal or iliac nodes, and then regional lymph nodes of the pelvis (Dewire & Lepor, 1992). Bilateral involvement of the lymph nodes is possible because of the crossover of the lymphatic vessels at the base of the penis (Crawford & Daneshgari, 1992).

More than 50% of men will have palpable groin lymphadenopathy at diagnosis; half caused by metastatic disease and half caused by inflammation (Sufrin & Huben, 1991). Of the patients with nonpalpable groin lymph nodes, about 20% will have metastatic disease. Lymph node metastases are more common when the primary lesion is the flat type, the majority of the penile shaft is involved, and the primary lesion is larger than 5 cm (Burgers et al., 1992). Distant metastasis occurs through hematologic spread of the tumor cells and is a late development in the disease. The most common sites of metastasis include the lungs and liver, with less common occurrences in the bone, brain, and skin (Micali, Nasca, Innocenzi, & Schwartz, 2004).

Diagnostic Studies

A biopsy to obtain a histologic diagnosis is the initial diagnostic study for penile cancer. It should be adequate enough to establish the grade or aggressiveness and depth of invasion of the tumor. The biopsy is usually a 1 cm elliptical wedge excision centered on the margin of the lesion (Micali, Nasca, et al., 2006). If, however, the biopsy is inadequate in determining the depth of tumor invasion, a full resection may be needed to establish the true grade of the lesion (Velazquez, Barreto, Rodriguez, Piris, & Cubilla, 2004). Figure 3-2 describes the Broders (1921) grading system to distinguish well-differentiated, moderately differentiated, and poorly differentiated higher-grade tumors.

Figure 3-2. Broders Grading System for Penile Cancer

Grade I
- Cells well differentiated with keratinization
- Prominent intercellular bridges
- Keratin pearls

Grade II–III
- Greater nuclear atypia
- Increased mitotic activity
- Fewer keratin pearls

Grade IV
- Marked nuclear pleomorphism
- Numerous mitoses
- Necrosis
- Lymphatic and perineural invasion
- No keratin pearls
- Deeply invasive

Note. Based on information from Broders, 1921; Lucia & Miller, 1992.

Lont, Besnard, Gallee, van Tinteren, and Horenblas (2003) compared the accuracy of physical examination, ultrasound, and MRI in determining the stage of the primary tumor. The results found that physical examination was the most accurate tool when measured against the actual stage identified at the time of surgery (Lont et al.). MRI enhanced with gadolinium can be helpful in determining soft tissue and lymph node involvement, as well as high-grade and high-stage lesion involvement of the corporal bodies of the penis, which may lead to partial or full penectomy (Razdan & Gomella, 2005).

Newer diagnostic techniques include MRI with artificial erection, which evaluates a rigid penis after intracorporeal injection of prostaglandin E to better visualize depth of invasion and determine tumor stage (Scardino et al., 2004). Autofluorescence and 5-aminolevulinic acid–induced fluorescence have been used to visualize superficial tumors, particularly those suitable for laser treatments. These methods use blue excitation light from a xenon arch lamp to illuminate the penis and are referred to as photodynamic diagnosis (PDD) (Frimberger et al., 2002). More recently, Frimberger et al. (2004) used PDD to guide and localize the treatment of metastatic lymphadenopathy in penile cancer.

Key to staging penile cancer is the identification of nodal involvement; this is crucial for predicting prognosis and survival. Clinical evaluation of inguinal nodes is the initial step in determining nodal involvement and, with a high grade/stage tumor, radiologic evaluation is essential. CT scan, ultrasound, and MRI with gadolinium enhancement are the recommended tests but do not always identify metastatic disease. Sentinel lymph node biopsy, intraoperative lymph node mapping, and fluorescence assay are feasible techniques to identify metastatic lymph nodes, but need further study (Busby & Pettaway,

2005). A sentinel lymph node biopsy is performed to determine the first lymph node that receives lymphatic drainage from the tumor. The node is identified by injecting either a blue dye or radioactive colloid around the tumor. The color blue identifies the lymph node to be biopsied intraoperatively (Cabanas, 1977).

Reliable identification of lymph node disease allows clinicians to adequately and aggressively treat this group of patients who are at a high risk for regional disease despite negative examination and negative radiographic study. In addition, reliable prediction of early lymph node disease will ensure that patients undergo a lymph node dissection early in the course of their disease (Mistry, Jones, Dannatt, Prasad, & Stockdale, 2007).

Tumor Markers

Standard, clinically reliable, and accepted tumor markers are not available for SCC of the penis. Recent studies evaluated the use of SCC antigen (SCCAg), a tumor-associated glycoprotein and a member of the serpin family as a tumor marker (Kommu, Hadway, & Watkin, 2005; Touloupidis et al., 2007). When SCCAg levels were measured in patients with SCC of the penis, levels were elevated preoperatively and declined after surgery, compared with negative levels in the control group without disease. This small, nonrandomized pilot study with promising results requires further study (Touloupidis et al.).

Tumor markers for penile cancer would be useful for disease surveillance, as well as valuable in predicting lymph node metastasis. A few molecular markers have been studied for their usefulness in the management of patients with penile cancer. Low E-cadherin immunoreactivity has been associated with lymph node metastases, and MMP-9 reactivity with risk of disease recurrence (Nelson, 2006). Loss of heterozygosity was found in six different chromosomes of more than 25% of 28 primary penile carcinomas thus supporting the possibility of tumor suppressor or metastasis suppressor gene involvement (Poetsch, Schuart, Schwesinger, Kleist, & Protzel, 2007). These findings were significantly related to stage ($p < 0.007$), metastasis ($p < 0.004$), and survival ($p < 0.007$). This small study may direct further investigation of E-cadherin, MMP-9, and other genes.

Staging

Two main staging systems are used to stage penile cancer: the original Jackson system (Jackson, 1966) presented in Table 3-4 and the widely accepted TNM system (Greene et al., 2002, 2006) presented in Table 3-5. These two systems do not adequately predict those patients who have regional lymph node metastases and require a lymphadenectomy. This information is crucial because it can dramatically increase survival and prevent unnecessary surgery with significant

Table 3-4. Jackson Staging System: Penile Cancer

Stage	Description
Stage I	Tumor confined to the glans or prepuce
Stage II	Tumor invades shaft or corpora with no palpable nodes or distant disease
Stage III	Tumor involves only the penis with resectable nodal disease in the groin
Stage IV	Tumor involves adjacent structures to the penis, groin nodes inoperable or distant metastasis

Note. Based on information from Jackson, 1966; Micali, Schwartz, et al., 2006.

Table 3-5. American Joint Committee on Cancer Staging System Squamous Cell Carcinoma of the Penis

Classification	Description
Tumor (T)	
TX	Not defined
T0	No evidence of primary tumor
Tis	Carcinoma in situ (Bowen disease, erythroplasia of Queyrat)
Ta	Noninvasive verrucous carcinoma
T1	Tumor invading the subepithelial connective tissue
T2	Tumor invading the corpus spongiosum or cavernosum
T3	Tumor invading urethra or prostate
T4	Tumor invading other adjacent structures
Node (N)	
NX	Not defined
N0	No evidence of regional node involvement
N1	Involvement of a single superficial inguinal node
N2	Involvement of multiple or bilateral superficial inguinal nodes
N3	Involvement of deep inguinal or pelvic nodes, unilateral or bilateral
Metastasis (M)	
MX	Not defined
M0	No evidence of distant metastasis
M1	Distant metastasis present
M1a	Occult metastasis (biochemical and/or other tests)
M1b	Single metastasis in a single organ
M1c	Multiple metastasis in a single organ
M1d	Metastasis in multiple organ sites

Note. From *AJCC Cancer Staging Manual* (6th ed., pp. 303–304), by F.L. Greene, D.L. Page, I.D. Fleming, A. Fritz, C.M. Balch, D.G. Haller, et al. (Eds.), 2002, New York: Springer. Copyright 2002 by American Joint Committee on Cancer. Adapted with permission.

long-term sequelae. Tabatabaei and McDougal (2006) have suggested a new system that incorporates stage with depth of invasion and grade to classify penile cancers according to the risk of groin metastasis (see Table 3-6).

With the TNM system, patients with stage I and IIA disease have a small chance of groin metastasis, whereas those with stage IIB and III disease have a greater chance and will require a lymph node dissection. According to Tabatabaei and McDougal (2006), patients with persistent palpable inguinal nodes are defined as
- Having received six weeks of antibiotics after removal of the primary tumor
- Having a wound that has adequately healed (stage 3 or maturation stage of wound healing).

The stage of penile cancer dictates proper treatment, and accurate staging of patients is imperative.

Table 3-6. Depth of Invasion/Grade Classification System for Penile Cancer

Stage	Description	T Stage
Stage I	Tumor is superficial with no extension into the subcutaneous tissue	T0, Tis, Ta, N0
Stage IIA	Locally invasive tumor without involvement of the corpora, well or moderately well differentiated	T1, N0
Stage IIB	Tumor invades the corpora or is poorly differentiated	T1, T2, N0
Stage III	Persistent palpable inguinal nodes	N1, N2
Stage IV	Bulky groin nodes with invasion extending outside the node, pelvic node involvement, distant metastases	N3, N4

Note. From "Penile Cancer: Clinical Signs and Symptoms" (p. 807), by S. Tabatabaei and W.S. McDougal in N. Vogelzang, P. Scardino, W. Shipley, F. Debruyne, and W. Linehan (Eds.), *Comprehensive Textbook of Genitourinary Oncology* (3rd ed.), 2006, Philadelphia: Lippincott Williams & Wilkins. Copyright 2006 by Lippincott Williams & Wilkins. Reprinted with permission.

Nursing History and Assessment

Early identification of penile cancer is imperative so that curative therapy can be initiated. A skilled interviewer can obtain information required for the clinician to better direct care. The nursing history focuses on high-risk populations and should include
- Skin abnormalities on the penis

- Sexually transmitted diseases
- Symptoms associated with urination and erection
- Erectile dysfunction
- Any other symptoms the patient may have related to his reproductive system.

The nursing assessment of high-risk patients includes examination of the penis including prepuce (foreskin) if applicable, glans, and shaft performed with and without retraction of the foreskin. The scrotal skin and urinary meatus also are examined. Careful inspection of the skin is performed to identify any lesions or abnormalities, and the meatus is inspected and gently pressed and observed for discharge. The penis and scrotum are palpated to identify any nodules, or subcutaneous or intracorporeal masses. The examination is performed with the client standing while the clinician is seated and wearing gloves. If latex gloves are used, assessment of latex allergy is needed.

History and physical examination of high-risk patients are important to detect early disease. They provide an opportunity for nurses to educate the patient regarding self-examination and safe sexual practices, and to establish a trust relationship with the patient. In particular, men who are at risk need to feel secure with their healthcare provider so that they report symptoms early. Delay in seeking medical care will lead to a higher stage of disease at the time of diagnosis.

Renal Cell Cancer

Introduction

Renal cell carcinoma (RCC) is a collection of malignant diseases. The recent explosion of discovery in the treatment of RCC has led to a more in-depth understanding of genetic and molecular changes, as well as treatments that are yielding positive results. RCCs are adenocarcinomas arising from renal tubular epithelium, the majority of which are located in the proximal region of the nephron (Campbell, Novick, & Bukowski, 2007; Zambrano et al., 1999).

Types of Renal Cell Carcinoma

In 1997, a team of urologic pathologists met to incorporate molecular genetics in the classification of RCCs. The term *conventional RCC* was based on genetics and selected to replace *clear cell carcinoma*, which indicated a cytologic and morphologic characteristic. As a result, the two names are used interchangeably in many references. In this chapter, the term *conventional* refers to the clear cell, granular, and mixed types of renal carcinoma as defined by the genetic deletion of chromosome 3p (Kovacs et al., 1997).

Table 3-7 lists the various types of RCC with conventional (which includes clear cell) as the most common type. Con-

Table 3-7. Renal Cell Carcinomas

Types of Renal Cell	Histologic Appearance	Incidence	Tumor Characteristics
Conventional • Clear	Round or polygonal with clear cytoplasm	70%–80%	• Derived from proximal tubule • Hypervascular and more aggressive than other types
• Granular	Eosinophilic cytoplasm with abundant mitochondria		
• Mixed	Both types of cells		
Chromophilic (Papillary)	Cells are arranged in a tubular configuration	10%–15%	• Derived from proximal tubule • Hypovascular • More common in acquired cystic disease associated with chronic dialysis • Type 2 has poorer prognosis of the two because of more genetic variation.
• Type 1	Basophilic cells with scant cytoplasm-small cells		
• Type 2	Eosinophilic cells and abundant granular cytoplasm-large cells		
Chromophobic	Tumors grow in large sheets of cells	3%–5%	• Derived from intercalated cells of the collecting duct • Although it is less aggressive than conventional renal cell carcinoma, there is an aggressive trait.
• Type 1	Classic—pale cytoplasm		
• Type 2	Eosinophilic—granular cytoplasm		
Collecting Duct	–	–	• Derived from collecting duct • Medullary renal cell carcinoma is a variant associated with sickle cell trait. • Poor prognosis • Lesion may be centrally located and infiltrating.
Unclassified	Includes a variety of tumors that do not fit into other categories	1%	• Poor prognosis

Note. Based on information from Campbell et al., 2007; Cohen & McGovern, 2005; Kovacs et al., 1997.

ventional RCC is derived from the proximal tube and is very vascular and more aggressive than any of the other types listed. Chromophilic (more commonly referred to as *papillary*) RCC, is the second most frequent. It is divided into two types based on histologic appearance, with type 2 designated as more aggressive. Both types have a less abundant vascular supply than conventional. Papillary RCC is associated with cystic disease and is most often seen in patients who are undergoing chronic dialysis for renal failure (Campbell et al., 2007; Cohen & McGovern, 2005; Kovacs et al., 1997).

Chromophobic RCC is uncommon and less aggressive than conventional RCC. Tumors appear to grow in large sheets and are derived from the intercalated cells of the collecting duct. Collecting duct RCC is even rarer than chromophobic. One variant, called medullary carcinoma of the kidney, is associated with the sickle cell trait. Medullary RCC usually manifests as a centrally located lesion and has a poor prognosis (Campbell et al., 2007).

Each of the various types of RCC may have a histologically distinct sarcomatoid variant. Before the Heidelberg classification was developed in 1999, sarcomatoid RCC was considered a distinct entity. However, the term applies to a histologic subtype that is poorly differentiated, more aggressive, and holds a poorer prognosis (Cangiano et al., 1999; Delahunt, 1999). It is seen in about 1%–5% of all cases of RCC, most often in conventional and chromophobic types (Cheville et al., 2004).

RCC can develop because of an inherited genetic defect that leads to a variety of hereditary syndromes. Table 3-8 lists these syndromes, their associated genetic aberration, and the type of RCC that can result. The most common hereditary syndrome is von Hippel-Lindau disease, an autosomal dominant disorder that is associated with clear cell RCC, pheochromocytoma, retinal angiomas, hemangioblastomas of the central nervous system, and cysts of the pancreas and inner ear. About half of patients with von Hippel-Lindau disease develop clear cell RCC, present at an earlier age, and have multifocal, bilateral disease (Neumann & Zbar, 1997).

Papillary RCC, or chromophilic type, is associated with two hereditary syndromes: hereditary papillary RCC

Table 3-8. Genetic Alterations With Inherited Syndromes Associated With Renal Cell Carcinoma

Hereditary Syndrome	Genetic Aberration	Renal Manifestation
von Hippel-Lindau (VHL)	Loss of function of VHL gene (tumor suppressor gene) on chromosome 3p	Clear cell renal cell carcinoma (RCC) multifocal/bilateral Pheochromocytoma
Hereditary papillary RCC	Inheritance of c-met gene on chromosome 7q. MET is a classic oncogene.	Type 1 papillary RCC multifocal/bilateral
Hereditary leiomyomatosis RCC	FH gene that encodes fumarate hydratase, a Krebs cycle enzyme is lost. This is a tumor suppressor gene.	Type 2 papillary RCC solitary and unilateral Collecting duct RCC
Birt-Hogg-Dubé (BHD) syndrome	Loss of function of BHD 1 gene on chromosome 17p that encodes a protein that is a tumor suppressor	Chromophobic RCC Oncocytomas (benign tumors) Tumors that are hybrids of the above Multifocal/bilateral

Note. Based on information from Campbell et al., 2007; Cohen & McGovern, 2005.

(HPRCC) and hereditary leiomyomatosis RCC (HLRCC). HPRCC is an autosomal dominant disorder causing inheritance and activation of the c-met proto-oncogene on chromosome 7. This pathway induces type 1 papillary RCC, which is multifocal and bilateral (Pavlovich, Schmidt, & Phillips, 2003; Schmidt et al., 1997).

HLRCC is also an autosomal dominant disorder involving the fumarate hydratase gene. Fumarate hydratase is an enzyme involved in oxidative metabolism in the Krebs cycle. The loss of this tumor suppressor gene is related to development of type 2 papillary RCC, which is unusually solitary and unilateral (Linehan, Walther, & Zbar, 2003; Pavlovich & Schmidt, 2004). An aggressive form of collecting duct RCC also is related to HLRCC, as well as cutaneous manifestations of leiomyomas and uterine fibroids in women (Linehan et al.). About 20% of patients with this hereditary syndrome develop RCC (Choyke, Glenn, Walther, Zbar, & Linehan, 2003).

Birt-Hogg-Dubé syndrome was named after the three Canadian physicians who first identified this hereditary syndrome, which is associated with cutaneous manifestations, fibrofolliculomas, and lung cysts (Linehan et al., 2003). Chromophobic RCC and oncocytomas, or a mixed histology of both, are the most common renal manifestations and occur in about 20%–30% of patients with Birt-Hogg-Dubé syndrome (Choyke et al., 2003).

The Fuhrman system of nuclear grading was established in 1982 to determine tumor aggressiveness and patient prognosis. It examines the size and shape of the nucleus and prominence of the nucleoli, subsequently assigning a number from 1 to 4 to the RCC type, with 4 being the most aggressive (Fuhrman, Lasky, & Limas, 1982). Delahunt, Bethwaite, and Nacey (2007) recently demonstrated that the Fuhrman grading system is useful with only clear cell renal carcinoma.

Carcinogenesis

Because of the genetic defects identified in the hereditary syndromes associated with RCC, many of the pathways involved in sporadic cases have been identified and targeted by various current therapies for RCC. Table 3-9 lists the genetic defects and mutations involved in the sporadic types of RCC. The most common pathway implicated in RCC, both sporadic and familial, is the role of hypoxia-inducible factors (HIF) (Rathmell, Martz, & Rini, 2007). HIF is the principal regulator in hypoxic conditions in multicellular organisms and is the prime target to promote RCC via the von Hippel-Lindau (VHL) gene and mammalian target of rapamycin (mTOR) pathways. This discussion will be directed toward the most central event in the tumorigenesis of RCC, HIF expression. How the tumor directs the pathway toward HIF overexpression will vary depending on the subtypes of RCC, but the genetic and molecular messages induce the same pathway leading to tumor growth and development.

Figure 3-3 illustrates HIF expression in the normoxic (normal levels of oxygen) state and in clear cell RCC. Under normoxic conditions, the VHL gene is responsible for tagging HIF for destruction by proteasomes when conditions are not stressful or hypoxic. When the VHL gene is mutated or methylated as in RCC or the patient is in a hypoxic state, HIF-alpha binds to HIF-beta. This activates the transcription of hypoxia-inducible genes, which promotes the production of vascular endothelial growth factor (VEGF), platelet-derived growth factor (PDGF), transforming growth factor (TGF), epidermal growth factor receptor (EGFR), and carbonic anhydrase (CA) IX or G250 (Rathmell, Wright, & Rini, 2005). The result is tumor cell growth and angiogenesis (Cohen & McGovern, 2005; George & Kaelin, 2003; Heng, Rini, Garcia, Wood, & Bukowski, 2007).

Table 3-9. Genetic Aberrations in Sporadic Cases of Renal Cell Carcinoma	
Type of Sporadic Renal Cell Carcinoma	Genetic Aberration
Conventional Clear cell Granular Mixed	• Deletions of chromosome 3p • von Hippel-Lindau gene mutations • Loss of chromosomes 8p, 9p, and 14q • Gain of chromosome 5q
Chromophilic	• Trisomy of chromosomes 7 and 17 • Mutation of met proto-oncogene that increases met protein that activates hepatocyte growth factor • Translocation of *TFE3* gene at chromosome Xp11.2
Chromophobic	• Loss of a variety of chromosomes
Collecting duct	• Loss and gain of various chromosomes

Note. Based on information from Campbell et al., 2007; Cohen & McGovern, 2005; Rathmell et al., 2005.

In addition to the mutated VHL gene initiating HIF, mTOR controls protein synthesis of HIF, which promotes the gene transcription for VEGF, PDGF, and EGFR. mTOR is a group of proteins that has been identified in multiple tumors. Its activation of HIF's protein synthesis and subsequent promotion of growth factor gene transcription results in tumor-promoting intracellular signaling pathways. In Figure 3-3, the agent temsirolimus downregulates HIF by inhibiting mTOR independent of the VHL mutations. Temsirolimus affects the phosphatidylinositol *P13* kinase pathway, which is particularly important in poorer prognosis RCC that is characterized by phosphatase and tensin homolog tumor suppressor (PTEN) loss (Rathmell et al., 2005).

The pathogenesis of papillary or chromophilic RCC is based on mutations of the hepatocyte growth factor and its receptor, met proto-oncogene. Hepatocyte growth factor is present in proximal tubular cells in the kidney and is increased in most patients with all types of RCC (Campbell et al., 2007).

Based on the biology of RCC, many pathways, proteins, receptors, and growth factors have been identified in recent years with the resulting development of effective therapies. In addition to the HIF pathway and its tumor promoting factors, the *Ras* family of proto-oncogenes also is implicated in RCC (Grandinetti & Goldspiel, 2007). The *Ras*-mediated signal transduction pathway involves TGF, EGFR, VEFG, and PDGF with their receptors on the cell surface. These factors activate *Ras*, which then binds to *Raf* and initiates the RAF/MEK/ERK pathway resulting in tumor cell proliferation, angiogenesis, and metastasis (Sridhar, Hedley, & Siu, 2005).

Signs and Symptoms

A triad of signs and symptoms heralds RCC: flank pain, hematuria, and palpable abdominal/renal mass. The presenting symptoms of more than 700 cases of RCC were reviewed in 1971, and the most common were the classic triad with weight loss (Skinner, Colvin, Vermillion, Pfister, & Leadbetter, 1971). Hematuria with clots occurs when tumor invades the collecting duct system, whereas flank pain and a palpable mass represent advanced local disease (Atkins, 2007). RCC involving the lower pole of the kidney and thin habitus leads to a more palpable tumor. Men can present with left scrotal varicocele if the tumor has invaded the junction of where the gonadal vein enters the renal vein. Inferior vena cava infiltration or compression can lead to lower extremity edema, ascites, hepatic dysfunction, or pulmonary embolism (Atkins).

Other presenting signs and symptoms are related to either metastatic disease or paraneoplastic syndromes. Because the kidneys secrete substances such as renin, erythropoietin, prostaglandins, and 1,25-dihydroxycholecalciferol, tumors of the kidney may secrete additional amounts of these, as well as hormone-like peptides or cytokines that function similarly to our natural hormones and cytokines. One such cytokine that is elevated in RCC is interleukin-6 (IL-6). These substances all have physiologic effects and are most likely the cause of symptoms such as hypertension, anemia, weight loss, and fever (Campbell et al., 2007; Gold, Fefer, & Thompson, 1996). Sufrin, Chasan, Golio, and Murphy (1989) proposed that hypertension may be caused not only by renin production from the tumor but also involvement of the renal artery or an arteriovenous fistula inside the tumor.

Anemia is present in approximately one-third of patients with advanced disease, may precede diagnosis, and is similar to anemia of chronic disease (McDougal & Garnick, 2006). Cachexia is found in about 30% of patients and predicts a poorer prognosis after controlling for factors such as grade, stage, and performance status (Kim et al., 2003). Thirty percent of patients will report fever that is usually intermittent, and may present with night sweats and fatigue (Atkins, 2007).

About 5% of patients with RCC develop hypercalcemia caused by malignancy. It is either a humoral hypercalcemia caused by a tumor-produced physiologically active bone-resorption factor or osteolytic hypercalcemia caused by bone metastases (Gold et al., 1996). Symptoms associated with hypercalcemia include nausea, anorexia, fatigue, constipation, confusion, and loss of deep tendon reflexes. Treatment is directed at reducing tumor burden, providing adequate hydration, and administering bisphosphonates.

Hepatic dysfunction not caused by tumor infiltration or Stauffer syndrome is another less common paraneoplastic syndrome (Rosenblum, 1987). Patients have elevated serum

Figure 3-3. Hypoxia-Inducible Factor Expression in the Normoxic State and in Clear Cell Renal Cell Carcinoma

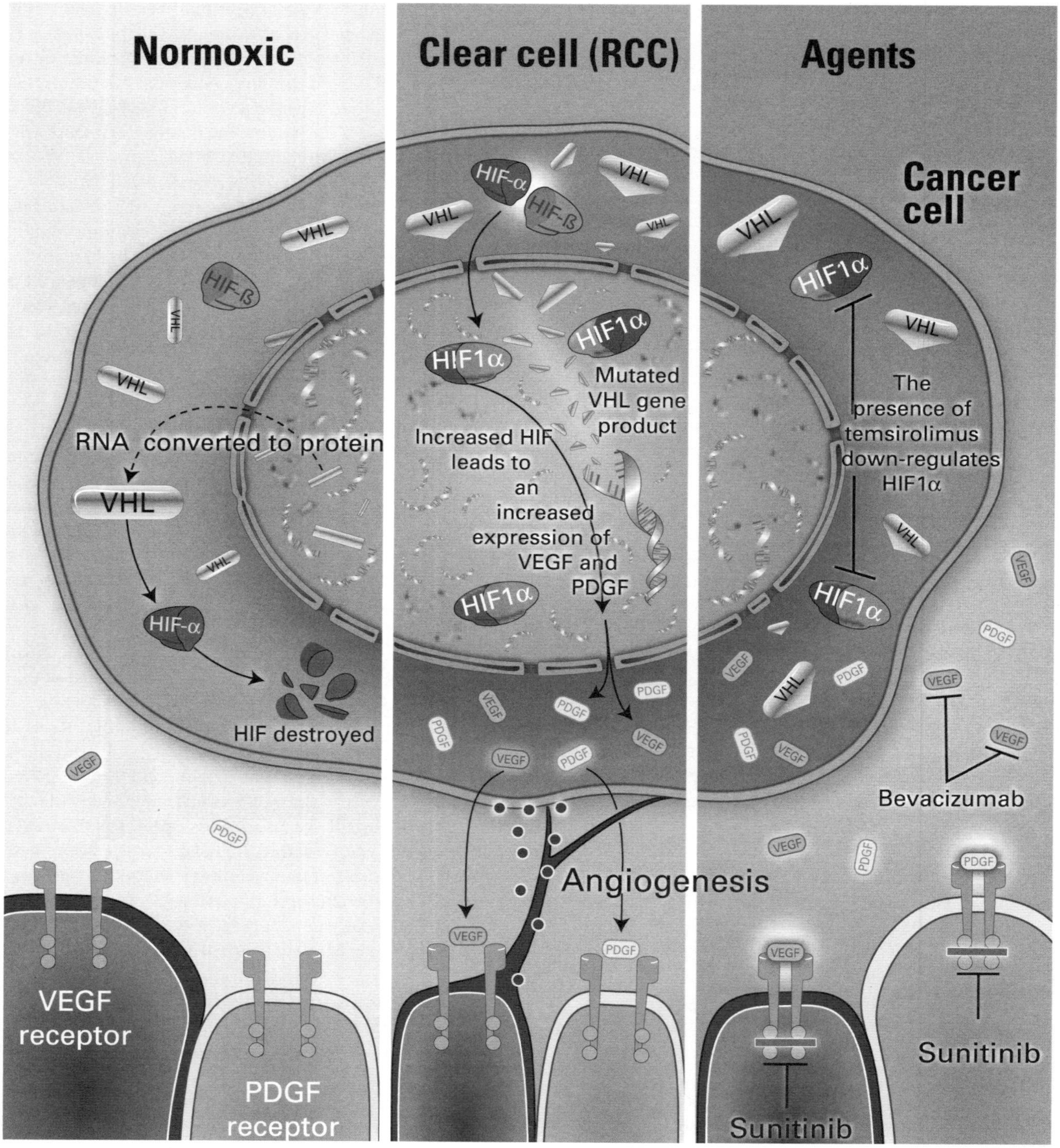

VHL pathway in clear-cell cancer of the kidney with examples of where agents (temsirolimus [or RAD001], bevacizumab, sunitinib [or sorafenib, pazopanib]) target the pathway.

Note. From "Targeted Therapy for Renal Cell Carcinoma," by R.J. Motzer and R.M. Bukowski, 2006, *Journal of Clinical Oncology, 24*(35), p. 5603. Copyright 2006 by American Society of Clinical Oncology. Reprinted with permission.

alkaline phosphatase, elevated prothrombin time, hypoalbuminemia, and elevated bilirubin or transaminases because of a nonspecific hepatitis caused by cytokines including IL-6 (Campbell et al., 2007; Gold et al., 1996; Sufrin et al., 1989). This can induce thrombocytopenia and neutropenia, with tumor resection being the only viable treatment.

Sites of Metastatic Disease

Approximately 25% of patients have locally advanced disease at the time of diagnosis, whereas 30% of patients have metastatic disease (Rodriguez & Sexton, 2006; Sachdeva, Makhoul, Javeed, & Curti, 2008). Table 3-10 lists the sites and incidence of metastasis, with lung as the most common followed by soft tissue, bone, and liver metastases. The pattern of dissemination follows lymphatic and hematogenous routes. RCC staging is also based on vascular and lymph node involvement. The hematogenous spread to the brain, skull, vertebrae, ribs, and sternum is via retrograde collateral flow by way of the lumbar veins into the Batson plexus (Scatarige, Sheth, Corl, & Fishman, 2001).

Table 3-10. Sites of Metastases With Renal Cell Carcinoma	
Site of Metastasis	**Incidence**
Lung	75%
Soft tissue	36%
Bone	20%
Liver	18%
Central nervous system	8%
Cutaneous sites	8%
Note. Based on information from Maldazys & deKernion, 1986.	

Diagnostic Studies

About 25% of all RCCs are identified incidentally on radiologic tests performed for another medical indication (Siow et al., 2000; Sweeney, Thornhill, Grainger, McDermott, & Butler, 1996). According to the National Comprehensive Cancer Network (NCCN, 2009) guidelines, if a renal mass is suspected, patients should have a complete history and physical examination; laboratory studies including complete blood count, comprehensive metabolic panel, lactate dehydrogenase (LDH), clotting studies, and urinalysis; and imaging studies, including abdominal/pelvic CT, and chest x-ray or CT. An abdominal MRI should be done if the CT suggests caval thrombosis, renal vein involvement, or renal insufficiency. If clinically indicated,

a needle biopsy should be performed. It will determine the level of extension of the caval thrombosis and better visualize the renal vein. A bone scan should be obtained if bone metastases are suspected or if the alkaline phosphatase is elevated. An MRI of the brain should be obtained only if clinically indicated. If a central renal mass is present and transitional cell carcinoma needs to be excluded, a urine cytology and ureteroscopy may be necessary to confirm the diagnosis (NCCN).

A current dilemma facing urologists is the small renal lesion, less than 1 cm, which is identified on a scan that was obtained for another reason. These have been referred to as a renal *incidentaloma* because they are an incidental finding and cause no clinical symptoms (Stone, 2006). Many benign conditions can present on a scan and appear similar to an early RCC. The benign diagnoses include benign cysts, pseudotumors, vascular malformations, angiomyolipomas, and oncocytomas. Malignant differential diagnoses include Wilms tumor, metastasis from another primary cancer, sarcoma, and lymphoma (Sachdeva et al., 2008).

Fine needle aspiration biopsy may not be possible because of the size or location of the lesion, complications with the procedure, and a high false-negative rate (Lane et al., 2008). Many patients have difficulty taking a wait-and-see attitude, leading to many unnecessary surgical procedures, including partial or total nephrectomy. These, in turn, can lead to renal insufficiency, hypertension, and other long-term medical sequelae.

The problem of clearly identifying the RCC prior to surgery has led the search for an imaging study to differentiate clear cell RCC, the most common and more aggressive type, from other malignant and benign tumors. Recently, a radiolabeled monoclonal antibody, G250, used with a positron-emission tomography (PET) scan, has been shown to target and bind to clear cell renal carcinoma. Additionally, G250 reacts against an enzyme, carbonic anhydrase IX (CAIX) antigen, which is present in 94% of renal carcinomas (Memorial Sloan-Kettering Cancer Center, 2007). PET scan has more than 94% sensitivity and may be used in the future to help to identify, stage, clinically manage, and determine response to treatment in clear cell RCC. This will help to reduce unnecessary surgery to remove benign and low-grade tumors such as oncocytoma and chromophobe.

Tumor Markers

Tumor markers are proteins released by cancer cells and are used to detect tumors, predict outcome, and determine response to therapy (National Cancer Institute, 2007). Currently, no reliable and sensitive tumor markers in RCC can perform these functions; however, much promising research is developing in this area. A number of proteins that have been identified in the carcinogenesis of RCC are being investigated, including G250/CAIX, and Ki-67 (Grabmaier et al., 2000). CAIX is expressed in 80%–90% of RCCs. Some studies have found that decreased expression of CAIX predicted a poorer prognosis, whereas another study showed that was not an independent predictor when the grade of the tumor was considered (Bui et al., 2003, 2004; Leibovich et al., 2007). Ki-67 is a ubiquitous nuclear antigen that is a marker for cellular proliferation. Increased Ki-67 expression has been associated with more aggressive cancers and a poorer prognosis (Bui et al., 2003, 2004; Grabmaier et al.; Li, Feng, Gentil-Perret, Genin, & Tostain, 2007).

Other potential tumor markers include CD70, a transmembrane protein of the tumor necrosis factor family that is present in clear cell RCC, cytokines IL-6 and IL-8, as well as C-reactive protein (CRP), an indicator of inflammation (Junker et al., 2005). Normal kidney tissue does not express CD70, whereas all clear cell RCCs highly express CD70 (Junker et al.). IL-6 historically has been found in high levels in clear cell RCC. Guida, Casamassima, Monticelli, Quaranta, and Colucci (2007) looked at IL-6, IL-8, CRP, and survival in patients with RCC and healthy volunteers. High levels of IL-6, IL-8, and CRP were associated with shorter survival, whereas high levels of IL-12 were associated with longer survival (Guida et al.).

Staging

Table 3-11 lists the current staging system used in RCC, which is the TNM system developed with input from the International Union Against Cancer and AJCC (Greene et al., 2002). It was most recently revised to incorporate current clinical evidence in the biology and prognosis of renal cell tumors (Greene et al., 2006).

The original staging system is the Flocks and Kadesky system that was developed in 1958 and revised by Robson, Churchill, and Anderson in 1969. These staging systems relied mainly on size of the tumor and presence or absence of vascular or lymph node involvement and metastases (Flocks & Kadesky, 1958; Robson, Churchill, & Anderson, 1969).

The TNM system incorporates specific, objective measurements, such as 7 cm being the cut off for stage T1. This is based on evidence that larger tumors had a poorer prognosis and smaller tumors had a similar prognosis (Greene et al., 2002). Invasion of Gerota fascia determines T3 versus T4, and three levels of T3 are defined by the presence or absence of adrenal or vascular involvement (Greene et al., 2002).

Currently, the following four areas of controversy exist concerning the TNM system (Nguyen & Campbell, 2006).
- Perinephric involvement
- Vascular tumor thrombus
- Adrenal involvement
- Invasion of the collecting duct

In the past, perirenal fat invasion carried a worse prognosis than organ-confined tumors. Recently, Siemer et al. (2005) showed that it does not hold any prognostic significance. Invasion of perisinus fat, however, reflects the more aggressive behavior of these tumors because of the close

proximity of the tumor to vascular and lymphatic structures with the hilum (Nguyen & Campbell, 2006).

The Mayo Clinic has used not only perinephric or perisinus fat invasion but also the level of venous tumor thrombi and presence of IVC invasion to stage renal tumors. Tumors

Table 3-11. American Joint Committee on Cancer Staging System for Renal Cell Carcinoma

Classification	Description
Primary Tumor (T)	
TX	Primary tumor cannot be assessed
T0	No evidence of primary tumor
T1	Tumor 7.0 cm or less in greatest dimension, limited to the kidney
T2	Tumor more than 7.0 cm in greatest dimension, limited to the kidney
T3	Tumor extends into major veins or invades adrenal gland or perinephric tissues but not beyond Gerota fascia
• T3a	• Tumor invades adrenal gland or perinephric tissues but not beyond Gerota fascia
• T3b	• Tumor grossly extends into renal vein(s) or vena cava below diaphragm
• T3c	• Tumor grossly extends into vena cava above diaphragm
T4	T4 Tumor invades beyond Gerota fascia
Regional Lymph Nodes (N) (Hilar, abdominal para-aortic, and paracaval nodes. Laterality has no effect)	
NX	Regional lymph nodes cannot be assessed
N0	No regional lymph node metastases
N1	Metastasis in a single regional lymph node
N2	Metastases in more than one regional lymph node
Distant Metastasis (M)	
MX	Distant metastasis cannot be assessed
M0	No distant metastases
M1	Distant metastases
TNM Grouping	
Stage I	T1 N0 M0
Stage II	T2 N0 M0
Stage III	T1 N1 M0 or T2 N1 M0 or T3 N0 or N1 M0
Stage IV	T4 N0, N1 M0 or any T N2 M0 or any T any N M1

Note. From *AJCC Cancer Staging Manual* (6th ed., pp. 323–325), by F.L. Greene, D.L. Page, I.D. Fleming, A. Fritz, C.M. Balch, D.G. Haller, et al. (Eds.), 2002, New York: Springer.

Copyright 2002 by American Joint Committee on Cancer. Adapted with permission.

with perisinus fat invasion and high IVC thrombus, and a level IV or high-level thrombus alone, hold a poorer prognosis (Leibovich et al., 2005). In the current TNM classification, adrenal involvement that is ipsilateral is considered T3a, and many feel that it holds a poor prognosis similar to T4 and metastatic disease. If the adrenal involvement is a result of direct extension, it is more positive and may be considered T4; however, all other adrenal involvement is considered metastatic disease (Nguyen & Campbell, 2006). Invasion of the collecting system has not been included in the current TNM system. It usually presents with other poor prognostic factors such as larger size, vascular invasion, and lymph node involvement. Because of this, it is doubtful that this parameter will be included in the TNM system (Nguyen & Campbell).

A useful tool to help predict survival is the *Motzer Score*, which is the sum of five prognostic factors that have been shown to predict survival from recurrence after nephrectomy (Eggener et al., 2006). The patient is assigned a point for each factor as follows.
- Hemoglobin less than lower limit of normal
- LDH > 1.5 times upper limit of normal
- Karnofsky performance status < 80%
- Serum calcium > 10 mg/dl
- Recurrence < 12 months after nephrectomy

Survival was greatest in the group that had a zero score and was poorest, less than six months, in the group scoring 3–5 points (Eggener et al., 2006).

Nursing History and Assessment

Initial assessment of the patient is directed by where in the diagnostic process a patient presents. During a general physical examination, nurses can encounter patients who present with symptoms that suggest a renal malignancy, or they may see patients who are looking for clarification of a lesion found on a radiologic evaluation. Nurses must perform a thorough history and assessment to identify those signs and symptoms that can suggest primary disease, metastatic disease, or related and paraneoplastic syndromes.

Family history is significant because a proportion of RCCs are related to genetic syndromes. Nurses need to be aware of syndromes such as HPRCC, HLRCC, and von Hippel-Lindau disease, as well as cystic disease of the kidneys and tubular sclerosis. Tubular sclerosis is an autosomal dominant disorder that is characterized by mental retardation, renal cysts, angiomyolipomas, seizure disorder, and a skin lesion referred to as adenoma sebaceum (Choyke et al., 2003).

Physical examination includes a thorough abdominal examination. A flank mass is palpable if it is in the lower pole of the kidney. The mass will not be tender but will feel firm and consolidated, and will change position with inspiration and expiration (Atkins, 2007). Constitutional symptoms also need to be assessed, and any bone pain or neurologic symptoms pursued.

Emotionally, the patient and family are dealing with a very serious cancer diagnosis and need education, support, and symptom management. The type of treatment will dictate the nursing plan and interventions, but presenting symptoms need to be addressed, especially if the patient is experiencing pain or any other urgent medical condition such as hypercalcemia.

Testicular Cancer

Introduction

Testicular cancers are the most common solid tumors in men between the ages of 15 and 35 and were estimated to be diagnosed in approximately 8,000 men in the United States in 2008 (American Cancer Society [ACS], 2008). Although testicular cancer is relatively rare, rates vary considerably by race and geographic locations. For instance, the disease occurs in white men five times more often than in black men (McGlynn et al., 2003). Several studies have demonstrated an increased incidence of testicular cancer over the past 40 years. Industrialized nations have the highest reported incidence and include Scandinavia, Switzerland, and Germany. The United States and Great Britain have an intermediate incidence, whereas countries in Africa and Asia have the lowest incidence (Huyghe, Matsuda, & Thonneau, 2003).

This section will present an overview of the pathophysiology of testicular cancer with a particular focus on germ cell tumors (GCTs), which comprise most testicular cancers. In addition, clinical nursing issues for testicular cancer, including signs and symptoms, sites of metastatic disease, diagnostic studies, workup, tumor markers, staging, and nursing history and assessment, will be addressed.

Origin of Testicular Cancer Cells

The two main types of testicular tumors are sex cord stromal tumors, which are rare and account for only about 5% of testicular tumors, and GCTs, which account for the vast majority (95%) of testicular tumors and are the focus of this chapter (Bahrami, Ro, & Ayala, 2007). Sex cord stromal tumors develop from the gonadal stroma. GCTs develop through malignant transformation of a fetal cell from the primordial germ cell line. Most GCTs originate in the testis from cells that would ordinarily develop into sperm (spermatogonia). A minority (10%) of GCTs originate outside the gonads (typically in the brain, chest, or abdomen) (Bosl & Motzer, 1997; Bosl, Sheinfeld, Bajorin, Motzer, & Chaganti, 2005).

Many features of the adult testes reflect their developmental origin in the abdomen. In utero, the testicles originate in the retroperitoneum and descend along the spermatic cord into the scrotum. Lymphatic drainage of the testes follows this same path back to the retroperitoneum. Therefore, the retroperitoneum is most often the first site of metastasis.

Almost all adult testicular GCTs begin as *intratubular germ cell neoplasia, unclassified* (IGCNU) and progress to become invasive. The average time from appearance of IGCNU to invasive carcinoma is five years (Bahrami et al., 2007; Skakkebaek, Berthelsen, & Muller, 1982).

Types of Germ Cell Tumors

GCTs are subdivided into two types: pure seminoma and nonseminoma. Approximately half of GCTs are classified as pure seminoma and half contain nonseminoma cell types. Because treatment options differ by tumor types, analysis of cell type is critical.

Seminomas

Seminomas present most frequently in the fourth decade of life. Pure seminomas retain germ cell characteristics and do not differentiate. They are slower growing than nonseminomas and are highly sensitive to radiation. In seminomas, the supporting stroma demonstrates lymphocytic infiltrate or granulomatous reaction. Infrequently, seminomas secrete human chorionic gonadotropin (HCG) (Bosl et al., 2005).

Some seminomas may show increased mitotic activity with atypia. This atypical variant of seminoma lacks the lymphocytic infiltrate and granulomatous reaction and is characterized by necrosis. These tumors should be distinguished from forms of embryonal carcinoma and yolk sac tumor, which are nonseminomatous and therefore require different treatment. Treatment and prognosis for atypical seminoma is the same as for any seminoma (Bosl et al., 2005).

Spermatocytic seminoma is a rare variant usually seen in men older than 40 years of age. Spermatocytic seminoma is not associated with IGCNU, carries a good prognosis, and has minimal metastatic potential (Sesterhenn & Davis, 2004).

Nonseminomas

Nonseminomatous GCTs (NSGCTs) peak in the third decade of life. They may be pure or, more commonly, they may consist of a mixture of two or more histologic subtypes. Nonseminomas are not sensitive to radiation. Types of nonseminomas include embryonal carcinoma, choriocarcinoma, yolk sac carcinoma, and teratoma (Bahrami et al., 2007; Bosl & Motzer, 1997).

Embryonal carcinoma is the most undifferentiated cell type and makes up 3%–4% of GCTs in its pure form. However, it is present in 40% of mixed GCTs. Embryonal carcinomas may secrete both alpha-fetoprotein (AFP) and HCG (Sesterhenn & Davis, 2004).

Choriocarcinoma in its pure form is rare is associated with high HCG levels, extensive hematogenous spread, and a poor prognosis. Most choriocarcinomas present with metastatic symptoms because of their propensity for rapid spread. Hemorrhage into metastatic tumor sites may be life threatening (Bahrami et al., 2007).

Yolk sac tumor, also known as endodermal sinus tumor, mimics the yolk sac of the embryo and produces AFP. Yolk sac tumor is most common in infants and children. Pure yolk sac tumor is rare in adults but is common in mixed GCTs (Sesterhenn & Davis, 2004).

Teratoma refers to a varied group of tumors that differentiate to form somatic-type tissues. Mature teratoma refers to adult-type elements such as cartilage or nerve tissue. Immature teratoma refers to partial differentiation of cells as seen in a fetus. Both are histologically benign and do not secrete markers. However, many cases of pure teratoma can develop the ability to metastasize. For this reason, any adult testicular pure teratoma should be considered fully malignant, and management should proceed as if malignant elements are present (Rabbani et al., 2003). See Figure 3-4 for the histologic classification of testicular tumors.

Risk Factors

The exact cause of testicular cancer is unknown, and few risk factors have been identified. Undescended testes, or cryptorchidism, is one known risk factor. Early orchiopexy performed before puberty has been shown to reduce the risk of GCTs (Herrinton, Zhao, & Husson, 2003). An increased

---

Figure 3-4. Histologic Classification of Testicular Neoplasms

Germ cell tumors
- Seminoma
  - Classic (typical)
  - Atypical
  - Spermatocytic
- Nonseminomatous
  - Embryonal carcinoma
  - Teratoma
  - Mature
  - Immature

Mature or immature, with malignant transformation
- Sex cord stromal tumors
  - Sertoli cell tumor
  - Leydig cell tumor
  - Granulosa cell tumor
  - Mixed types (e.g., Sertoli-Leydig cell tumor)
  - Unclassified
- Mixed germ cell and stromal elements
  - Gonadoblastoma
- Adnexal and paratesticular tumors
  - Adenocarcinoma of rete testis
  - Mesothelioma
- Miscellaneous tumors
  - Carcinoid
  - Lymphoma
  - Testicular metastases

Note. From "Testicular Germ-Cell Cancer," by G.J. Bosl and R.J. Motzer, 1997, *New England Journal of Medicine, 337*(4), p. 242. Copyright 1997 by Massachusetts Medical Society. All rights reserved. Adapted with permission.

incidence of mediastinal GCT has been found in boys and men with Klinefelter syndrome, a condition characterized by small, firm testes, azoospermia, gynecomastia, and elevated levels of plasma gonadotropins (Nichols et al., 1987). Familial clustering of GCT, particularly among siblings, has been observed, but recent studies have yet to reveal linkage to a specific gene (Bridges & Hussain, 2007).

Despite recognition of some risk factors for GCTs, the etiology of GCTs, including the contributing role of environmental factors such as diethylstilbestrol exposure, vasectomy, trauma, viral infection, or genetic susceptibility, remains unknown (Dieckmann & Pichlmeier, 2004).

Carcinogenesis

Testicular GCT is a disease of the post-pubescent male. One or more copies of an isochromosome of the short arm of chromosome 12 (i12p) or other forms of 12p amplification are found in all GCTs (Bosl & Motzer, 1997; Reuter, 2005). Gene expression profiling studies have identified the target genes mapped to 12p and overexpressed in both IGCNU and GCTs. These studies revealed several genes (*CCND2, GLUT3, NANOG, DPPA3,* and *GDF3*) involved in cell growth, self-renewal, and pluripotency (Korkola et al., 2005). Older studies have linked cisplatin chemotherapy resistance to a genetic mutation of *TP53* (Houldsworth et al., 1998). The understanding and identification of the biology of GCTs is still in an early phase, and further understanding may help improve treatment for this and other cancers.

Signs and Symptoms

Most patients present with testicular swelling and discomfort. A minority of patients present with a painless testicular mass. A trial of antibiotics can be undertaken for presumed orchitis or epididymitis, but if symptoms are not relieved within two to four weeks, a testicular ultrasound should be performed. Testicular trauma may prompt an evaluation by a healthcare provider. Rarely, testicular cancer is discovered during an infertility workup. The differential diagnosis for a testicular mass includes hydrocele, testicular torsion, hernia, hematoma, and spermatocele.

Almost half of patients present with symptoms of metastatic disease, including (Bosl et al., 1981, 2005)
- Neck mass from supraclavicular lymph node metastasis
- Cough
- Hemoptysis or dyspnea from pulmonary metastasis
- Lumbar back pain from retroperitoneal lymph node metastasis involving the psoas muscle or nerve roots
- Bone pain from skeletal metastasis (varies with the site of metastasis)
- Rarely, gynecomastia occurs as a result of elevated HCG (Tseng et al., 1985).

A small percentage of patients present with extragonadal GCTs. The most common sites for extragonadal GCTs are the mediastinum, the retroperitoneum, and rarely, the pineal gland. Presenting symptoms for extragonadal GCTs include chest pain, shortness of breath, and back pain. Very rarely, patients present with cord compression from vertebral metastasis. The workup for extragonadal GCTs should always include a scrotal ultrasound to rule out an occult testicular primary tumor or a burned-out primary tumor (a testicular tumor that has completely regressed). Determining that the testis is the organ of an extragonadal GCT origin is crucial as the patient's prognosis and treatment may differ based on site of origin (Bosl et al., 2005).

Sites of Metastatic Disease

Testicular cancer generally spreads in a predictable, step-wise fashion. The testicular arteries arise directly from the abdominal aorta. The right testicular vein drains into the inferior vena cava, and the left testicular vein drains into the left renal vein. Testicular lymphatic drainage follows the testicular vessels in the spermatic cord back to the retroperitoneal lymph nodes. The primary site for metastasis from a right testicular tumor is the interaortocaval lymph nodes between the aorta and the inferior vena cava. The primary site of metastasis from a left testicular tumor is the preaortic and para-aortic lymph nodes lateral to the aorta (Donohue, Zachary, & Maynard, 1982). Superior to the renal vessels, the lymphatic drainage continues to the retrocrural and posterior mediastinal lymph nodes. Rarely, metastatic spread will skip the retroperitoneum and present as left supraclavicular and/or pulmonary metastases. Metastatic spread to the liver, bone, or brain may occur in advanced disease (Bosl & Motzer, 1997).

Diagnostic Studies

Workup for testicular cancer should include a physical examination of
- Neck for supraclavicular or cervical lymphadenopathy
- Lungs
- Breasts for gynecomastia
- Abdomen for retroperitoneal masses
- Testicles.

Scrotal ultrasound is a noninvasive and reliable tool used to exclude hydrocele or epididymitis and should be obtained if any suspicion of testicular tumor exists. When positive, the ultrasound shows a mass inside the testicle. One or more hypoechoic masses may be present (Bosl & Motzer, 1997). Fine needle biopsy of a testicular mass is contraindicated because of an increased risk of local spread from tumor seeding (Bosl & Motzer). Instead, radical inguinal orchiectomy is the only acceptable diagnostic and therapeutic procedure. The use of an inguinal incision with high ligation of the spermatic cord decreases the risk of local recurrence and lymphatic spread (Fung & Garnick, 1988). A trans-scrotal orchiectomy is contraindicated because it may alter the lymphatic drainage of the inguinal and pelvic lymph nodes, thus predisposing the patient to scrotal, inguinal, and pelvic nodal metastases (Bosl et al., 2005).

Staging includes reviewing CT scans with contrast of the chest, abdomen, and pelvis to evaluate for metastatic disease. PET scanning fails to detect small-volume lymphadenopathy and does not improve staging (Huddart et al., 2007). However, PET scanning has been shown to be a useful predictor of viable tumor in cases of postchemotherapy residual disease involving pure seminoma, especially with residual masses larger than 3 cm (DeSantis et al., 2001).

Tumor Markers

Alpha-Fetoprotein

AFP is a glycoprotein normally produced by the fetal yolk sac. Nonseminomatous GCTs, specifically embryonal carcinoma and yolk sac tumor, also may produce AFP. Elevated levels also may occur in liver disease, hepatocellular carcinoma, or other gastrointestinal cancers, but are never seen in pure seminoma.

The normal adult serum concentration of AFP usually is less than 15 ng/ml. Elevations in serum AFP occur in 20%–40% of clinical stage II and 40%–60% of advanced NSGCTs (Bosl et al., 2005).

Human Chorionic Gonadotropin

A smaller glycoprotein molecule than AFP, HCG normally is produced by the embryo soon after conception and by syncytiotrophoblasts (part of the placenta) later in pregnancy. With GCTs, an increased concentration of HCG may occur in both seminomas and nonseminomatous tumors. Human chorionic gonadotropin consists of an alpha and beta subunit. The alpha subunit of HCG is common to several pituitary hormones, including luteinizing hormone, follicle-stimulating hormone, and thyroid-stimulating hormone. The beta subunits of HCG are similar to the alpha subunits but have different amino-acid sequences. Most commercial laboratories use the World Health Organization's standard code and are able to detect the beta subunit. Normal levels in men or nonpregnant women are less than 5 IU/ml. False-positive elevations may occur in hypogonadal states related to treatment (Bosl & Motzer, 1997).

Lactate Dehydrogenase

LDH is a less specific tumor marker that adds prognostic value for patients with advanced GCTs. A marker of tumor burden, growth rate, and cellular proliferation, LDH is elevated in approximately 60% of patients with advanced NSGCT. In 80% of patients with advanced seminoma, the LDH may be elevated, and in patients with advanced nonseminomatous disease, a significantly elevated serum LDH is associated with a worse prognosis. However, serum LDH is not a sensitive or specific early marker of disease recurrence (Bosl et al., 2005).

Tumor Marker Evaluation

Serum tumor markers should be evaluated before, during, and after treatment and throughout long-term follow-up. The half-life of AFP is 5–7 days, and the half-life of HCG is approximately 30 hours. A slow decline or plateau during treatment may suggest residual active disease (Toner, Geller, Tan, Nisselbaum, & Bosl, 1990). A rise in serum tumor markers during the post-treatment follow-up period is often the first sign of disease recurrence (Toner et al.).

Staging

Revised TNM and stage groupings of the AJCC and the International Union Against Cancer were adopted in 1997. In the TNM system, assessments of primary tumor (T), lymph node (N), and distant metastasis (M) are combined with those of serum tumor markers to define stage groupings from I to III. The serum concentrations of tumor markers are incorporated into an "S" category because of their independent prognostic value (Greene et al., 2002).

Stage I germ cell testicular cancer is defined as disease confined to the testis. Pathologic stage II disease involves metastases to the retroperitoneal lymph nodes with either microscopic (IIA) or macroscopic disease (IIB). Stage III disease involves metastases to nonretroperitoneal lymph nodes (e.g., pelvic, supradiaphragmatic), lung, visceral sites, or increased serum tumor markers (Bosl et al., 2005). See Table 3-12 for TNM staging.

Nursing History and Assessment

A nursing history includes obtaining information regarding a family history of testicular cancer and a personal history of undescended testes, recurrent orchitis or epididymitis, trauma, gynecomastia, or infertility. Nursing assessment includes evaluation for signs or symptoms of progressive disease such as back pain, shortness of breath, or hemoptysis.

A psychosocial history should include personal or family history of depression or anxiety disorders, as these conditions may be exacerbated by cancer diagnosis and treatment. Counseling, social service, and/or a psychiatric consult should be offered when appropriate. Practical issues such as lack of transportation or disruptions in work, school, and family life may weaken and interfere with acceptance and compliance with therapy.

A diagnosis of testicular cancer can be extremely stressful for patients and their families. Assessment for patient and family knowledge deficits regarding disease process and treatment effects should be ongoing.

In summary, testicular GCTs are the most common neoplasm in young adult males. The etiology of GCTs remains largely unknown. GCTs are classified by their histology and divided into two types: pure seminoma and nonseminoma.

Table 3-12. American Joint Committee on Cancer Staging System for Testis Tumors	
Classification	**Description**
Primary Tumor (PT)	
pTX	Primary tumor cannot be assessed (if no radical orchiectomy has been performed, TX is used)
pT0	No evidence of primary tumor (e.g., histologic scar in testis)
pTis	Intratubular germ cell neoplasia (carcinoma in situ)
pT1	Tumor limited to the testis and epididymis without vascular/lymphatic invasion. Tumor may invade into the tunica albuginea but not the tunica vaginalis
pT2	Tumor limited to the testis and epididymis with vascular/lymphatic invasion or tumor extending through the tunica albuginea with involvement of the tunica vaginalis
pT3	Tumor invades the spermatic cord with or without vascular/lymphatic invasion
pT4	Tumor invades the scrotum with or without vascular/lymphatic invasion
Regional Lymph Nodes (N)	
Clinical	
NX	Regional lymph nodes cannot be assessed
N0	No regional lymph node metastasis
N1	Metastasis with a lymph node mass ≤ 2 cm in greatest dimension; or multiple lymph nodes, none > 2 cm in greatest dimension
N2	Metastasis with a lymph node mass > 2 cm but not > 5 cm in greatest dimension; or multiple lymph nodes, any one mass > 2 cm but not > 5 cm in greatest dimension
N3	Metastasis with a lymph node mass > 5 cm in greatest dimension
Pathologic (pN)	
pNX	Regional lymph nodes cannot be assessed
pN0	No evidence of tumor in lymph nodes
pN1	Metastasis with a lymph node mass ≤ 2 cm in greatest dimension and ≤ 5 nodes positive, none > 2 cm in greatest dimension
pN2	Metastasis with a lymph node mass > 2 cm but not > 5 cm in greatest dimension; or > 5 nodes positive, none > 5 cm; or evidence of extranodal extension of tumor
pN3	Metastasis with a lymph node mass > 5 cm in greatest dimension
Distant Metastases (M)	
MX	Distant metastasis cannot be assessed
M0	No distant metastasis
M1	Distant metastasis
M1a	Nonregional nodal or pulmonary metastases
M1b	Distant metastasis other than to nonregional lymph nodes and lungs

(Continued on next page)

Table 3-12. American Joint Committee on Cancer Staging System for Testis Tumors *(Continued)*			
Serum Tumor Markers (S)			
	LDH	**HCG (mIU/ml)**	**AFP (ng/ml)**
S1	< 1.5 × N†	< 5,000	< 1,000
S2	1.510 × N†	5,000–50,000	1,000–10,000
S3	> 10 × N†	> 50,000	> 10,000

Stage Grouping	**T**	**N**	**M**	**S**
Stage I				
IA	pT1	N0	M0	S0
IB	pT2	N0	M0	S0
	pT3	N0	M0	S0
	pT4	N0	M0	S0
IS	Any pT/Tx	N0	M0	S1–3
Stage II				
IIA	Any pT/Tx	N1	M0	S0
	Any pT/Tx	N1	M0	S1
IIB	Any pT/Tx	N2	M0	S0
	Any pT/Tx	N2	M0	S1
IIC	Any pT/Tx	N3	M0	S0
	Any pT/Tx	N3	M0	S1
Stage III				
IIIA	Any pT/Tx	Any N	M1a	S0
	Any pT/Tx	Any N	M1a	S1
IIIB	Any pT/Tx	N1–3	M0	S2
	Any pT/Tx	Any N	M1a	S2
IIIC	Any pT/Tx	N1–3	M0	S3
	Any pT/Tx	Any N	M1a	S3
	Any pT/Tx	Any N	M1b	Any S

† N indicates the upper limit of normal for the LDH assay.
AFP—alpha-fetoprotein; HCG—human chorionic gonadotropin; LDH—lactate dehydrogenase

Note. From *AJCC Cancer Staging Manual* (6th ed., pp. 317–322), by F.L. Greene, D.L. Page, I.D. Fleming, A. Fritz, C.M. Balch, D.G. Haller, et al. (Eds.), 2002, New York: Springer. Copyright 2002 by American Joint Committee on Cancer. Reprinted with permission.

Seminomas are slower growing and highly sensitive to radiation. NSGCTs are further subdivided into embryonal carcinoma, choriocarcinoma, yolk sac carcinoma, and teratoma. With appropriate therapy, the majority of GCTs are curable.

Summary

Care of patients with a GU malignancy requires in-depth and updated knowledge of cancer pathophysiology, staging, carcinogenesis, and diagnostic testing so that an individualized treatment plan can be developed for each patient. This chapter reviews the background information in order to prepare nurses to provide patient care and a better understanding of the patient treatment options in the following chapters. Therefore, nurses will be able to deliver comprehensive patient care and patient teaching.

References

Albani, J.M., Ciaschini, M.W., Streem, S.B., Herts, B.R., & Angermeier, K.W. (2007). The role of computerized tomographic urography in the initial evaluation of hematuria. *Journal of Urology, 177*(2), 644–648.

American Cancer Society. (2008). *Cancer facts and figures 2008.* Atlanta, GA: Author.

Amiel, G.E., Shu, T., & Lerner, S.P. (2004). Alternatives to cytology in the management of non–muscle invasive bladder cancer. *Current Treatment Options in Oncology, 5*(5), 377–389.

Ammin, B., Tamboli, P., & Cubilla, A. (2003). Penis and scrotum. In N. Weidner, R. Cote, S. Suster, & L. Weiss (Eds.), *Modern surgical pathology* (pp. 1197–1214). Philadelphia: Elsevier.

Andriole, G. (2008). *Carcinoma of the penis: Epidemiology, risk factors and clinical presentation* [UpToDate]. Retrieved February 5, 2009, from http://www.utdol.com/utd/content/topic.do?topicKey=gucancer/9552&selectedTitle=2~13&source=search_result

Atkins, M.B. (2007). *Clinical manifestations, evaluation, and staging of renal cell carcinoma* [UpToDate]. Retrieved August 19, 2007, from http://www.utdol.com/utd/content/topic.do?topicKey=gucancer/4484

Bahrami, A., Ro, J.Y., & Ayala, A.G. (2007). An overview of testicular germ cell tumors. *Archives of Pathology and Laboratory Medicine, 131*(8), 1267–1280.

Bajaj, A., Sokhi, H., & Rajesh, A. (2007). Intravenous urography for diagnosing synchronous upper-tract tumours in patients with newly diagnosed bladder carcinoma can be restricted to patients with high-risk superficial disease. *Clinical Radiology, 62*(9), 854–857.

Barnholtz-Sloan, J., Maldonado, J., Pow-sang, J., & Guiliano, A. (2007). Incidence trends in primary malignant penile cancer. *Urologic Oncology, 25*(5), 361–367.

Bassi, P., De Marco, V., De Lisa, A., Mancini, M., Pinto, F., Bertoloni, R., et al. (2005). Non-invasive diagnostic tests for bladder cancer: A review of the literature. *Urologia Internationalis, 75*(3), 193–200.

Bleeker, M., Heideman, D., Snijders, P., Horenblas, S., Dillner, J., & Meijer, C.J. (2009). Penile cancer: Epidemiology, pathogenesis, and prevention. *World Journal of Urology, 27*(2), 141–150.

Borden, L.S., Jr., Clark, P.E., & Hall, M.C. (2005). Bladder cancer. *Current Opinion in Oncology, 17*(3), 275–280.

Bosl, G.J., & Motzer R.J. (1997). Testicular germ-cell cancer. *New England Journal of Medicine, 337*(4), 242–254.

Bosl, G.J., Sheinfeld, J., Bajorin, D.F., Motzer, R.J., & Chaganti, R.S.K. (2005). Cancer of the testis. In V.T. DeVita Jr., S. Hellman, & S.A. Rosenberg (Eds.), *Cancer: Principles and practice of oncology* (7th ed., pp. 1269–1293). Philadelphia: Lippincott Williams & Wilkins.

Bosl, G.J., Vogelzang, N.J., Goldman, A., Fraley, E.E., Lange, P.H., Levitt, S.H., et al. (1981). Impact of delay in diagnosis on clinical stage of testicular cancer. *Lancet, 318*(8253), 970–973.

Botteman, M.F., Pashos, C.L., Redaelli, A., Laskin, B., & Hauser, R. (2003). The health economics of bladder cancer: A comprehensive review of the published literature. *Pharmacoeconomics, 21*(18), 1315–1330.

Brauers, A., Buettner, R., & Jakse, G. (2001). Second resection and prognosis of primary high risk superficial bladder cancer: Is cystectomy often too early? *Journal of Urology, 165*(3), 808–810.

Brosman, S. (2008, December). *Penile cancer.* Retrieved February 5, 2008, from http://emedicine.medscape.com/article/446554-overview

Bridges, B., & Hussain, A. (2007). Testicular germ cell tumors. *Current Opinion in Oncology, 19*(3), 222–228.

Broders, A.C. (1921). Squamous-cell epithelioma of the skin: A study of 256 cases. *Annals of Surgery, 73*(2), 141–143.

Bui, M.H., Seligson, D., Han, K.R., Pantuck, A.J., Dorey, F.J., Huang,Y., et al. (2003). Carbonic anhydrase IX is an independent predictor of survival in advanced renal clear cell carcinoma: Implications for prognosis and therapy. *Clinical Cancer Research, 9*(2), 802–811.

Bui, M.H., Visapaa, H., Seligson, D., Kim, H., Han, K.R., Huang, Y., et al. (2004). Prognostic value of carbonic anhydrase IX and KI67 as predictors of survival for renal clear cell carcinoma. *Journal of Urology, 171*(6, Pt.1), 2461–2466.

Burgers, J.K., Badalament, R.A., & Drago, J.R. (1992). Penile cancer. Clinical presentation, diagnosis and staging. *Urologic Clinics of North America, 19*(2), 247–256.

Busby, J.E., & Pettaway, C.A. (2005). What's new in the management of penile cancer? *Current Opinion in Urology, 15*(5), 350–357.

Cabanas, R.M. (1977). An approach for the treatment of penile carcinoma. *Cancer, 39*(2), 456–466.

Campbell, S.C., Novick, A.C., & Bukowski, R.M. (2007). Renal tumors. In A.J. Wein, L.R. Kavoussi, A.N. Partin, & C.A. Peters (Eds.), *Campbell-Walsh urology* (9th ed., pp. 1567–1637). Philadelphia: Saunders.

Campos, R.S., Lopes, A., Guimares, G.C., Carvalho, A.L., & Soares, F.A. (2006). E-cadherin, MMP-2 and MMP-9 as prognostic markers in penile cancer: Analysis of 125 patients. *Urology, 67*(4), 797–802.

Cangiano, T., Liao, J., Naitoh, J., Dorey, F., Figlin, R., & Belldegrun, A. (1999). Sarcomatoid renal cell carcinoma: Biologic behavior, prognosis, and response to combined surgical resection and immunotherapy. *Journal of Clinical Oncology, 17*(2), 523–528.

Cheng, L., Neumann, R.M., Nehra, A., Spotts, B.E., Weaver, A.L., & Bostwick, D.G. (2000). Cancer heterogeneity and its biologic implications in the grading of urothelial carcinoma. *Cancer, 88*(7), 1663–1670.

Cheng, L., Pan, C.X., Yang, X.J., Lopez-Beltran, A., MacLennan, G.T., Lin, H., et al. (2004). Small cell carcinoma of the urinary bladder: A clinicopathologic analysis of 64 patients. *Cancer, 101*(5), 957–962.

Cheville, J.C., Lohse, C.M., Zincke, H., Weaver, A.L., Leibovich, B.C., Frank, I., et al. (2004). Sarcomatoid renal cell carcinoma: An examination of underlying histologic subtype and an analysis of associations with patient outcome. *American Journal of Surgical Pathology, 28*(4), 435–441.

Choyke, P.L., Glenn, G.M., Walther, M.M., Zbar, B., & Linehan, W.M. (2003). Hereditary renal cancers. *Radiology, 226*(1), 33–46.

Cohen, H.T., & McGovern, F.J. (2005). Renal-cell carcinoma. *New England Journal of Medicine, 353*(23), 2477–2490.

Comperat, E., Bieche, I., Dargere, D., Ferlicot, S., Laurendeau, I., Benoit, G., et al. (2007). p63 gene expression study and early bladder carcinogenesis. *Urology, 70*(3), 459–462.

Crawford, E.D., & Daneshgari, F. (1992). Management of regional lymphatic drainage in carcinoma of the penis. *Urologic Clinics of North America, 19*(2), 305–317.

Cruz Guerra, N., Saenz Medina, J., Ursua Sarmiento, I., Zamora Martinez, T., Madrigal Montero, R., Diego Pinto, D., et al. (2005). Recidiva malignizada de cuerno cutáneo peneano. [Malignant recurrence of a penile cutaneous horn.] *Archivos Españoles de Urología, 58*(1), 61–63.

Cubilla, A., Piris, A., Pfannl, R., Rodriguez, I., Aguero, F., & Young, R.H. (2001). Anatomic levels: Important landmarks in penectomy specimens: A detailed anatomic and histologic study based on examination of 44 cases. *American Journal of Surgical Pathology, 25*(8), 1091–1094.

Cubilla, A.L., Reuter, V., Velazquez, P., Piris, A., Saito, S., & Young, R.H. (2001). Histologic classification of penile carcinoma and its relation to outcome in 61 patients with primary resection. *International Journal of Surgical Pathology, 9*(2), 111–120.

Daling, J.R., Madeleine, M.M., Johnson, L.G., Schwartz, S.M., Shera, K.A., Wurscher, M.A., et al. (2005). Penile cancer: Importance of circumcision, human papillomavirus and smoking in in situ and invasive disease. *International Journal of Cancer, 116*(4), 606–616.

Datta, S.N., Allen, G.M., Evans, R., Vaughton, K.C., & Lucas, M.G. (2002). Urinary tract ultrasonography in the evaluation of haematuria—report of over 1,000 cases. *Annals of the Royal College of Surgeons England, 84*(3), 203–205.

Delahunt, B. (1999). Sarcomatoid renal carcinoma: The final common dedifferentiation pathway of renal epithelial malignancies. *Pathology, 31*(3), 185–190.

Delahunt, B., Bethwaite, P.B., & Nacey, J.N. (2007). Outcome prediction for renal cell carcinoma: Evaluation of prognostic factors for tumours divided according to histological subtype. *Pathology, 39*(5), 459–465.

DeSantis, M., Bokemeyer, C., Becherer, A., Stoiber, F., Oechsle, K., Kletter, K., et al. (2001). Predictive impact of 2-18fluoro-2-deoxy-D-glucose positron emission tomography for residual postchemotherapy masses in patients with bulky seminoma. *Journal of Clinical Oncology, 19*(17), 3740–3744.

Dewire, D., & Lepor, H. (1992). Anatomic consideration of the penis and its lymphatic drainage. *Urologic Clinics of North America, 19*(2), 211–219.

Dieckmann, K.P., & Pichlmeier, U. (2004). Clinical epidemiology of testicular germ cell tumors. *World Journal of Urology, 22*(1), 2–14.

Donat, S.M. (2003). Evaluation and follow-up strategies for superficial bladder cancer. *Urologic Clinics of North America, 30*(4), 765–776.

Donohue, J.P., Zachary, J.M., & Maynard, B.R. (1982). Distribution of nodal metastases in nonseminomatous testis cancer. *Journal of Urology, 128*(2), 315–320.

Droller, M.J. (2005). Diagnosis and staging of bladder cancer. In J.P. Richie & A.V. D'Amico (Eds.), *Urologic oncology* (pp. 301–316). St. Louis, MO: Elsevier Saunders.

Eggener, S.E., Yossepowitch, O., Pettus, J.A., Snyder, M.E., Motzer, R.J., & Russo, P. (2006). Renal cell carcinoma recurrence after nephrectomy for localized disease: Predicting survival from time of recurrence. *Journal of Clinical Oncology, 24*(19), 3101–3106.

Epstein, J.I., Amin, M.B., Reuter, V.R., & Mostofi, F.K. (1998). The World Health Organization/International Society of Urological Pathology consensus classification of urothelial (transitional cell) neoplasms of the urinary bladder. Bladder Consensus Conference Committee. *American Journal of Surgical Pathology, 22*(12), 1435–1448.

Fassett, R. (1984). Exercise haematuria. *Australian Family Physician, 13*(7), 518–519.

Flocks, R.H., & Kadesky, M.C. (1958). Malignant neoplasms of the kidney: An analysis of 353 patients followed five years or more. *Journal of Urology, 79*(2), 196–201.

Frimberger, D., Linke, R., Meissner, H., Stepp, H., Zaak, D., Hungerhuber, E., et al. (2004). Fluorescence diagnosis: A novel method to guide radical inguinal lymph node dissection in penile cancer. *World Journal of Urology, 22*(2), 150–154.

Frimberger, D., Schneede, P., Hungerhuber, E., Sroka, R., Zaak, D., Siebels, M., et al. (2002). Autofluorescence and 5-aminolevulinic acid induced fluorescence diagnosis of penile carcinoma—new techniques to monitor Nd:YAG laser therapy. *Urological Research, 30*(5), 295–300.

Fuhrman, S.A., Lasky, L.C., & Limas, C. (1982). Prognostic significance of morphologic parameters in renal cell carcinoma. *American Journal of Surgical Pathology, 6*(7), 655–663.

Fung, C.Y., & Garnick, M.B. (1988). Clinical stage I carcinoma of the testis: A review. *Journal of Clinical Oncology, 6*(4), 734–750.

Gallucci, M., Guadagni, F., Marzano, R., Leonardo, C., Merola, R., Sentinelli, S., et al. (2005). Status of the *p53, p16, RB1,* and *HER-2* genes and chromosomes 3, 7, 9, and 17 in advanced bladder cancer: Correlation with adjacent mucosa and pathological parameters. *Journal of Clinical Pathology, 58*(4), 367–371.

Geisse, L.J., & Tweeddale, D.N. (1978). Pre-clinical cytological diagnosis of bladder cancer. *Journal of Urology, 120*(1), 51–56.

George, D.J., & Kaelin, W.G., Jr. (2003). The von Hippel-Lindau protein, vascular endothelial growth factor and kidney cancer. *New England Journal of Medicine, 349*(5), 419–421.

Gibanel, R., Ribal, M.J., Filella, X., Ballesta, A.M., Molina, R., Alcaraz, A., et al. (2002). BTA TRAK urine test increases the efficacy of cytology in the diagnosis of low-grade transitional cell carcinoma of the bladder. *Anticancer Research, 22*(2B), 1157–1160.

Gilligan, T., & Dreicer, R. (2007). The atypical urothelial cancer patient: Management of bladder cancers of non-transitional cell histology and cancers of the ureters and renal pelvis. *Seminars in Oncology, 34*(2), 145–153.

Goessl, C., Knispel, H.H., Miller, K., & Klan, R. (1997). Is routine excretory urography necessary at first diagnosis of bladder cancer? *Journal of Urology, 157*(2), 480–481.

Gold, P.J., Fefer, A., & Thompson, J.A. (1996). Paraneoplastic manifestations of renal cell carcinoma. *Seminars in Urologic Oncology, 14*(4), 216–222.

Golijanin, D., Tan, J.Y., Kazior, A., Cohen, E.G., Russo, P., Dalbagni, G., et al. (2004). Cyclooxygenase-2 and microsomal prostaglandin E synthase-1 are overexpressed in squamous cell carcinoma of the penis. *Clinical Cancer Research, 10*(3), 1024–1031.

Grabmaier, K., Vissers, J.L., De Weijert, M.C.A., Oosterwijk-Wakka, J.C., Van Bokhoven, A., Brakenhoff, R.H., et al. (2000). Molecular cloning and immunogenicity of renal cell carcinoma-associated antigen G250. *International Journal of Cancer, 85*(6), 865–870.

Grandinetti, C.A., & Goldspiel, B.R. (2007). Sorafenib and sunitinib: Novel targeted therapies for renal cell cancer. *Pharmacotherapy, 27*(8), 1125–1144.

Greene, F.L., Compton, C.C., Fritz, A.G., Shah, J.P., & Winchester, D.P. (Eds.). (2006). *AJCC cancer staging atlas.* New York: Springer.

Greene, F.L., Page, D.L., Fleming, I.D., Fritz, A., Balch, C.M., Haller, D.G., et al. (Eds.). (2002). *AJCC cancer staging manual* (6th ed.). New York: Springer.

Grossman, H.B., Gomella, L., Fradet, Y., Morales, A., Presti, J., Ritenour, C., et al. (2007). A phase III, multicenter comparison of hexaminolevulinate fluorescence cystoscopy and white light cystoscopy for the detection of superficial papillary lesions in patients with bladder cancer. *Journal of Urology, 178*(1), 62–67.

Grossman, H.B., Messing, E., Soloway, M., Tomera, K., Katz, G., Berger, Y., et al. (2005). Detection of bladder cancer using a point-of-care proteomic assay. *JAMA, 293*(7), 810–816.

Guida, M., Casamassima, A., Monticelli, G., Quaranta, M., & Colucci, G. (2007). Basal cytokines profile in metastatic renal cell carcinoma patients treated with subcutaneous IL-2–based therapy compared with that of healthy donors. *Journal of Translational Medicine, 5,* 51–55.

Guimaraes, A.R., & Harisinghani, M.G. (2006). Imaging of transitional cell carcinoma. In N.J. Vogelzang, P.T. Scardino, W.U. Shipley, F.M.J. Debruyne, & W.M. Linehan (Eds.), *Comprehensive textbook of genitourinary oncology* (3rd ed., pp. 417–434). Philadelphia: Lippincott Williams & Wilkins.

Hassan, J.M., Cookson, M.S., Smith, J.A., Jr., & Chang, S.S. (2006). Patterns of initial transitional cell recurrence in patients after cystectomy. *Journal of Urology, 175*(6), 2054–2057.

Heney, N.M. (2006). Clinical signs and symptoms of bladder cancer. In N.J. Vogelzang, P.T. Scardino, W.U. Shipley, F.M.J. Debruyne, & W.M. Linehan (Eds.), *Comprehensive textbook of genitourinary oncology* (3rd ed., pp. 355–356). Philadelphia: Lippincott Williams & Wilkins.

Heng, D.Y., Rini, B.I., Garcia, J., Wood, L., & Bukowski, R.M. (2007). Prolonged complete responses and near-complete responses to sunitinib in metastatic renal cell carcinoma. *Clinical Genitourinary Cancer, 5*(7), 446–451.

Herr, H.W. (2000). Tumor progression and survival of patients with high grade, noninvasive papillary (TaG3) bladder tumors: 15-year outcome. *Journal of Urology, 163*(1), 60–62.

Herrinton, L.J., Zhao, W., & Husson, G. (2003). Management of cryptorchidism and risk of testicular cancer. *American Journal of Epidemiology, 157*(7), 602–605.

Hirao, S., Hirao, T., Marsit, C.J., Hirao, Y., Schned, A., Devi-Ashok, T., et al. (2005). Loss of heterozygosity of chromosome *9q* and *p53* alterations in human bladder cancer. *Cancer, 104*(9), 1918–1923.

Hoglund, M. (2007). Bladder cancer, a two phased disease? *Seminars in Cancer Biology, 17*(3), 225–232.

Houldsworth, J., Xiao, H., Murty, V.V., Chen, W., Ray, B., Bosl, G., et al. (1998). Human male germ cell tumor resistance to cisplatin in linked to TP53 gene mutation. *Oncogene, 16*(18), 2345–2349.

Huddart, R.A., O'Doherty, M.J., Padhani, A., Rustin G.J., Mead, G.M., Joffe, J.K., et al. (2007). 18fluorodeoxyglucose positron emission tomography in the prediction of relapse in patients with high-risk, clinical stage I nonseminomatous germ cell tumors: Preliminary report of MRC Trial TE22—the NCRI Testis Tumour Clinical Study Group. *Journal of Clinical Oncology, 25*(21), 3090–3095.

Hudson, M.A., & Herr, H.W. (1995). Carcinoma in situ of the bladder [Review]. *Journal of Urology, 153*(3, Pt. 1), 564–572.

Huyghe, E., Matsuda, T., & Thonneau, P. (2003). Increasing incidence of testicular cancer worldwide: A review. *Journal of Urology, 170*(1), 5–11.

Jackson, S.M. (1966). The treatment of carcinoma of the penis. *British Journal of Surgery, 53*(1), 33–35.

Jemal, A., Siegel, R., Ward, E., Murray, T., Hao, Y., Xu, J., et al. (2008). Cancer statistics, 2008. *CA: A Cancer Journal for Clinicians, 58*(2), 71–96.

Jones, G.R., & Newhouse, I. (1997). Sport-related hematuria: A review. *Clinical Journal of Sport Medicine, 7*(2), 119–125.

Jones, T.D., & Cheng, C. (2006). Papillary urothelial neoplasm of low malignant potential: Evolving terminology and concepts [Review]. *Journal of Urology, 175*(6), 1995–2003.

Jordan, A.M., Weingarten, J., & Murphy, W.M. (1987). Transitional cell neoplasms of the urinary bladder: Can biologic potential be predicted from histologic grading? *Cancer, 60*(11), 2766–2774.

Junker, K., Hindermann, W., von Eggeling, F., Diegmann, J., Haessler, K., & Schubert, J. (2005). CD70: A new tumor specific biomarker for renal cell carcinoma. *Journal of Urology, 173*(6), 2150–2153.

Kakizoe, T. (2006). Development and progression of urothelial carcinoma. *Cancer Science, 97*(9), 821–828.

Kayes, O., Ahmed, H.U., Arya, M., & Minhas, S. (2007). Molecular and genetic pathways in penile cancer. *Lancet Oncology, 8*(5), 420–429.

Kim, B., Semelka, R.C., Ascher, S.M., Chalpin, D.B., Carroll, P.R., & Hricak, H. (1994). Bladder tumor staging: Comparison of contrast-enhanced CT, T1- and T2-weighted MR imaging, dynamic gadolinium-enhanced imaging, and late gadolinium-enhanced imaging. *Radiology, 193*(1), 239–245.

Kim, H.L., Belldegrun, A.S., Freitas, D.G., Bui, M.H., Han, K.R., & Figlin, R.A. (2003). Paraneoplastic signs and symptoms of renal cell carcinoma: Implications for prognosis. *Journal of Urology, 170*(5), 1742–1746.

Kirkali, Z., Chan, T., Manoharan, M., Algaba, F., Busch, C., Cheng, L., et al. (2005). Bladder cancer: Epidemiology, staffing and grading, and diagnosis. *Urology, 66*(6, Suppl. 1), 4–34.

Kommu, S., Hadway, P., & Watkin, N. (2005). Squamous cell carcinoma antigen as a biomarker for penile cancer. *BJU International, 95*(4), 478–479.

Korkola, J.E., Houldsworth, J., Dobrzynski, D., Olshen, A.B., Reuter, V.E., Bosl, G.J., et al. (2005). Gene expression-based classification of nonseminomatous male germ cell tumors. *Oncogene, 24*(32), 5101–5107.

Koss, L.G., Tiamson, E.M., & Robbins, M.A. (1974). Mapping cancerous and precancerous bladder changes: A study of the urothelium in ten surgically removed bladders. *JAMA, 227*(3), 281–286.

Kovacs, G., Akhtar, M., Beckwith, B.J., Bugert, P., Cooper, C.S., Delahunt, B., et al. (1997). The Heidelberg classification of renal cell tumours. *Journal of Pathology, 183*(2), 131–133.

Lane, B.R., Samplaski, M.K., Herts, B.R., Zhou, M., Novick, A.C., & Campbell, S.C. (2008). Renal mass biopsy—a renaissance? *Journal of Urology, 179*(1), 20–27.

Leibovich, B.C., Cheville, J.C., Lohse, C.M., Zincke, H., Kwon, E.D., Frank, I., et al. (2005). Cancer specific survival for patients with pT3 renal cell carcinoma-can the 2002 primary tumor classification be improved? *Journal of Urology, 173*(3), 716–719.

Leibovich, B.C., Sheinin, Y., Lohse, C.M., Thompson, R.H., Cheville, J.C., Zavada, J., et al. (2007). Carbonic anhydrase IX is not an independent predictor of outcome for patients with clear cell renal cell carcinoma. *Journal of Clinical Oncology, 25*(30), 4757–4764.

Leibovitch, I., & Mor, Y. (2005). The vicious cycling: Bicycling related urogenital disorders. *European Urology, 47*(3), 277–286.

Li, G., Feng, G., Gentil-Perret, A., Genin, C., & Tostain, J. (2007). *CA9* gene expression in conventional renal cell carcinoma: A potential marker for prediction of early metastasis after nephrectomy. *Clinical and Experimental Metastasis, 24*(3), 149–155.

Lindgren, D., Liedberg, F., Andersson, A., Chebil, G., Gudjonsson, S., Borg, A., et al. (2006). Molecular characterization of early-stage bladder carcinomas by expression profiles, *FGFR3* mutation status, and loss of 9q. *Oncogene, 25*(18), 2685–2696.

Linehan, W.M., Walther, M.M., & Zbar, B. (2003). The genetic basis of cancer of the kidney. *Journal of Urology, 170*(6, Pt. 1), 2163–2172.

Lont, A.P., Besnard, A.P., Gallee, M., van Tinteren, H., & Horenblas, S. (2003). A comparison of physical examination and imaging in determining the extent of primary penile cancer. *BJU International, 91*(6), 493–495.

Lott, S., Lopez-Beltran, A., Montironi, R., MacLennan, G.T., & Cheng, L. (2007). Soft tissue tumors of the urinary bladder part II: Malignant neoplasms. *Human Pathology, 38*(7), 963–977.

Lucia, M.S., & Miller, G.J. (1992). Histopathology of malignant lesions of the penis. *Urologic Clinics of North America, 19*(2), 227–246.

Maldazys, J.D., & deKernion, J.B. (1986). Prognostic factors in metastatic renal carcinoma. *Journal of Urology, 136*(2), 376–381.

McDougal, W.S., & Garnick, M.B. (2006). Signs and symptoms of renal cell carcinoma and paraneoplastic syndromes. In N.J. Vogelzang, P.T. Scardino, W.U. Shipley, F.M.J. Debruyne, & W.M. Linehan (Eds.), *Comprehensive textbook of genitourinary oncology* (3rd ed., pp. 661–667). Philadelphia: Lippincott Williams & Wilkins.

McGlynn, K.A., Devesa, S.S., Sigurdson, A.J., Brown, L.M., Tsao, L., & Tarone, R.E. (2003). Trends in the incidence of testicular germ cell tumors in the United States. *Cancer, 97*(1), 63–70.

Memorial Sloan-Kettering Cancer Center. (2007, March 9). PET imaging identifies aggressive kidney cancers that require surgery. *Science Daily.* Retrieved November 24, 2007, from http://www.sciencedaily.com/releases/2007/03/070307075512.htm

Mhawech-Fauceglia, P., Cheney, R.T., & Schwaller, J. (2006). Genetic alterations in urothelial bladder carcinoma: An updated review. *Cancer, 106*(6), 1205–1216.

Micali, G., Nasca, M.R., Innocenzi, D., & Schwartz, R.A. (2004). Invasive penile carcinoma: A review. *Dermatologic Surgery, 30*(4), 311–320.

Micali, G., Nasca, M., Innocenzi, D., & Schwartz, R. (2006). Penile cancer. *Journal of the American Academy of Dermatology, 54*(3), 369–391.

Micali, G., Schwartz, R., & Nasca, M. (2006, October 19). *Penile squamous cell carcinoma.* Retrieved August 25, 2007, from http://www.emedicine.com/derm/TOPIC919.HTM

Mistry, T., Jones, R.W., Dannatt, E., Prasad, K.K., & Stockdale, A.D. (2007). A 10-year retrospective audit of penile cancer management in the UK. *BJU International, 100*(6), 1277–1281.

Nasca, M., Innocenzi, D., & Micali, G. (1999). Penile cancer among patients with genital lichen sclerosis. *Journal of the American Academy of Dermatology, 41*(6), 911–914.

National Cancer Institute. (2007). *Dictionary of terms.* Retrieved December 31, 2007, from http://www.cancer.gov/Templates/db_alpha.aspx?CdrID=46636

National Comprehensive Cancer Network. (2009). *NCCN Clinical Practice Guidelines in Oncology™: Kidney cancer* [v.1.2009]. Retrieved April 6, 2009, from http://www.nccn.org/professionals/physician_gls/PDF/kidney.pdf

Nelson, R. (2006). Potential prognostic markers in penile cancer. *Lancet Oncology, 7*(5), 369.

Neumann, H.P., & Zbar, B. (1997). Renal cysts, renal cancer, and von Hippel-Lindau disease. *Kidney International, 51*(1), 16–26.

Nguyen, C.T., & Campbell, S.C. (2006). Staging of renal cell carcinoma: Past, present, and future. *Clinical Genitourinary Cancer, 5*(3), 190–197.

Nichols, C.R., Heerema, N.A., Palmer, C., Loehrer, P.J., Sr., Williams, S.D., & Einhorn, L.H. (1987). Klinefelter's syndrome associated with mediastinal germ cell neoplasms. *Journal of Clinical Oncology, 5*(8), 1290–1294.

O'Donnell, M.A. (2007). Advances in the management of superficial bladder cancer. *Seminars in Oncology, 34*(2), 85–97.

Papadopoulos, O., Betsi, E., Tsakistou, G., Frangoulis, M., Kouvatseas, G., Anagnostakis, D., et al. (2007). Expression of cyclin D1 and Ki-67 in squamous cell carcinoma of the penis. *Anticancer Research, 27*(4B), 2167–2174.

Pashos, C.L., Botteman, M.F., Laskin, B.L., & Redaelli, A. (2002). Bladder cancer: Epidemiology, diagnosis, and management. *Cancer Practice, 10*(6), 311–322.

Pavlovich, C.P., & Schmidt, L.S. (2004). Searching for the hereditary causes of renal-cell carcinoma. *Nature Reviews Cancer, 4*(5), 381–393.

Pavlovich, P.C., Schmidt, L.S., & Phillips, J.L. (2003). The genetic basis of renal cell carcinoma. *Urologic Clinics of North America, 30*(3), 437–454.

Pettaway, C., Lynch, D., & Davis, J. (2007). Tumors of the penis. In A. Wein (Ed.), *Campbell-Walsh textbook of urology* (9th ed., pp. 959–966). Philadelphia: Elsevier Saunders.

Pietrzak, P., Hadway, P., Corbishley, C.M., & Watkin, N.A. (2006). Is the association between balanitis xerotica obliterans and penile carcinoma underestimated? *BJU International, 98*(1), 74–76.

Planz, B., Jochims, E., Deix, T., Caspers, H.P., Jakse, G., & Boecking, A. (2005). The role of urinary cytology for detection of bladder cancer. *European Journal of Surgical Oncology, 31*(3), 304–308.

Poetsch, M., Schuart, B., Schwesinger, G., Kleist, B., & Protzel, C. (2007). Screening of microsatellite markers in penile cancer reveals differences between metastatic and non metastatic carcinomas. *Modern Pathology, 20*(10), 1069–1077.

Rabbani, F., Farivar-Mohseni, H., Leon, A., Motzer, R.J., Bosl, G.J., & Sheinfeld, J. (2003). Clinical outcomes after retroperitoneal lymphadenectomy of patients with pure testicular teratoma. *Urology, 62*(6), 1092–1096.

Rathmell, W.K., Martz, C.A., & Rini, B.I. (2007). Renal cell carcinoma. *Current Opinion in Oncology, 19*(3), 234–240.

Rathmell, W.K., Wright, T.M., & Rini, B.I. (2005). Molecularly targeted therapy in renal cell carcinoma. *Expert Review of Anticancer Therapy, 5*(6), 1031–1040.

Razdan, S., & Gomella, L. (2005). Cancers of the genitourinary system: Cancer of the penis. In V.T. DeVita Jr., S. Hellman, & S.A. Rosenberg (Eds.), *Cancer: Principles and practice of oncology* (7th ed., pp. 1263–1267). Philadelphia: Lippincott Williams & Wilkins.

Reddy, C., Devendranath, V., & Pratap, S. (1984). Carcinoma of the penis—role of phimosis. *Urology, 24*(1), 85–89.

Reuter, V.E. (2005). Origins and molecular biology of testicular germ cell tumors. *Modern Pathology, 18*(Suppl. 2), S51–S60.

Robson, C.J., Churchill, B.M., & Anderson, W. (1969). The results of radical nephrectomy for renal cell carcinoma. *Journal of Urology, 101*(3), 297–301.

Rodriguez, A., & Sexton, W.J. (2006). Management of locally advanced renal cell carcinoma. *Cancer Control, 13*(3), 199–210. Retrieved March 1, 2009, from http://www.medscape.com/viewarticle/543004

Rosenblum, S.L. (1987). Paraneoplastic syndromes associated with renal cell carcinoma. *Journal of South Carolina Medical Association, 83*(7), 375–378.

Ross, R.K., Yu, M.C., & Yuan, J.-M. (2006). The epidemiology of bladder cancer. In N.J. Vogelzang, P.T. Scardino, W.U. Shipley, F.M.J. Debruyne, & W.M. Linehan (Eds.), *Comprehensive textbook of genitourinary oncology* (3rd ed., pp. 357–363). Philadelphia: Lippincott Williams & Wilkins.

Rubin, M., Kleter, B., Zhou, M., Ayala, G., Cubilla, A.L., Quint, W.G., et al. (2001). Detection and typing of human papillomavirus DNA in penile carcinoma: Evidence for multiple independent pathways of penile carcinogenesis. *American Journal of Pathology, 159*(4), 1211–1218.

Sachdeva, K., Makhoul, I., Javeed, M., & Curti, B. (2008). *Renal cell carcinoma.* Retrieved March 1, 2009, from http://emedicine.medscape.com/article/281340-overview

Scardino, E., Villa, G., Bonomo, G., Matei, D.V., Verweij, F., & Rooco, B. (2004). Magnetic resonance imaging combined with artificial erection for local staging of penile cancer. *Urology, 63*(6), 1158–1162.

Scatarige, J.C., Sheth, S., Corl, F.M., & Fishman, E.K. (2001). Patterns of recurrence in renal cell carcinoma: Manifestations on helical CT. *American Journal of Roentgenology, 177*(3), 653–658.

Schmidt, L., Duh, F.M., Chen, F., Kishida, T., Glenn, G., Choyke, P., et al. (1997). Germline and somatic mutations in the tyrosine kinase domain of the MET proto-oncogene in papillary renal carcinomas. *Nature Genetics, 16*(1), 68–73.

Sesterhenn, I.A., & Davis, C.J., Jr. (2004). Pathology of germ cell tumors of the testis. *Cancer Control, 11*(6), 374–387.

Shipley, W.U., Kaufman, D.S., McDougal, W.S., Dahl, D.M., Michaelson, M.D., & Zietman, A.L. (2005). Cancer of the bladder, ureter, and renal pelvis. In V.T. DeVita Jr., S. Hellman, & S.A. Rosenberg (Eds.), *Cancer: Principles and practice of oncology* (7th ed., pp. 1168–1192). Philadelphia: Lippincott Williams & Wilkins.

Siemer, S., Lehmann, J., Loch, A., Becker, F., Stein, U., Schneider, G., et al. (2005). Current TNM classification of renal cell carcinoma evaluated: Revising stage T3a. *Journal of Urology, 173*(1), 33–37.

Siow, W.Y., Yip, S.K., Ng, L.G., Tan, P.H., Cheng, W.S., & Foo, K.T. (2000). Renal cell carcinoma: Incidental detection and pathological staging. *Journal of the Royal College of Surgeons of Edinburgh, 45*(5), 291–295. Retrieved March 1, 2009, from http://www.rcsed.ac.uk/journal/vol45_5/4550005.htm

Skakkebaek, N.E., Berthelsen, J.G., & Muller, J. (1982). Carcinoma-in-situ of the undescended testes. *Urologic Clinics of North America, 9*(3), 377–385.

Skinner, D.G., Colvin, R.B., Vermillion, C.D., Pfister, R.C., & Leadbetter, W.F. (1971). Diagnosis and management of renal cell carcinoma. A clinical and pathologic study of 309 cases. *Cancer, 28*(5), 1165–1177.

Slack, N.H., & Prout, G.R., Jr. (1980). Heterogeneity of invasive bladder carcinoma and different responses to treatment. *Journal of Urology, 123*(5), 644–652.

Soloway, M.S., Lee, C.T., Steinberg, G.D., Ghandi, A.A., & Jewett, M.A. (2007). Difficult decisions in urologic oncology: Management of high grade T1 transitional cell carcinoma of the bladder. *Urologic Oncology, 25*(4), 338–340.

Sridhar, S.S., Hedley, D., & Siu, L.L. (2005). Raf kinase as a target for anticancer therapeutics. *Molecular Cancer Therapeutics, 4*(4), 667–685.

Stancik, I., & Holtl, W. (2003). Penile cancer: Review of the recent literature. *Current Opinion in Urology, 13*(6), 467–472.

Stone, J.H. (2006). Incidentalomas—clinical correlation and translational science required. *New England Journal of Medicine, 354*(26), 2748–2749.

Sufrin, G., Chasan, S., Golio, A., & Murphy, G.P. (1989). Paraneoplastic and serologic syndromes of renal adenocarcinoma. *Seminars in Urology, 7*(3), 158–171.

Sufrin, G., & Huben, R. (1991). Benign and malignant lesions of the penis. In J. Gillenwater (Ed.), *Adult and pediatric urology* (2nd ed., pp. 375–388). Chicago: Yearbook Medical.

Sweeney, J.P., Thornhill, J.A., Grainger, R., McDermott, T.E., & Butler, M.R. (1996). Incidentally detected renal cell carcinoma: Pathological features, survival trends and implications for treatment. *British Journal of Urology, 78*(3), 351–353.

Sylvester, R.J., van der Meijden, A., Witjes, J.A., Jakse, G., Nonomura, N., Cheng, C., et al. (2005). High-grade Ta urothelial carcinoma and carcinoma in situ of the bladder. *Urology, 66*(6, Suppl. 1), 90–107.

Tabatabaei, S., & McDougal, S. (2006). Penile cancer: Clinical signs and symptoms. In N.J. Vogelzang, P.T. Scardino, W.U. Shipley, F.M.J. Debruyne, & W.M. Linehan (Eds.), *Comprehensive textbook of genitourinary oncology* (3rd ed., pp. 805–808). Philadelphia: Lippincott Williams & Wilkins.

Tanimoto, A., Yuasa, Y., Imai, Y., Izutsu, M., Hiramatsu, K., Tachibana, M., et al. (1992). Bladder tumor staging: Comparison of conventional and gadolinium-enhanced dynamic MR imaging and CT. *Radiology, 185*(3), 741–747.

Tekes, A., Kamel, I., Imam, K., Szarf, G., Schoenberg, M., Nasir, K., et al. (2005). Dynamic MRI of bladder cancer: Evaluation of staging accuracy. *American Journal of Roentgenology, 184*(1), 121–127.

Toner, G.C., Geller, N.L., Tan, C., Nisselbaum, J., & Bosl, G.J. (1990). Serum tumor marker half-life during chemotherapy allows early prediction of complete response and survival in nonseminomatous germ cell tumors. *Cancer Research, 50*(18), 5904–5910.

Touloupidis, S., Zisimopoulos, A., Giannokopoulos, S., Papatsoris, A.G., Kalaitzis, C., & Thanos, A. (2007). Clinical usage of the squamous cell carcinoma antigen in patients with penile cancer. *International Journal of Urology, 14*(2), 174–176.

Tseng, A., Jr., Horning, S.J., Freiha, F.S., Resser, K.J., Hannigan, J.F., & Torti, F.M. (1985). Gynecomastia in testicular cancer patients. Prognostic and therapeutic implications. *Cancer, 56*(10), 2534–2538.

Tseng, H.-F., Morgenstern, H., Mack, T., & Peters, R.K. (2001). Risk factors for penile cancer: Results of a population-based case-control study in Los Angeles County (United States). *Cancer Causes and Control, 12*(3), 267–277.

Varella-Garcia, M., Akduman, B., Sunpaweravong, P., Di Maria, M.V., & Crawford, E.D. (2004). The UroVysion fluorescence in situ hybridization assay is an effective tool for monitoring recurrence of bladder cancer. *Urologic Oncology, 22*(1), 16–19.

van Oers, J.M., Adam, C., Denzinger, S., Stoehr, R., Bertz, S., Zaak, D., et al. (2006). Chromosome 9 deletions are more frequent than *FGFR3* mutations in flat urothelial hyperplasias of the bladder. *International Journal of Cancer, 119*(5), 1212–1215.

Velazquez, E.F., Barreto, J.E., Rodriguez, I., Piris, A., & Cubilla, A. (2004). Limitations in the interpretation of biopsies in patients with penile squamous cell carcinoma. *International Journal of Surgical Pathology, 12*(2), 139–146.

Vineis, P., & Pirastu, R. (1997). Aromatic amines and cancer. *Cancer Causes and Control, 8*(3), 346–355.

Walboomers, J., Jacobs, M., Manos, M., Bosch, F., Lummer, J., Shah, K., et al. (1999). Human papillomavirus is a necessary cause of invasive cervical cancer worldwide. *Journal of Pathology, 189*(1), 12–19.

Wallmeroth, A., Wagner, U., Moch, H., Gasser, T.C., Sauter, G., & Mihatsch, M.J. (1999). Patterns of metastasis in muscle-invasive bladder cancer (pT2-4): An autopsy study on 367 patients. *Urology International, 62*(2), 69–75.

Wijkstrom, H., Cohen, S.M., Gardiner, R.A., Kakizoe, T., Schoenberg, M., Steineck, G., et al. (2000). Prevention and treatment of urothelial premalignant and malignant lesions. *Scandinavian Journal of Urology Nephrology Supplement, 205,* 116–135.

Young, R.H., & McKee, G.T. (2006). Cytology and pathology of carcinomas of the urinary tract. In N.J. Vogelzang, P.T. Scardino, W.U. Shipley, F.M.J. Debruyne, & W.M. Linehan (Eds.), *Comprehensive textbook of genitourinary oncology* (3rd ed., pp. 365–384). Philadelphia: Lippincott Williams & Wilkins.

Zambrano, N.R., Lubensky, I.A., Merino, M.J., Linehan, W., Marston, W., McClellan, M., et al. (1999). Histopathology and molecular genetics of renal tumors: Toward unification of a classification system. *Journal of Urology, 162*(4), 1246–1258.

Zeegers, M.P.A., Tan, F.E.S., Dorant, E., & van den Brandt, P.A. (2000). The impact of characteristics of cigarette smoking on urinary tract cancer risk: A meta-analysis of epidemiologic studies. *Cancer, 89*(3), 630–639.

Zhang, J., Gerst, S., Lefkowitz, R.A., & Bach, A. (2007). Imaging of bladder cancer. *Radiologic Clinics of North America, 45*(1), 183–205.

Zhu, Y., Ye, D.W., Yao, X.D., Zhang, S.L., Dai, B., Zhang, H.L., et al. (2008). The value of squamous cell carcinoma antigen in the prognostic evaluation, treatment monitoring, and follow-up of patients with penile cancer. *Journal of Urology, 180*(5), 2019–2023.

Zigeuner, R., Tsybrovskyy, O., Ratschek, M., Rehak, P., Lipsky, K., & Langner, C. (2004). Prognostic impact of *p63* and *p53* expression in upper urinary tract transitional cell carcinoma. *Urology, 63*(6), 1079–1083.

CHAPTER 4

Prevention, Screening, and Early Detection for Genitourinary Malignancies

Tara S. Baney, RN, MS, AOCN®

Introduction

Prevention, early detection, and screening are important components in the management of urologic cancers. Nurses with awareness of the causes of specific cancers can provide information to patients so they may limit their exposure to risk factors linked to carcinogenesis. Ongoing research has identified specific genetic factors that are linked to an increased risk for some urologic cancers. In this at-risk patient population, strict screening criteria to detect tumors early and institute the necessary treatment can be lifesaving.

Renal Cancer

Risk Factors

Research has shown a link between renal carcinoma and environmental, chemical, hormonal, and genetic factors.

Environment

Cigarette smoke is one of the most likely causes of renal cancer, especially in males. Estimations conclude that 30% of renal cancers in men and 24% of renal cancers in women are associated with smoking (Linehan, Bates, & Yang, 2005). In a meta-analysis of 24 studies, smoking cessation more significantly reduced the risk of renal cancer in those who had quit for 10 years or more as compared to those who had quit for less than 10 years. A correlation exists between the number of cigarettes smoked per day and the risk for developing renal cancer. As the number of daily cigarette usage increases, the risk increases as well (Hunt, van der Hel, McMillan, Boffetta, & Brennan, 2005).

Acquired polycystic renal disease may develop in renal failure patients who are treated with long-term dialysis. As many as 30%–40% of patients who receive long-term dialysis will develop acquired polycystic disease (Linehan et al., 2005). It can develop at any time, even in patients who have undergone renal transplantations. Acquired polycystic disease is found in equal rates in both patients who receive hemodialysis and those who receive peritoneal dialysis. Those who have developed polycystic renal disease because of end-stage renal disease are at a 100-fold greater risk for developing renal cancers; of those patients who have polycystic disease, approximately 5.8% will develop a renal cancer (Doublet, Peraldi, Gattegno, Thibault, & Sraer, 1997; Linehan et al.). The pathophysiology is thought to be caused by papillary hyperplasia found in the epithelium of the cyst in the kidney that progresses to cancer (Linehan et al.).

Chemical

Although in the past analgesic use, primarily phenacetin-containing analgesics, was linked to an increased risk of renal cancer, a review of several studies showed no association with those medications that are currently available for use (Dhote, Thiounn, Debre, & Vidal-Trecan, 2004). Studies concluded that paracetamol and aspirin use do not support an increased risk of renal cancer; the risk was only seen in those who had taken phenacetin-containing analgesics on a regular basis (Dhote et al.). The U.S. Food and Drug Administration (FDA) removed phenacetin from the market in 1983 because of its carcinogenic properties.

The role of diuretics in the development of renal cancer is still debated. Currently, the only link has been found in women. A significant increase in the risk of developing renal cancer was observed in women who use diuretics, even after adjusting for the presence of hypertension (Hiatt, Tolan, & Quesenberry, 1994; Kreiger, Marrett, Dodds, Hilditch, & Darlington, 1993). Data from pooled statistics of three studies showed that the age-adjusted risk for fatal renal cell carcinoma in women related to diuretic use had a risk ratio of 2.43 (95% confidence interval [CI], 2.13–2.78), whereas men had a risk ratio of 1.29 (95% CI, 0.42–3.97) (Grossman, Messerli, & Goldbourt, 2001; Heath, Lally, Calle, McLaughlin, & Thun, 1997; Mellemgaard, Moller, & Olsen, 1992; Prineas, Folsom, Zhang, Sellers, & Potter, 1997). Two other studies showed an association between renal cell carcinoma and thiazide diuretic use with ratios of 2.3 (95% CI, 1.3–4) and 4 (95% CI, 1.5–10.8) (Dhote et al., 2004; Hiatt et al.; Kreiger et al.).

At one time, antihypertensives other than thiazide diuretics were thought to cause renal cancer, but it appears that hypertension is the causative factor (McLaughlin, Lipworth, & Tarone, 2006; Zucchetto et al., 2007). The biologic mechanism by which hypertension affects risk is unclear. Lipid peroxidation, which is increased in hypertensive individuals, has been hypothesized to be a causative factor in development of tumors (Gago-Dominguez & Castelao, 2006).

Trichloroethylene is a chemical solvent that has been implicated in the cause of renal cancer with long-term exposure (Brauch et al., 1999). Those employed in the iron and steel industries and firefighters have an increased risk of developing renal carcinoma because of the exposure to hydrocarbons and its derivatives such as petroleum and solvents. However, the duration of exposure was over a long time period, greater than 30 years (Dhote et al., 2004).

Hormonal

An increased risk of developing renal cancer, especially in women and those with a high body mass index, is linked to obesity. Some of the potential mechanisms may be higher estrogen levels, elevated insulin levels, greater concentrations of growth factors in adipose tissue, hypertension, cholesterol metabolism abnormalities, and immunosuppression. Obese individuals also may have lower serum levels of vitamin D and engage in less physical activity, which has been shown to have a correlation with a higher risk of renal cancer (Moyad, 2001).

Hereditary

Renal cancer occurs in nonhereditary and hereditary forms. Four hereditary forms have been identified: von Hippel-Lindau (VHL) disease, hereditary papillary renal carcinoma (HPRC), hereditary leiomyomatosis renal cancer (HLRCC), and Birt-Hogg-Dubé (BHD) syndrome. VHL is an autosomal dominant inherited disorder that predisposes carriers of the disease for specific signs and symptoms. People with VHL may develop one or more of the following characteristics (Middelton & Lessick, 2003).
- Central nervous system benign hemangioblastomas
- Retinal angiomas
- Pheochromocytomas
- Clear cell cancers
- Endolymphatic sac tumors

Forty percent of patients with VHL develop multiple bilateral renal tumors or cysts. These renal tumors often occur early in life and can metastasize (Linehan et al., 2005). Patients undergo multiple nephron-sparing surgeries but over time may require bilateral nephrectomies and dialysis. HPRC is caused by a mutation of the *MET* gene. These patients are predisposed to papillary tumors of the kidney, which are often less aggressive, less vascular, and with a lower histologic grade than the more common types of renal cancer such as clear cell (Zbar et al., 1995). In the past decade, HLRCC was identified as a predominantly inherited cancer syndrome. It was discovered that several families having members affected by cutaneous and/or uterine leiomyomas also were found to have kidney cancers of papillary histology. The fumarate hydratase gene was found to be the responsible link in these families (Middelton & Lessick, 2003). BHD is another autosomal dominantly inherited condition with multiple manifestations, including hair follicle tumors, pulmonary cysts, and bilateral multifocal chromophobe renal cell carcinomas. The gene responsible for this disorder is located on chromosome 17 and produces a novel protein called folliculin (Middelton & Lessick). It is thought that folliculin functions as a tumor suppressor, although its exact function is still uncertain (Adley, Smith, Nayar, & Yang, 2006; Schmidt et al., 2005).

Prevention

Smoking is clearly the one risk factor that can be eliminated to reduce the risk of renal cancer. Other health problems such as hypertension and obesity have been associated with a higher risk of renal cancer. These health problems often can be eliminated or controlled by a healthy diet and routine exercise. By adopting healthy lifestyle behaviors, the risk of renal cancer may be reduced (Dhote et al., 2004).

Screening and Early Detection

Most early-stage renal cancers are discovered incidentally. The classic presentation of pain, hematuria, and flank mass is usually an indication of advanced disease. In the general population with no known genetic disorder related to the development of renal cancer or end-stage renal disease, no recommended screening guidelines are available at the present time.

Patients who have family members affected with the clinical features associated with VHL, HPRC, HLRCC, or BHD or who exhibit the clinical features themselves should undergo genetic testing for the appropriate mutation (see Table 4-1). Those who have one of the renal cancer–associated genetic disorders should have routine abdominal/pelvic computed tomography (CT) scans with and without contrast to evaluate for renal masses. CT scan is the preferred method when evaluating for renal masses because of the suboptimal detection of papillary tumors when using renal ultrasound (Linehan et al., 2005; Middelton & Lessick, 2003).

Bladder Cancer

Bladder (urothelial) cancer is diagnosed more commonly in men than in women. The risk factors associated with bladder cancer are genetic abnormalities, chemical exposure, and chronic irritation.

Table 4-1. Hereditary Renal Cancer Syndromes

Genetic Disorder	Clinical Manifestations	Genetic Evaluation
Hereditary papillary renal carcinoma	Bilateral multifocal papillary renal cancers	c-*Met* germ-line mutation testing
Hereditary leiomyomatosis renal cancer	Cutaneous nodules (leiomyomas) Uterine fibroids Renal tumors (solitary, aggressive)	Fumarate hydratase
Von Hippel-Lindau (VHL) disease	Renal cyst/tumors (clear cell) Pheochromocytomas Retinal hemangiomas Central nervous system hemangioblastomas	*VHL* gene germ-line mutation testing
Birt-Hogg-Dubé (BHD) syndrome	Hair follicle tumors Pulmonary cyst Renal tumors (bilateral, multifocal)	*BHD* gene germ-line mutation testing

Note. Based on information from Middelton & Lessick, 2003.

Risk Factors

Genetic

Mutations, such as the loss of heterozygosity of chromosome 17 with the mutation of *TP53* suppressor gene, have been linked to the evolution of invasive disease and metastatic disease. The loss of heterozygosity of chromosome 9 has been linked with the development of superficial bladder cancer (American Joint Committee on Cancer, 2002). Not only are genetic mutations linked to the development of bladder cancer, but certain mutations, such as *P16*, retinoblastoma gene (*pRB*), and chromosome 17, also are responsible for the aggressiveness and invasiveness of the disease. Other tumor suppressor genes that have been linked to bladder cancer are *p21* and *p27* (Shipley et al., 2005).

Chemical

Chemical exposure has a very strong link to the development of bladder cancer. Individuals who smoke are at a threefold increased risk of developing bladder cancer and even ex-smokers have a twofold risk (Zeegers, Goldbohm, & van den Brandt, 2002). Chemicals associated with plastics, coal, tar, asphalt, aromatic amines, aniline dyes, nitrites, and nitrates also are associated with bladder cancer development (Band, Le, MacArthur, Fang, & Gallagher, 2005; Shipley et al., 2005). Retired firefighters may be a group with higher risk factors related to cigarette smoking and exposure to unknown chemicals (Greene, Konety, & Stoller, 2008). Although coffee, tea, and artificial sweetener consumption was thought to be a risk factor for bladder cancer, research has failed to support this hypothesis (Shipley et al.).

Patients who have received cyclophosphamide chemotherapy over a long time period for malignant and nonmalignant diseases have an increased risk of developing bladder cancer. The mechanism responsible for this increased risk is the cyclophosphamide metabolite acrolein (Vlaovic & Jewett, 1999). During the administration of this agent, it is important to hydrate the patient to limit exposure of the metabolite on the bladder mucosa and encourage frequent voiding. Treatment with cyclophosphamide places survivors of childhood malignancies at higher risk for bladder cancer (Gurung, Frobisher, Leiper, Woodhouse, & Hawkins, 2008).

Inflammation

Chronic inflammation and irritation have been attributed to a risk of bladder cancer. Irritants include indwelling catheters, parasites, and irradiation. Chronic use of indwelling urinary bladder catheters is associated with an increased risk of urinary tract infections (UTIs) (Cochran, 2007; Hart, 2008). Patients with chronic indwelling urinary catheters associated with UTI are at great risk for bladder cancer because of the chronic inflammation from infection (Shipley et al., 2005). Certain populations, such as spinal cord injury patients, who require long-term indwelling urinary catheters have shown an increase (16–28-times greater risk) in the incidence of bladder cancer compared to the general population (Groah et al., 2002; Hess, Zhan, Foo, & Yalla, 2003). The parasitic worm *Schistosoma haematobium* is found in water sources in tropical Africa, Central and South America, Australia, and Asia. Infection with this parasite is associated with an increased risk of both squamous cell carcinoma and transitional cell carcinoma of the bladder (Shipley et al., 2005). Patients who receive pelvic irradiation, such as for prostate and cervical cancers, are at a greater risk for bladder cancer because of the inflammatory process that follows radiation therapy.

Prevention

The biggest risk-reducing behavior to prevent bladder cancer is to not smoke or to stop smoking. Smoking triples the risk for developing bladder cancer over time. Limiting exposure to the chemicals listed as cancer-promoting agents is another way to cut the risk of developing bladder cancer. If this is impossible, as with patients who require cyclophosphamide for cancer therapy, steps such as increasing hydration can help to reduce the risk. Healthcare providers should attempt to limit the use of indwelling catheters, and if catheter use is absolutely necessary, they should use measures to reduce the risk of UTIs. Those who travel to areas where water supplies are infested with *Schistosoma haematobium* need to take precautions to reduce or eliminate exposure. Retired firefighters and survivors of childhood cancers treated with cyclophosphamide may be groups that could benefit from screening (Greene et al., 2008; Gurung et al., 2008). Finally, increased water consumption, intake of vitamins such as selenium or folate, and various diets that are high in soy protein and low in fat may be beneficial for the prevention of bladder cancer (Ashughyan, Marihart, & Djavan, 2006; Brinkman, Buntinx, Muls, & Zeegers, 2006; Brock et al., 2006; Schabath et al., 2005).

Screening and Early Detection

Anyone with hematuria should undergo a workup for a bladder tumor, including urine culture, urinalysis, urine cytology, and possible cystoscopy (American Urological Association [AUA], 2007). However, screening of the general population for microhematuria has not proved to be useful in the detection of bladder tumors because hematuria often is intermittent and can be missed on single or occasional testing (Messing, 2007). Of the patients who are screened and found to have microhematuria, only 0.1%–6.6% have a bladder tumor (Shipley et al., 2005). This translates into a bladder cancer detection rate of 0.005%–0.2% in the general population (Shipley et al.). In one study that looked at newly detected bladder cancers, one of the patients with noninvasive papillary tumors (Ta) showed disease progression or died of the disease at the five-year interval. However, 32% of those with T1 tumors progressed to muscle-invasive disease within five years. Finally, 68% of those found to have muscle-invasive disease at diagnosis died within five years (Larsson et al., 2003).

Routine screening in high-risk populations may be warranted because of the detection of high-grade tumors. The rationale is that patients with high-grade tumors would be found prior to muscle invasion by the cancer, and patients could be treated with transurethral resection and intravesical therapy (Shipley et al., 2005). Most patients (65%–90%) who have muscle-invasive (or deeper) disease have it at the time of diagnosis (Messing, 2007). Because of the high rate of false positives for low-grade tumors, screening for bladder cancer is not currently utilized. Nevertheless, questions regarding episodes of hematuria and irritative symptoms should be included in the history component of a physical assessment for patients who have risk factors, such as smoking (AUA, 2007).

Over the past few years, several noninvasive urine tests have been developed and approved by FDA for use in the detection and surveillance of noninvasive bladder cancers. These tests look for cancer cells using techniques such as nuclear matrix protein 22 assay detection, detection of chromosomal abnormalities by fluorescence in situ hybridization, and immunocytofluorescence assay based on a combination of monoclonal antibodies labeled with fluorescent markers (Gray & Sims, 2004). The sensitivities and specificities vary between tests. Many of the available markers have a reduced sensitivity for small cancers that would be found on cystoscopy. Because of the low sensitivity of these markers, other noninvasive screening tests, specifically urine cytology and

cystoscopy, still are considered the gold standard for screening patients for bladder cancer. One study that surveyed patients regarding the use of a noninvasive urine test versus cystoscopy concluded that patients would only want to replace cystoscopy if the test was capable of detecting more than 90% of cancers (AUA, 2007; Yossepowitch, Herr, & Donat, 2007).

Penile Cancer

Penile cancer is relatively rare in the Western world but remains a disease with severe morbidity and mortality and significant psychological ramifications. In other countries, such as those in Asia, Africa, and South America, it is a major health problem where it may represent 10% of all malignancies (Razdan & Gomella, 2005). Rates of penile cancer may vary from different geographical areas in the same country. Whether the differences are caused by social factors or environmental factors is unclear (Micali, Nasca, Innocenzi, & Schwartz, 2006).

Risk Factors

The implementation of universal circumcision could significantly decrease the incidence of invasive penile cancer (Schoen, 2006). Several theories exist regarding why circumcision has this protective effect. Especially in the presence of poor hygiene, the buildup of smegma (exfoliated foreskin cells) has been shown to be carcinogenic. In circumcised males, smegma buildup does not occur because the foreskin has been removed. The smegma buildup may cause inflammation and recurrent infections, thus leading to phimosis, which is a risk factor for penile cancer. In patients with penile cancer, more than half were found to also have phimosis. Phimosis is much more common in males that are uncircumcised. This is demonstrated by the rarity of penile cancer in religious groups such as Muslims, Jews, and the Ibos of Nigeria that perform circumcision as a religious ritual, whereas a higher rate is seen in Hindus, who do not practice circumcision (Micali et al., 2006).

The human papillomavirus (HPV) has been implicated as a risk factor in the development of invasive penile cancer. Men with anogenital warts caused by HPV have a sixfold risk of developing penile cancer (Maden et al., 1993). The prevalence of HPV infection in penile cancer ranges from 15%–71% (Gross & Pfister, 2004; Micali et al., 2006). However, not all penile cancers are positive for HPV. Possibly, two different pathways contribute to the development of penile cancer: one that may be related to HPV in younger adults, and the other unrelated to HPV and found in older adults (Micali et al.).

Smoking also has been shown to be a risk factor for the development of penile cancer, especially invasive penile cancer (Daling et al., 2005). Tobacco may be a promoter of malignant transformation in the setting of infection or chronic inflammation caused by poor hygiene (Razdan & Gomella, 2005). In summary, good hygiene, circumcision, and the avoidance of tobacco use and infection with HPV can reduce the risk of penile cancer.

Screening and Early Detection

Currently, no official guidelines exist for the screening of penile cancer. However, patients who have risk factors should be aware of their risk. They should be taught the signs and symptoms of penile cancer so that if a penile lesion develops, they can seek medical attention promptly.

Penile cancer can manifest in a wide variety of lesions from a reddened area to ulceration. Men at high risk also should be aware of specific premalignant lesions. Leukoplakia is a whitish plaque involving the glans or prepuce associated with chronic inflammation (Razdan & Gomella, 2005). Balanitis xerotic obliterans (BXO) is a chronic sclerosing inflammatory disorder that often causes phimosis. The phimosis is most likely the causative factor rather than the BXO itself (Macali et al., 2006). These lesions usually are removed via surgical resection and correction of the phimosis.

Testicular Cancer

Risk Factors

The cause of testicular cancer is not well understood. Several factors are associated with a higher risk of testicular cancer. The incidence is higher in whites than in blacks. The incidence is highest in Scandinavia, Switzerland, Germany, and New Zealand; intermediate in the United States and Great Britain; and the lowest in Africa and Asia. The ratio of whites to blacks who develop testicular cancer is approximately 4:1 (Bosl, Bajorin, Sheinfeld, Motzer, & Chiganti, 2005). In addition, men who have had one testicular cancer are also at a higher risk for developing a second testicular cancer (Stotts, 2004).

Although the reason is unclear, cryptorchidism (undescended testicle) has been found to increase the risk of testicular cancer. Approximately 2% of patients with inguinal cryptorchid testes develop a germ cell tumor (GCT), whereas 5%–20% of males with a cryptorchid testis will develop a GCT in the normally descended testis (Bosl et al., 2005). An abdominal cryptorchid testis poses a higher risk than an inguinal cryptorchid testis in the development of a GCT. The timing of performing orchiopexy is controversial, but the risk of developing a GCT seems to be reduced if orchiopexy is performed before puberty (Bosl et al.). Men with Klinefelter syndrome 47, XXY karyotype, have testicular atrophy, absence of spermatogenesis, eunuchoid habitus, and gynecomastia. Men with this genetic syndrome are at greater risk for germ cell tumors, especially of the mediastinum.

Finally, men who have a brother with testicular cancer are more likely to develop testicular cancer (McCullagh & Lewis, 2005). A tenfold risk when a sibling has had a testis tumor and a four- to sixfold risk when a father has had a testis tumor have been reported (Rapley, 2007). With this strong link between relatives, a genetic component to the development of testicular cancer has been hypothesized. Ongoing exploration for a causative gene continues (Rapley).

Prevention

The only preventive measure that can be implemented to reduce the risk of testicular cancer is to perform orchiopexy on a cryptorchid testicle before the onset of puberty. All the other known risk factors are genetic or cellular in nature and cannot be altered at this time.

Screening and Early Detection

Testicular examinations by healthcare providers should be implemented during routine physical examinations on all males, particularly those who are 15–35 years of age. Currently, the American Cancer Society (ACS, 2008) does not recommend testicular self-examination as a routine screening technique because of the lack of research supporting such behavior. However, it is an easy and inexpensive way to detect tumors for a highly curable disease, especially if caught early. Teenage males should be given the opportunity to learn how to perform a self-examination (ACS). The best time for it to be performed is after a warm bath or in the shower on a monthly basis. The testicle should be held in one hand while palpated with the other hand, gently rolling the testicle between the thumb and fingers. The testicle should feel smooth and have no lumps. A tubular structure will be felt on the posterior aspect of the testicle, which is the epididymis.

Although testicular cancer is the most common solid tumor among young males, public awareness campaigns in the United States have been lacking because of the rare nature of the disease. To assist in the promotion of self-examination, oncology nurses may partner with schools and other groups that work with teenage males to develop awareness programs of testicular self-examination. This will give young males the information necessary so that they can make an informed decision regarding whether to perform self-examination and what action to take in the event that something unusual is discovered.

Summary

Smoking tobacco is a risk factor for many of the urologic cancers. Quitting smoking or never starting could prevent many urologic cancers. No strongly evidence-based screening or early detection techniques are available for these cancers. Ongoing research is focused on finding better ways to screen for bladder cancer. Therefore, prevention measures such as smoking cessation are important for the general population to implement.

References

Adley, B.P., Smith, N.D., Nayar, R., & Yang, X.J. (2006). Birt-Hogg-Dubé syndrome: Clinicopathologic findings and genetic alterations. *Archives of Pathology and Laboratory Medicine, 130*(12), 1865–1870.

American Cancer Society. (2008). *Can testicular cancer be found early?* Retrieved June 27, 2008, from http://www.cancer.org/docroot/CRI/content/CRI_2_4_3X_Can_Testicular_Cancer_Be_Found_Early_41.asp

American Joint Committee on Cancer. (2002). *Cancer staging handbook* (6th ed.). New York: Springer.

American Urological Association. (2007). *Bladder cancer clinical guideline.* Retrieved June 27, 2008, from http://www.auanet.org/content/guidelines-and-quality-care/clinical-guidelines.cfm?sub=bc

Ashughyan, V.R., Marihart, S., & Djavan, B. (2006). Chemopreventive trials in urologic cancer. *Reviews in Urology, 8*(1), 8–13.

Band, P.R., Le, N.D., MacArthur, A.C., Fang, R., & Gallagher, R.P. (2005). Identification of occupational cancer risks in British Columbia: A population-based case-control study of 1,129 cases of bladder cancer. *Journal of Occupational and Environmental Medicine, 47*(8), 854–858.

Bosl, G.J., Bajorin, D.F., Sheinfeld, J., Motzer, R.J., & Chaganti, R.S.K. (2005). Cancer of the testis. In V.T. DeVita Jr., S. Hellman, & S.A. Rosenberg (Eds.), *Cancer: Principles and practice of oncology* (7th ed., pp. 1269–1293). Philadelphia: Lippincott Williams & Wilkins.

Brauch, H., Weirich, G., Hornauer, M.A., Storkel, S., Wohl, T., & Bruning, T. (1999). Trichloroethylene exposure and specific somatic mutations in patients with renal cell carcinoma. *Journal of the National Cancer Institute, 91*(10), 854–861.

Brinkman, M., Buntinx, F., Muls, E., & Zeegers, M.P. (2006). Use of selenium in chemoprevention of bladder cancer. *Lancet Oncology, 7*(9), 766–774.

Brock, K.E., Gridley, G., Brown, L.M., Yu, M.C., Schoenberg, J.B., Lynch, C.F., et al. (2006). Dietary factors and cancers of the renal pelvis and ureter. *Cancer Epidemiology, Biomarkers and Prevention, 15*(5), 1051–1053.

Cochran, S. (2007). Care of the indwelling urinary catheter: Is it evidence based? *Journal of Wound, Ostomy, and Continence Nursing, 34*(3), 282–288.

Daling, J.R., Madeleine, M.M., Johnson, L.G., Schwartz, S.M., Shera, K.A., Wurscher, M.A., et al. (2005). Penile cancer: Importance of circumcision, human papillomavirus and smoking in in situ and invasive disease. *International Journal of Cancer, 116*(4), 606–616.

Dhote, R., Thiounn, N., Debre, B., & Vidal-Trecan, G. (2004). Risk factors for adult renal carcinoma. *Urologic Clinics of North America, 31*(2), 237–247.

Doublet, J.D., Peraldi, M.N., Gattegno, B., Thibault, P., & Sraer, J.D. (1997). Renal cell carcinoma of native kidneys: Prospective study of 129 renal transplant patients. *Journal of Urology, 158*(1), 42–44.

Gago-Dominguez, M., & Castelao, J.E. (2006). Lipid peroxidation and renal cell carcinoma: Further supportive evidence and new mechanistic insights. *Free Radical Biology and Medicine, 40*(4), 721–733.

Gray, M., & Sims, T.W. (2004). NMP-22 for bladder cancer screening and surveillance. *Urologic Nursing, 24*(3), 171–172, 177–179, 186.

Greene, K.L., Konety, B., & Stoller, M. (2008, May). *Results from the San Francisco Firefighters Bladder Cancer Screening Study* [Abstract]. Poster session presented at the annual meeting of the American Urological Association, Orlando, FL. Retrieved July 29, 2008, from http://www.abstracts2view.com/aua/view.php?nu=AUA08_93782

Groah, S.L., Weitzenkamp, D.A., Lammertse, D.P., Whiteneck, G.G., Lezotte, D.C., & Hamman, R.F. (2002). Excess risk of bladder cancer in spinal cord injury: Evidence for an association between indwelling catheter use and bladder cancer. *Archives of Physical Medicine and Rehabilitation, 83*(3), 346–351.

Gross, G., & Pfister, H. (2004). Role of human papillomavirus in penile cancer, penile intraepithelial squamous cell neoplasias and in genital warts. *Medical Microbiology and Immunology, 193*(1), 35–44.

Grossman, E., Messerli, F.H., & Goldbourt, U. (2001). Antihypertensive therapy and the risk of malignancies. *European Heart Journal, 22*(15), 1343–1352.

Gurung, P.M., Frobisher, C., Leiper, A., Woodhouse, C.R.J., & Hawkins, M.M. (2008, May). *Risk of bladder cancer after childhood cancer* [Abstract]. Poster session presented at the annual meeting of the American Urological Association, Orland, FL. Retrieved July 29, 2008, from http://www.abstracts2view.com/aua/view.php?nu=AUA08_93442

Hart, S. (2008). Urinary catheterization. *Nursing Standard, 22*(27), 44–48.

Heath, C.W., Jr., Lally, C.A., Calle, E.E., McLaughlin, J.K., & Thun, M.J. (1997). Hypertension, diuretics, and antihypertensive medications as possible risk factors for renal cell cancer. *American Journal of Epidemiology, 145*(7), 607–613.

Hess, M.J., Zhan, E.H., Foo, D.K., & Yalla, S.V. (2003). Bladder cancer in patients with spinal cord injury. *Journal of Spinal Cord Medicine, 26*(4), 335–338.

Hiatt, R.A., Tolan, K., & Quesenberry, C.P., Jr. (1994). Renal cell carcinoma and thiazide use: A historical, case control study (California, U.S.A.). *Cancer Causes and Control, 5*(4), 319–325.

Hunt, J.D., van der Hel, O.L., McMillan, G.P., Boffetta, P., & Brennan, P. (2005). Renal cell carcinoma in relation to cigarette smoking: Meta-analysis of 24 studies. *International Journal of Cancer, 114*(1), 101–108.

Larsson, P., Wijkstrom, H., Thorstenson, A., Adolfsson, J., Norming, U., Wicklund, P., et al. (2003). A population-based study of 538 patients with newly detected urinary bladder neoplasms followed during 5 years. *Scandinavian Journal of Urology and Nephrology, 37*(3), 195–201.

Linehan, W.M., Bates, S.E., & Yang, J.C. (2005). Cancer of the genitourinary system: Kidney cancer. In V.T. DeVita Jr., S. Hellman, & S.A. Rosenberg (Eds.), *Cancer: Principles and practice of oncology* (7th ed., pp. 1139–1168). Philadelphia: Lippincott Williams & Wilkins.

Kreiger, N., Marrett, L.D., Dodds, L., Hilditch, S., & Darlington, G.A. (1993). Risk factors for renal cell carcinoma: Results of a population-based case-control study. *Cancer Causes and Control, 4*(2), 101–110.

Maden, C., Sherman K.J., Beckmann, A.M., Hislop, T.G., Teh, C.Z., Ashley, R.L., et al. (1993). History of circumcision, medical conditions, and sexual activity and risk of penile cancer. *Journal of the National Cancer Institute, 85*(1), 19–24.

McCullagh, J., & Lewis, G. (2005). Testicular cancer: Epidemiology, assessment and management. *Nursing Standard, 19*(25), 45–53.

McLaughlin, J.K., Lipworth, L., & Tarone, R.E. (2006). Epidemiologic aspects of renal cell carcinoma. *Seminars in Oncology, 33*(5), 527–533.

Mellemgaard, A., Moller, H., & Olsen, J.H. (1992). Diuretics may increase risk of renal cell carcinoma. *Cancer Causes and Control, 3*(4), 309–312.

Messing, E. (2007). Markers of detection. *Urologic Oncology, 25*(4), 344–347.

Micali, G., Nasca, M.R., Innocenzi, D., & Schwartz, R.A. (2006). Penile cancer. *Journal of the American Academy of Dermatology, 54*(3), 369–391.

Middelton, L., & Lessick, M. (2003). Inherited urologic malignant disorders: Nursing implications. *Urologic Nursing, 23*(1), 15–18, 23–30.

Moyad, M.A. (2001). Obesity, interrelated mechanisms, and exposures and kidney cancer. *Seminars in Urologic Oncology, 19*(4), 270–279.

Prineas, R.J., Folsom, A.R., Zhang, Z.M., Sellers, T.A., & Potter, J. (1997). Nutrition and other risk factors for renal cell carcinoma in postmenopausal women. *Epidemiology, 8*(1), 31–36.

Rapley, E. (2007). Susceptibility alleles for testicular germ cell tumour: A review. *International Journal of Andrology, 30*(4), 242–250.

Razdan, S., & Gomella, L.G. (2005). Cancers of the genitourinary system: Cancer of the urethra and penis. In V.T. DeVita Jr., S. Hellman, & S.A Rosenberg (Eds.), *Cancer: Principles and practice of oncology* (7th ed., pp. 1260–1267). Philadelphia: Lippincott Williams & Wilkins.

Schabath M.B., Spitz, M.R., Lerner S.P., Pillow, P.C., Hernandez, L.M., Delclos, G.L., et al. (2005). Case-control analysis of dietary folate and risk of bladder cancer. *Nutrition and Cancer, 53*(2), 144–151.

Schoen, E.J. (2006). Ignoring evidence of circumcision benefit. *Pediatrics, 118*(1), 385–387.

Schmidt, L.S., Nickerson, M.L., Warren, M.B., Glenn, G.M., Toro, J.R., Merino, M., et al. (2005). Germline BHD-mutation spectrum and phenotype analysis of a large cohort of families with Birt-Hogg-Dubé syndrome. *American Journal of Human Genetics, 76*(6), 1023–1033.

Shipley, W.U., Kaufman, D.S., McDougal, W.S., Dahl, D.M., Michaelson, M.D., & Zietman, A.L. (2005). Cancer of the genitourinary system: Cancer of the bladder, ureter, and renal pelvis. In V.T. DeVita Jr., S. Hellman, & S.A. Rosenberg (Eds.), *Cancer: Principles and practice* (7th ed., pp. 1168–1192). Philadelphia: Lippincott Williams & Wilkins.

Stotts, R.C. (2004). Cancers of the prostate, penis, and testicles: Epidemiology, prevention, and treatment. *Nursing Clinics of North America, 39*(2), 327–340.

Vlaovic, P., & Jewett, M.A. (1999). Cyclophosphamide-induced bladder cancer. *Canadian Journal of Urology, 6*(2), 745–748.

Yossepowitch, O., Herr, H.W., & Donat, S.M. (2007). Use of urinary biomarkers for bladder cancer surveillance: Patient perspective. *Journal of Urology, 177*(4), 1277–1282.

Zbar, B., Glenn, G., Lubensky, I., Choyke, P., Walther, M.M., Magnusson, G., et al. (1995). Hereditary papillary renal cell carcinoma: Clinical studies in 10 families. *Journal of Urology, 153*(3, Pt. 2), 907–912.

Zeegers, M.P., Goldbohm, R.A., & van den Brandt, P.A. (2002). A prospective study on active and environmental tobacco smoking and bladder cancer risk (The Netherlands). *Cancer Causes and Control, 13*(1), 83–90.

Zucchetto, A., Dal Maso, L., Tavani, A., Montella, M., Ramazzotti, V., Talamini, R., et al. (2007). History of treated hypertension and diabetes mellitus and risk of renal cell cancer. *Annals of Oncology, 18*(3), 596–600.

CHAPTER 5

Treatment of Bladder Cancer

Dana L. Overstreet, RN, MSN, FNP-BC, Hong Zhao, MSN, ACNP-BC, CCRN,
Terran W. Sims, RN, MSN, ACNP-BC, COCN, and Jennifer Cash, ARNP, MS, OCN®

Introduction

The majority of bladder cancers are termed *superficial* (or non–muscle invasive) because they do not invade the bladder muscle; approximately one-third are invasive into the bladder muscle. Superficial tumors respond well to local therapy, but recurrence rates can be as high as 30%–70%, with the risk of progression to invasive cancer as high as 10%–30% (Messing, 2007). Approximately 68,810 new cases of bladder cancer were diagnosed and more than 14,100 Americans died of bladder cancer in the United States in 2008 (Jemal et al., 2008). The expected prognosis once bladder cancer has spread to other organs is less than one year (Dreicer, 2001). Understanding the differences in treatment approaches is important when caring for patients with bladder cancer and when helping them and their families decide on treatment options (Overstreet & Sims, 2006).

Surgery

Several surgical options are available to treat both superficial and muscle-invasive bladder cancer. Surgical interventions include tumor biopsy, local resection, and fulguration of the tumor, laser therapy, and total cystectomy with urinary diversion.

Superficial Bladder Cancer

Transurethral Resection of the Bladder Tumor

The initial surgical management of superficial low-grade papillary bladder cancer is transurethral resection of the bladder tumor (TURBT). After either spinal or general anesthesia is induced, a cystoscope is placed through the urethra into the bladder (Bernier, 2005), and a cystoscopic examination of the bladder is performed. After this examination, a resectoscope is inserted to remove the tumor. A fluid such as glycine is infused into the bladder during both the cystoscopy and resec-

tion to remove blood and tissue and aid visualization during the procedures. Electrocautery is used to resect the tumor and control bleeding. The goals of TURBT are to
- Resect all lesions that can be visualized
- Obtain specimens for pathology to diagnose the tumor type and grade
- Stage the tumor (Jones & Campbell, 2007).

At the end of the procedure, specimens are taken to identify any muscle invasion at the tumor base to determine if the entire tumor has been removed. This is performed by the use of a final "pass of the cutting loop or a cold cup biopsy" into the tumor bed (Jones & Campbell, 2007, p. 2451). All abnormal or suspicious areas are biopsied (Jones & Campbell). An indwelling urinary bladder catheter may be placed after bleeding is controlled. This may be a two-way or a three-way catheter that allows for continuous bladder irrigation (CBI) using saline. CBI is used to clear the bladder of clots or debris. In this case, the patient would require hospitalization. Patients with large tumors may have repeated TURBT four to six weeks after the first procedure to examine the bladder and to remove any residual tumor (Nieh & Marshall, 2007).

Risks of TURBT include (Chambers, 2002; Jones & Campbell, 2007)
- Bleeding
- Infection
- Bladder perforation
- Pain
- Damage to the urethra
- Need for more surgery or procedures
- Transurethral resection syndrome (rare) (intraoperative absorption of excess water producing acid-base disturbances and hyponatremia).

The risks of anesthesia include changes in vital signs; injury to eyes, gums, teeth, and dental work; pulmonary embolism; and death. TURBT generally is performed on an outpatient basis and requires 30 minutes to several hours to resect the tumor depending on its size. Patients receive an IV antibiotic such as ciprofloxacin 400 mg prior to the procedure.

They are discharged on a course of antibiotics, a bladder analgesic (e.g., phenazopyridine), and an oral narcotic such as acetaminophen with oxycodone. Patients are instructed that they may experience irritative voiding symptoms in the immediate postoperative period and hematuria for several days. If bleeding or clots are a concern, the patient may be admitted for CBI. Nurses instruct patients to call and report symptoms of fever, urinary clot retention (such as pain, bladder spasms, dark urine, seeping of clots through the urethra), dysuria, or severe bladder pain. Patients are seen a few weeks postoperatively to discuss the pathology report and to discuss additional treatment planning, as needed.

Laser Therapy

Laser therapy is more expensive than TURBT because of the cost of laser fibers (Jones & Campbell, 2007). Tumors up to 2.5 cm in size may be managed using this approach (Jones & Campbell). The neodymium:yttrium-aluminum-garnet (Nd:YAG) laser often is used to treat bladder tumors (Jones & Campbell). The YAG laser minimizes bleeding, and obturator reflex (leg rotation and adduction during procedure) is not a risk. Laser therapy coagulates the tissues, so no tissue is available for pathologic analysis after therapy. Patients undergoing YAG laser treatment usually have "recurrent, low-grade lesions whose biology is already known" (Jones & Campbell, p. 2453). The scatter of laser energy to normal tissue is a potential complication that could damage or perforate normal surrounding organs (Jones & Campbell).

Invasive Bladder Cancer

Treatment for invasive bladder cancer includes surgery, radiation, radiation plus chemotherapy, and chemotherapy alone. Radical cystectomy or cystoprostatectomy with urinary diversion is the gold standard for the treatment of muscle-invasive bladder cancer. When treating bladder cancer with radical cystectomy, pelvic lesion recurrence rates of 5%–30% and overall five-year survival rates of 45%–60% is the standard outcome to which bladder preservation regimens must be compared (Coen et al., 2006; Shipley et al., 2002). Cystectomy also may be used to manage radiation fibrosis or cystitis arising from exposure to external beam radiation or interstitial radiation for cancers such as pelvic or gynecologic cancers. The factors to consider when choosing a treatment option include patient age, overall health and comorbidities, the grade and stage of the cancer, and the risks and benefits of each treatment (National Cancer Institute [NCI], 2002).

Radical Cystectomy

Radical cystectomy may be performed through an open laparotomy incision or by a robotic-assisted laparoscopic approach. Because of the risk of intraoperative and postoperative complications, a surgeon trained in cystectomy and urinary diversion is required. Cystectomy is a complicated surgery that removes the bladder and bilateral pelvic lymph nodes. In females, the uterus and ovaries are removed, and in males, the prostate is removed via a midline incision. Advances in laparoscopy, robotic surgery, and urologic oncology surgery have made it possible for surgeons to perform nerve-sparing robotic-assisted laparoscopic radical cystoprostatectomy, which may allow for the preservation of erectile function (Menon et al., 2003). Not every patient is a candidate for robotic-assisted surgery, nor is each patient a candidate for each type of urinary diversion. Patient variables influence the type of surgical approach and procedure performed. In addition to the routine management of patients undergoing major abdominal surgery, management of urinary diversion is a major component of the patients' preoperative and postoperative care. Part of the intestine (small or large bowel) is used to create a route for urinary drainage. An ileal conduit (urostomy) drains effluent through a stoma or an internal pouch (Indiana pouch or neobladder) created with a section of intestine to allow for catheterization of urine (Indiana) or normal voiding (neobladder). Important factors requiring consideration are the cancer stage, extent of the cancer involving the ureters or urethra, previous radiation, surgery involving the bowel or fibrosis, and other cancers. The urologist, with input from the patient, prepares an individualized patient plan of care and selects the most appropriate urinary diversion for each patient. Information about the surgical options presented both orally and in writing along with educational diagrams of each type of procedure is provided prior to the final determination of the type of surgery to be performed. Patients are encouraged to discuss their options with family, the ostomy nurse, and nursing staff. The ostomy nurse is helpful with assessment of the patient in order to assist with determination of the best type of diversion for a particular patient, selection of the optimal placement of the urinary diversion and initiation of ostomy or diversion preoperative teaching (Colwell, Goldberg, & Carmel, 2004). Additional issues of concern include the current health situation, patient age, mental status, presence of physical dexterity required to perform self-care, assistance available in the home, mental preparedness for altered body image, and patient motivation to learn care (Colwell et al.). Preoperative teaching includes the role of the certified wound, ostomy, and continence nurse, surgical procedure, stoma creation, appearance and care, incisions, expected outcomes for each surgery, recovery time, drain and tube placement, surgical supplies, appliances, clothing options, and discharge planning including home care. Routine preoperative teaching includes pulmonary hygiene, early ambulation, prevention of deep vein thromboembolic (DVT) events, return of gastrointestinal (GI) function, prevention of pressure sites on the skin, and pain management.

Robotic-Assisted Laparoscopic Cystectomy

Robotic-assisted laparoscopic cystectomy has gained attention in the recent years and can offer patients many advantages, including minimal blood loss, shorter hospital stay and quicker recovery, and possibly more precise and rapid removal of the bladder and possibly nerve preservation, depending on the experience and expertise of the surgeon (Menon et al., 2003; Steers, LeBeau, Cardella, & Fulmer, 2004). Understanding patient variables, selection, risks, potential complications, and benefits of robotic-assisted surgery helps nurses to care for patients through the preoperative and postoperative course to achieve a successful surgical outcome (Anvari, Birch, Bamehriz, Gryfe, & Chapman, 2004; Overstreet & Sims, 2006).

A variety of patient variables may influence surgical procedure selection. Because of the length of the laparoscopes and the robotic instruments along with configuration of the robot, the height and weight of the patient must be considered (Overstreet & Sims, 2006). Obese patients may not be candidates because of body size in relationship to the length and configuration of the laparoscopic instruments. A complete medical and surgical history is obtained from the patient and evaluated in relationship to the planned urinary diversion (Overstreet & Sims). Contraindications to laparoscopic robotic surgery include prior radiation therapy (RT) to the abdomen because scarring, adhesions, and friable tissue may be present in the abdomen (Overstreet & Sims). Other contraindications include previous abdominal hernia repairs with mesh placement or a history of colon resection, which would narrow the selection of urinary diversion procedures that could be performed (Overstreet & Sims).

In addition to a thorough review of the patient's medical and surgical history, other "red flags" that can have an adverse impact on surgical outcomes also are considered. These include a history of ruptured viscera and peritonitis, obesity, body mass index greater than 40, previous RT, a history of transurethral or suprapubic prostatectomy, large-volume prostates, large median or lateral lobes, and a narrow pelvis (Menon et al., 2004). The presence of a red flag does not make the patient ineligible for a robotic-assisted laparoscopic surgery. Rather, it should be addressed when discussing surgical options with the patient, especially the topics of patient expectations and postoperative outcomes.

Both general and laparoscopic robotic surgeries may require 8–12 hours of operative time. After the induction of general anesthesia, the operating room table is adjusted so the patient is placed in an extended lithotomy with a 45° Trendelenburg position tilt (Menon et al., 2003). As with any major surgical procedure involving the abdomen, a nasogastric tube (NGT) is placed for the management of GI secretions, and an indwelling urinary bladder catheter is placed to monitor renal function via urinary output. The robotic procedure approach includes the use of the robot, the laparoscopic instrument ports, and the console where the surgeon sits. The abdomen is marked for optimal placement of the insertion of the ports and instruments and so the robot can work with ease without one arm interfering with the function of another. Marking the abdomen also allows for accurate positioning of the robot. Other members of the surgical support team stand at the operating room table on either side of the patient to provide the surgeon with support during the procedure. The surgeon operates the laparoscopic arms through the console. The majority of the dissection is completed using forceps and a cautery hook (Menon et al., 2003). The other team members use grasping forceps and suction to provide retraction of surrounding organs and to provide adequate exposure (Menon et al., 2003). Bilateral pelvic lymphadenectomy is completed, and the bladder is removed. Pelvic drains and a urinary catheter are placed based on the type of urinary diversion chosen. The urinary diversion is completed using the open 5–6 cm surgical incision (Menon et al., 2003).

Preoperative Patient Care

The routine preoperative evaluation of cystectomy patients considers the patient history and physical examination, height and weight, vital signs, pulse, oximetry, the type of surgery and diversion planned, and whether the surgery is elective or emergency. The age of the patient, smoking history, bleeding history, and probable length of the surgical procedure are considered in relation to the patient's functional status (including manual dexterity), exercise tolerance, and cardiopulmonary systems. Psychosocial factors are considered, including the presence of help in the home or need for placement in a skilled facility after surgery, the diagnosis of dementia or other cognitive impairment, and the level of patient preparedness and acceptance of the procedure, as these variables can impair self-care and adjustment to the diversion. Routine laboratory studies performed include complete blood count (CBC), chemistry, and coagulation studies and a type and hold for at least three units of packed red blood cells.

Cardiac Concerns

Many patients with bladder cancer have an extensive smoking history and are at risk for both intraoperative and postoperative cardiac events. This is in addition to the prolonged intraoperative immobility and the patient's age, which may prompt a more extensive preoperative cardiac evaluation. An electrocardiogram is recommended for men older than 40 years old and women older than 50 years old or anyone with a cardiac history, cardiac surgery, hypertension, shortness of breath, smoking history, or cardiac symptoms such as chest pain (Girard, 2005; Shurpin & DeSimone, 1998). A preoperative echocardiogram or stress test may be needed in patients with a heart murmur or other cardiac history, and a cardiology consult should be obtained in patients with heart disease or multiple comorbidities. Patients with heart valve disease will need antibiotic prophylaxis to reduce the risk of endocarditis (Overstreet & Sims, 2006).

Pulmonary Concerns

A chest x-ray is routinely performed on all preoperative patients. A smoking history, prolonged operating room time, exaggerated Trendelenburg positioning, and insufflation of the abdomen with air may require that patients at risk for or with a history of pulmonary disease such as chronic obstructive pulmonary disease (COPD) have a preoperative pulmonary consult, pulmonary function tests, and arterial blood gases. These will evaluate lung capacity and function and determine the patient's risk of requiring postoperative ventilator support. All patients are instructed to stop smoking immediately at the first preoperative consultation.

Medication Review

Routine preoperative care includes a review of medications, both prescribed and over the counter, alcohol consumption, smoking, use of herbs, vitamins, and illegal substances, and provision of instructions on how the patient should take medications prior to surgery. Patients continue to take routine medications such as those prescribed for heart disease, seizures, or hypertension with a small sip of water the morning of surgery. Diabetic patients who take metformin should be instructed to stop taking the drug 48 hours before surgery to decrease the risk of lactic acidosis (Overstreet & Sims, 2006). Additionally, diabetic patients taking insulin are instructed to take 2/3 of their usual bedtime insulin dose and to not take insulin on the morning of their surgery (Overstreet & Sims). Many medications increase the risk of bleeding during surgery and in the postoperative period. To reduce the risk of drug-associated bleeding, aspirin is stopped one to two weeks prior to surgery and vitamin E is stopped one week prior to surgery (Nieh & Marshall, 2007; Overstreet & Sims). Warfarin is stopped five days before surgery with approval from the prescriber. Patients may require anticoagulant replacement with continuous infusion of unfractionated heparin or enoxaparin. Consultation with a hematologist may be required (Overstreet & Sims).

Gastrointestinal Concerns

Bowel preparation is required prior to cystectomy to clean the bowel. Two days before surgery, a clear liquid diet is initiated. The bowel prep is started the day before surgery with laxatives and nonabsorbable antibiotics. This is needed not only because a bowel segment is needed for the reconstruction or diversion but also to reduce the risk of infection should the bowel be accidently perforated during the surgical procedure. Both oral and written instructions on the bowel preparation and clear liquid diet are provided to patients. Patients at risk for dehydration, nausea and vomiting, or intolerance to the bowel preparation regimen may require hospitalization for IV hydration during preparation.

Prior to surgery, the patient receives warm IV hydration such as lactated Ringer's (2,000 ml) and IV antibiotic such as cefotetan (2 g). Clindamycin (900 mg) and aztreonam (2 g) may be substituted for patients with a penicillin allergy (Overstreet & Sims, 2006). To reduce the risk of DVT from prolonged immobility, thromboembolic stockings are applied prior to surgery and sequential compression devices are used intraoperatively and in the recovery room (Overstreet & Sims). The use of subcutaneous heparin for DVT prevention varies by facility policy.

Postoperative Nursing Care

Routine postoperative nursing care is provided to all patients who have undergone a cystectomy. A complete nursing assessment is performed on all body systems with a focus on the drains and catheters specific to the diversion; early ambulation; GI, cardiac, and pulmonary function; and prevention of postoperative complications associated with prolonged immobility during surgery. Paralytic ileus prolongs the hospital stay in patients undergoing a radical cystectomy (Baumgartner, Wells, Chang, Cookson, & Smith, 2002) (see Table 5-1 for information related to the postoperative care of the patient).

Early Ambulation

Getting patients out of bed into the chair and ambulating is crucial to their recovery. Ambulation reduces the risk of DVT and pressure ulcer formation and improves lung, cardiovascular, and GI function, as well as general overall well-being. Ambulation is so important in prevention that some surgeons initiate it as early as the first postoperative day. All the drainage tubes and catheters must be held in place securely to prevent dislodgement and so that they do not interfere with walking. DVT prophylaxis is important because of the long surgical time with prolonged immobility. Subcutaneous heparin and compression stockings are used routinely for any abdominal surgery, and use is continued until discharge. Patients who undergo pelvic surgery are at risk for lower-extremity edema and may want to wear the support/compression stockings at home. Ambulation also will assist with mobilization of postoperative fluid retention.

Cardiac and Pulmonary Concerns

All patients who undergo surgery may develop cardiac and pulmonary complications. Vital signs are assessed frequently along with pulse oximetry readings. Depending on the patient's condition, supplemental oxygen may be needed. Atelectasis is common in the postoperative period and may manifest itself as an early postoperative fever (Girard, 2005). Therefore, pulmonary hygiene with incentive spirometry, coughing, deep breathing, and turning are extremely important in helping to prevent respiratory complications. Good pain management is needed to promote patient cooperation with these activities. Pneumonia is a postoperative complication that will prolong the hospital admission. Prompt removal of the NGT when bowel function returns will help to reduce this risk, as will good pulmonary hygiene. Nurses monitor for these problems and also administer blood products to manage anemia.

Table 5-1. Postoperative Assessment and Nursing Interventions

Assessment	Nursing Intervention
Knowledge deficit related to surgery and urinary diversion	Patient education for an incontinent diversion includes • Normal appearance of stoma • Care of stoma and peristomal skin and incisional care • Signs and symptoms of infection and methods to reduce risk • Purpose of urethral stents that are removed (usually) at the first postoperative visit in the doctor's office or clinic visit • Expected effluent, including presence of mucus and, in the early postoperative period, possible presence of blood • Emptying of pouch, connecting and disconnecting of night bag • Cleansing of night bag • Application of appliance and basic appliance problem solving such as achieving a good seal • General clothing options • Activity restrictions such as no heavy lifting for four to six weeks after surgery and no driving for at least two weeks • Pain management and bowel management, diet, and hydration. Patient education for a continent diversion includes • Management of the tubes and drains • Signs and symptoms of infection • Signs and symptoms requiring physician notification after discharge • Necessary supplies and equipment • Incision management.
Malecot tube or catheter and indwelling urinary catheters	• Keep drains, tubes, and catheters straight (not kinked), patent, and functioning at all times. • Monitor urine output frequently as per policy. Notify the physician of urine output less than 30 ml/hour. • Investigate the cause if urine output decreases. Examine tubes for kinks and twists. Check urinary appliance for leaks underneath. • Gently irrigate the Malecot as per physician order as preferences vary to establish and maintain open drainage. If urine does not drain after gentle irrigation to flush mucous plugs, notify the surgical team. If not corrected, this could lead to undue tension on surgical anastomoses secondary to obstruction. • Assess patient for dehydration, which also may be a cause of inadequate urine drainage. Compare intake and output with total fluid balance. • Monitor serum lab markers for renal function. • Weigh patient daily.
Surgical drains	• Notify the surgical team if the Jackson Pratt or Penrose drainage increases in volume. This could represent a urine leak or bleeding. • Send a sample of fluid to the lab to determine if it is urine.
Pain	• Administer epidural narcotics per institutional policy to effectively manage immediate postoperative pain. • Administer parenteral narcotics for breakthrough pain. • Administer oral pain medication after the patient's gastrointestinal (GI) motility is established. • Notify the surgeon if patient's pain relief is inadequate.
Cardiovascular and pulmonary systems	• Support deep vein thrombosis (DVT) prophylaxis with heparin, compression stockings, and early ambulation. Some centers use sequential compression devices instead of stockings. Post-cystectomy patients are at high risk for DVT. • Assist patient with ambulation to prevent both cardiovascular and pulmonary complications such as pulmonary embolus, atelectasis, pleural effusions, and pneumonia. • Administer IV fluids. • Assist patient with pulmonary hygiene.
Self-care, catheterizing and irrigation of the Malecot	• Instruct the patient and family members to irrigate the Malecot and indwelling urinary bladder catheters as directed by the physician for consistent drainage and removal/flushing of any mucous plugs prior to discharge.
Security of ureteral stents	• Notify the surgeon immediately if a ureteral stent dislodges.
Infection	• Monitor vital signs as per policy. • Monitor complete blood count (CBC) results. • Notify surgeon of patient temperature over 100.5°F, abdominal pain, abdominal rigidity, change in wound appearance, change in breath sounds, redness or swelling of legs, tachycardia, or hypotension.

(Continued on next page)

Table 5-1. Postoperative Assessment and Nursing Interventions *(Continued)*	
Assessment	**Nursing Intervention**
Bleeding	• Monitor CBC. • Monitor patient for pallor or signs of active bleeding. • Monitor color and quantity of output from drains. • Report increase in heart rate or decrease in blood pressure immediately to physician.
GI tract function	• Maintain patency of nasogastric tube (NGT). • Monitor NGT output. • Monitor GI tract function by listening for bowel sounds and asking patient to report passage of flatus or small stools.
Stoma or diversion	• Assess color of stoma. Stoma should be red and moist with possible edema. Report changes in color to blue, gray, or black immediately to surgical team, as this may be evidence of tissue hypoxia. If present, these color changes may be a surgical emergency to repair. • Assess functioning of diversion. • Monitor output from diversion catheter and drains. Report changes in color and output to surgeon.
Incontinence related to diversion	• Consult certified wound, ostomy, and continence nurse, advanced practice nurse, or ostomy clinical nurse specialist for assistance with managing a patient's incontinence.

Note. Based on information from Bernier, 2005; Chu & DeVita, 2006; Colwell et al., 2004; Langerak & Dreisbach, 2001; National Comprehensive Cancer Network, 2009.

From "Care of the Patient Undergoing Radical Cystectomy With a Robotic Approach," by D.L. Overstreet and T.W. Sims, 2006, *Urologic Nursing, 26*(2), p. 121. Copyright 2006 by Society of Urologic Nurses and Associates, Inc. Adapted with permission.

Pain Management

Pain is managed with an epidural catheter and patient-controlled analgesia (PCA) for the first several days (usually 24–48 hours) after surgery. Pain is assessed every two hours, and the physician is notified of inadequate pain relief so that the dose or rate of the PCA can be increased. After several days, the epidural catheter may be removed and IV PCA used. Once bowel function returns, oral medications are used.

Gastrointestinal Function

The bowel stops peristalsis when the abdomen is opened. Therefore, to manage GI secretions and reduce the risk of vomiting, the patient will have an NGT. The NGT is kept secured, patent, and draining. The amount of drainage is recorded, and the patient is assessed for nausea and vomiting. Patients may require antiemetics in spite of the NGT to manage nausea. The tube may need to be flushed to remain patent. The nurse monitors daily serum chemistry levels. IV fluids are administered for hydration, and electrolytes may need replacement depending on electrolyte levels. When the NGT is removed after the patient starts to pass flatus, the nurse monitors the patient's tolerance to clear liquids and an advancing diet. A stool softener is used to reduce the risk of constipation developing.

Renal Function

Monitoring renal function is a critical function of nurses. The creatinine and blood urea nitrogen levels are checked along with electrolyte and ion levels. Urine output is monitored every hour for the first postoperative day and then every eight hours, and the physician is notified of a volume output of less than 30 ml/hour (Bernier, 2005). All tubes must be kept straight (not kinked) and patent, and the output must be recorded. If a stoma was created, its function must be monitored closely. Nurses must watch for leakage and urine seepage from under a urinary appliance.

Wound Care

The incisions and abdomen are monitored for infection and bleeding. If drainage is suspicious for an infection, a culture may be ordered and sent to the laboratory. The patient's CBC is monitored for a rising white blood cell count, and the vital signs are monitored for evidence of an infection or bleeding. Output from drains and tubes also is monitored, and any increase in output or change in color is reported to the surgeon. The color of the stoma is monitored, and if it is not red and moist (its normal condition), the surgeon is notified (Bernier, 2005).

Hospital Discharge

The hospital stay ranges from 7–10 days with discharge depending on diet tolerance, bowel function, and ability to perform some self-care related to management of the diversion and to ambulate (Overstreet & Sims, 2006). Patient education includes management of the wound, care of the urinary diversion, and any drains or catheters the patient has at the time of discharge. Activity, diet, and signs and symptoms to report to the surgeon are taught to the patient and family. Both written and oral instructions are provided. Sexual concerns are addressed because men may experience erectile dysfunction (caused by the removal of the prostate and nerves), and women may experience menopause (prompted by the removal of the ovaries) as a result of the surgery (Nieh & Marshall, 2007).

Complications

Complications associated with cystectomy include DVT, pneumonia, wound infection, blood loss, ureteral anastomosis stricture, stenosis, alteration in acid-base balance, altered electrolytes, and cancer recurrence (Nieh & Marshall, 2007; Overstreet & Sims, 2006). Urethral stricture (with neobladder) may present as urinary retention and overflow incontinence. A reservoir rupture (neobladder) may result from an untreated urethral stricture. In addition, sphincter failure presents as incontinence (Overstreet & Sims). Failure to catheterize an Indiana pouch as directed can lead to pouch rupture. Patients may develop skin problems from the urinary diversion appliance. The ostomy nurse should be consulted to assist with the management of skin issues. Patient education includes the risk of a parastomal hernia with a urostomy. Prevention strategies are discussed, as surgical repair usually is not an option because of the high rate of recurrence and need for additional surgery. Management includes the use of a hernia support belt and the application of an appropriate appliance that allows for a good fit dependent on the anatomic changes in the stoma due to the hernia. Other stomal complications may occur after a urinary diversion. The most common include stenosis or retraction, prolapse, and necrosis (Colwell et al., 2004). Long-term complications may include formation of renal or urinary reservoir calculi, urinary tract infection, pyelonephritis, or pouchitis.

Nursing Implications for Surgical Patients

Nursing care of surgical patients begins with a complete preoperative physical assessment; continues with instructing and counseling patients regarding their particular type of surgery and reservoir, postoperative nursing care, and side effects and possible complications of the surgery; and exploring patients' expectations of the surgery. When nurses have an understanding of the types of surgery used to treat bladder cancer, they are able to provide total care to their patients.

Radiation Therapy

Over the past two decades, the use of traditional external beam RT as a single-modality treatment of bladder cancer has decreased (Petrovich, Stein, Jozsef, & Formenti, 2004). Contemporary management of bladder cancer using RT, either external beam or internal brachytherapy, has become multifaceted. Goals of treatment include (Coen, Zietman, Kaufman, & Shipley, 2007; National Comprehensive Cancer Network [NCCN], 2009; Petrovich et al.)

- Organ-sparing regimens
- Postsurgical adjuvant therapy, with or without chemotherapy, to decrease the risk of local or incisional recurrence
- Palliation of locally advanced or metastatic disease to alleviate obstruction, bleeding, or pain.

A combination of advances in imaging modalities, RT delivery systems, and planning techniques have allowed for more precise definition of treatment fields. These advances have enabled the delivery of higher doses to the tumor while sparing critical surrounding targets for greater control of disease with anticipated better quality of life.

Treatment of Early-Stage (T1) Disease and Tumor In Situ (Tis)

Management of newly diagnosed bladder cancer is based on the pathology of the biopsy specimen, more specifically, the histology, grade, and depth of invasion of the tumor. Seventy to eighty percent of newly diagnosed bladder tumors are low grade (Ta, T1) and confined to the mucosa (Kaufman, 2006; NCCN, 2009). RT is not indicated in the treatment of superficial (Ta) papillomas, T1 carcinomas (grade 1 or 2), or a T1-associated in situ component (Tis) because of a low risk of progression to a more advanced stage, although local recurrence rates are approximately 70% (NCCN; Petrovich et al., 2004). NCCN guidelines for patients with high-grade (G3) Ta papillary or T1 solid tumors, although considered to have a relatively high risk (25%–70%) for recurrence and progression of disease, have not integrated RT into their management regimen. Prior to the development of the NCCN guidelines, studies conducted in Israel (Gofrit et al., 2004) and the Netherlands (van der Heijden et al., 2004) evaluated the efficacy of local microwave or radio frequency hyperthermia (thermal energy) and adjuvant intravesical chemotherapy for patients prophylactically or with multiple or recurrent G3, Ta or T1 bladder tumors. Approximately 80% of patients were reported as recurrence-free at 20–24 months.

Treatment of Muscle-Invasive Disease (Organ-Confined T2a, T2b)

Radical cystectomy has been considered the gold standard in the treatment of patients with invasive bladder cancer (NCCN, 2009; Petrovich et al., 2004; Rodel, 2004; Shipley, Kaufman, Tester, Pilepich, & Sandler, 2003). However, since the early 1990s, organ preservation with multimodality treatment regimens of limited surgery, chemotherapy, and RT have been recommended as reasonable alternatives to standard radical cystectomy and urinary diversion with comparable or higher survival rates (Kaufman, 2006; NCCN; Petrovich et al.; Rodel; Shipley et al., 2003).

The primary goal of therapy for organ-confined invasive lesions is to determine if the bladder should be preserved or removed immediately, and to assess the risk for regional or distant spread that requires adjuvant systemic therapies. For patients with T2 disease without evidence of hydronephrosis, bladder-sparing regimens include complete TURBT with consideration of adjuvant RT, with or without chemotherapy given concurrently for radiosensitization (NCCN, 2009). RT also may be utilized in patients who had a segmental cystectomy with a subsequently identified increased pathologic risk of positive lymph nodes, positive margins, or the identification of higher-grade disease. RT may be the sole modality used for patients with extensive comorbid disease and poor performance status (NCCN; Petrovich et al., 2004). Five-year survival rates for patients receiving multimodality therapy were higher (50% or greater) than for those receiving RT as a single treatment modality (50% or less) (NCI, 2008; NCCN; Petrovich et al.).

Common radiation dosing and treatment schedules consist of delivering 60–66 gray (Gy), given in equally divided fractions of 1.8–2 Gy per day, 5 days per week, over 6–8 weeks (Petrovich et al., 2004). External beam radiation therapy (EBRT) delivers high-energy beams directed from a machine outside the body with treatment fields that commonly include the bladder, proximal urethra, and in male patients, the prostate with the prostatic urethra and the regional lymphatics. See Table 5-2 for a guide to bladder symptom management for patients receiving RT. Treatment planning considerations for decreasing side effects of therapy include boosting a smaller treatment volume to the highest doses, treating patients with an empty bladder to reduce the overall size of the smaller target volume, as well as the use of sophisticated delivery systems (e.g., image-guided intensity-modulated radiotherapy [IMRT] or TomoTherapy®) that utilize real-time monitoring systems to account for bladder movement for increased treatment accuracy (McBain & Logue, 2005; NCCN, 2009; Petrovich et al.).

Trimodality therapy, using a combination of chemotherapy and radiation after maximal TURBT, has been extensively studied over the past 20 years. Researchers from many prominent groups and institutions, including Massachusetts General Hospital and the Radiation Therapy Oncology Group (RTOG) developed six prospective phase I–III protocols (Kaufman, 2006; NCCN, 2009; Petrovich et al., 2004; Rodel, 2004; Shipley et al., 2003). The most studied chemoradiation protocol reported by NCCN is the delivery of 40 Gy EBRT in equally divided daily fractions with two doses of concurrent cisplatin, followed by an additional 25 Gy of EBRT with one additional dose of cisplatin if no evidence of residual disease is demonstrated on endoscopic reevaluation. Of the patients who received this protocol, 70% were disease-free in the bladder on initial post-treatment cystoscopic examination. However,

nearly one-quarter of the patients developed recurrence or progression of their disease. The addition of chemotherapy to EBRT results in an overall increased complete response (CR) of 40%–80% (Petrovich et al.). A prospective randomized clinical trial by Naslund, Nilsson, and Littbrand (1994) in 168 patients with T2 to T4 tumors used hyperfractionation treatment schedules (e.g., two or three times daily radiation dosing with lower daily doses) to higher cumulative doses greater than 84 Gy, with comparable bladder toxicity, increased local-control benefit, and higher 5-year and 10-year survival rates than conventional single-day dosing (NCCN; Petrovich et al.).

Internal radiation, or brachytherapy, is not a common part of bladder cancer management in the United States. However, for stages T1–T3 disease, combination treatment with EBRT and interstitial brachytherapy has been used primarily in Europe and Japan. For example, an interstitial therapy protocol for bladder cancer delivers 40 Gy of EBRT at 2 Gy per day. This is followed by a boost of 20–30 Gy of afterloaded interstitial therapy with iridium-192 sources with or without associated partial cystectomy and/or lymphadenectomy with five-year survival rates of 48%–74% (Petrovich et al., 2004).

The use of preoperative RT for T2 bladder cancer is controversial. Treatment goals in this setting are to (Huncharek, Muscat, & Geschwind, 1998; NCI, 2008; Petrovich et al., 2004)
- Reduce the tumor size in an attempt to downstage the cancer, thus making the surgery easier
- Decrease the incidence of local recurrence following radical cystectomy
- Decrease the incidence of distant metastasis
- Improve survival
- Lessen the incidence of surgical complications.

A meta-analysis by these same authors examining the role of preoperative radiation (16 Gy to upwards of 40–50 Gy) versus radical cystectomy alone concluded that the routine use of preoperative radiation produced no significantly improved treatment outcomes (Huncharek et al., 1998; NCI, 2008; Petrovich et al., 2004). Petrovich et al. also reported that the disadvantage of preoperative RT is the unavailability of a complete pathologic staging, which may contribute to unnecessary adjuvant therapy for those patients inaccurately identified with having a lower probability of tumor recurrence.

Treatment of Muscle-Invasive Disease (Non–Organ-Confined, T3a, T3b, T4)

According to NCCN (2009) guidelines, considerations for RT, with or without chemotherapy, are given to those patients with disease that has spread beyond the confines of the bladder wall, with nodal involvement, with or without vascular invasion because of a greater than 50% risk of systemic relapse. Bladder-sparing regimens generally are not recommended for this group of patients; however, they still may be utilized

Table 5-2. Bladder Symptom Management for Patients Receiving Radiation Therapy

Side Effect	Symptoms	Interventions (for Duration of Symptoms)

Urinary bladder, acute	• Frequency
	• Urgency
	• Hesitancy
	• Hematuria
	• Dysuria
	• Bladder spasms (uncommon)
	• Incomplete bladder emptying
	• Nocturia
		• Alpha-blockers (titrate dose)
		  – Tamsulosin 0.4 mg, 1–2 times/day
		  – Doxazosin 1–8 mg daily
		  – Terazosin 1–10 mg daily
		  – Alfuzosin 10 mg once daily
		  – Educate patient about potential hypotensive episodes, dizziness, GI upset, and peripheral edema.
		• Steroids; NSAIDs (ibuprofen, naproxen)
		• Antispasmodics (as needed for bladder spasms)
		  – Tolterodine tartrate 2–4 mg daily
		  – Oxybutynin chloride 5–15 mg
		  – Belladonna and opium suppository every 12 hours
		  – Educate the patient about dry mouth, constipation, somnolence, and risks of urinary retention and infection.
		• Urinary antiseptics (combination products that include methylene blue)
		  – Educate patient about discoloration of urine, possible appearance of rash, flushing of skin, dizziness.
		• Urinary alkalinizers
		  – Potassium citrate
		  – Sodium bicarbonate tablets, baking soda
		  – Educate patient about GI upset, bowel changes, electrolyte disturbance, and the need to reduce dietary salt intake.
		  – Remind patient that smoking is a major bladder irritant.

	• Urinary retention	• Perform voiding trial, urodynamics
		  – Phenoxybenzamine hydrochloride or bethanecol chloride three times daily orally to increase urine flow.
		  – Educate patient about hypotensive episodes, bowel changes, flushing of skin.
		  – Indwelling catheter may be used or patient may be taught intermittent self-catherization, if indicated.

Urinary bladder, late	• Dysuria
	• Hematuria
		• Avoid dietary bladder irritants
		• Avoid urinary alkalinizers
		• Increase fluid intake
		• Pentosan polysulfate sodium 100 mg tid for 6–12 months to reduce symptoms of chronic dysuria. Educate patient about GI upset, bowel changes.
		• Antidepressants/anxiolytic
		  – Amitriptyline hydrochloride 25–50 mg at bedtime
		  – Alprazolam 0.25–0.5 mg at bedtime
		  – Educate patient about drowsiness, dizziness, and caution with driving and operating heavy equipment.
		• Dimethyl sulfoxide (DMSO) bladder installations for chronic dysuria/cystitis *not* remedied by other medications. Educate patient about garlic odor on breath and skin and possible transient discomfort during installation.
		• Other workup: urine cytology, IVP, cystoscopy, FISH test to determine etiology and source of chronic hematuria.

Rectal, acute	• Bowel changes • Diarrhea/constipation • Frequency • Urgency • Painless rectal bleeding • Rectal irritation	• Low-residue diet • Sitz baths as needed • Sucralfate 1 g, 4–6 time/day to regulate bowel consistency and protect rectal mucosa. Educate patient about GI upset, bloating. • Hydrocortisone or mesalamine suppository 1–2 times/day to reduce rectal discomfort. Not to exceed six weeks of use. Educate patient about bowel changes. • Non-prescriptive fiber laxatives to reduce incidence of diarrhea or constipation

(Continued on next page)

Table 5-2. Bladder Symptom Management for Patients Receiving Radiation Therapy *(Continued)*

Side Effect	Symptoms	Interventions (for Duration of Symptoms)
Rectal, late	• Proctitis • Bleeding • Rectal discomfort	• Mesalamine suppository daily at bedtime for 6–8 weeks • Sucralfate 1 g 4–6 times/day for 3 months • Pentoxifylline 400 mg 3 times/day for 3 months to reduce incidence of rectal bleeding and aid in healing of tissue. Educate patient about GI upset, dizziness, and headache. • Colonoscopy to evaluate chronic rectal bleeding not remedied by medications after 3 months use. • Laser coagulation to remedy chronic rectal bleeding not resolved by medications.
Erectile dysfunction, acute and late	• Decreased ability to maintain erection	• Address psychogenic and other causes (e.g., stress, marital problems, job responsibilities, age, smoking, comorbid illness) • PDE5 inhibitors (e.g., sildenafil, vardenafil, tadalafil). Educate patient about contraindications of nitrates, visual changes, headache, nasal stuffiness, possible interaction with alpha-blockers, and prolonged erection. • Alprostadil intraurethral suppositories. Educate patient about penile irritation, urethritis. • Intracavernosal alprostadil self-injections. Educate patient about penile pain, prolonged erection, and hematoma. • Vacuum erection device • Over-the-counter supplements (no testosterone derivatives)

FISH—fluorescence in situ hybridization; GI—gastrointestinal; IVP—intravenous pyelography; NSAIDs—nonsteroidal anti-inflammatory drugs; PDE5—phosphodiesterase type-5

Note. Based on information from Krause et al., 2006; McMahon et al., 2006; Yamanouchi Pharmaceutical Co., 2004. Table courtesy of the Dattoli Cancer Center, Sarasota, FL. Reprinted with permission.

for those patients with extensive comorbid disease or poor performance status. Treatment for patients with unresectable disease includes palliative therapy if they have already undergone previous surgery, or consolidative therapy with radiation with or without chemotherapy with treatment courses as outlined in the previous section. Five-year survival rates for patients with T3 bladder cancer range from 10%–50%, with the addition of concurrent chemotherapy increasing disease-free survival to 50% or greater (NCI, 2008; Petrovich et al., 2004). Unfortunately, combination therapies have not improved overall survival or decreased the incidence of distant metastasis (Petrovich et al.; Raghavan, 2006).

For patients who are not candidates for cystectomy, well-recognized prognostic factors for overall and disease-free survival include tumor stage, tumor morphology, presence of solitary versus multiple tumors, presence of ureteral obstruction, presence of intravesical versus extravesical tumor, and completeness of TURBT, if performed (NCCN, 2009; Petrovich et al., 2004). Over the past two decades, major developments in molecular biology have identified other prognostic factors that may better represent tumor behavior and possible resistance to treatment with radiation and chemotherapy. Prospective RTOG trials using cisplatin-based chemoradiation protocols investigated the clinical significance of epidermal growth factor receptor (EGFR) and *HER2* ex-

pression (Chakravarti et al., 2005). Results from these trials indicated that EGFR expression significantly correlated with improved outcomes, whereas *HER2* expression was associated more specifically with reduced CR rates after chemoradiation. Lara et al. (1998) assessed tumor proliferation, measured by Ki67 immunostaining, to predict local control in patients treated with RT. Lower expression of Ki67 demonstrated better local control (69% at five years) after fractionated radiotherapy in those patients with very low proliferating tumors versus those with higher proliferation (31.5% at five years). Zhang et al. (2003) demonstrated that gene therapy with cytosine deaminase/5-fluorocytosine combined with RT enhanced cell killing of human bladder cancer cells in vitro and in vivo animal models. Additional studies must be completed to verify these results.

RT, alone or in combination with chemotherapy, is considered for patients with a fixed bladder mass or positive lymph nodes prior to laparotomy and who have unresectable disease (T4), according to NCCN (2009) guidelines. The prognosis is poor in patients with stage IV disease, with 10-year survival rates reported at 20% or less (NCI, 2008). In patients with no computed tomography (CT) transaxial imaging-identified nodal disease, RT may be combined with chemotherapy as a consolidative measure. Patients with pelvic lymph nodes larger than 2 cm as shown by CT imaging and who have a good performance status also may be considered for radiotherapy in a combination protocol with chemotherapy.

Treatment of Metastatic or Recurrent Disease

For patients with recurrent or progressive disease to distant sites, treatment considerations for the use of RT are based on prior therapy, sites of recurrence, performance status, and individual patient considerations. High-risk patients with poor performance status or visceral disease (e.g., liver, lung), with or without bone disease, have the lowest survival (median 12–18 months), and enrollment in a clinical trial is highly recommended when possible (NCI, 2008; NCCN, 2009; Raghavan, 2006). RT may be a consideration in patients who achieved a significant partial response after two to three cycles of chemotherapy in an unresectable tumor, or those with a solitary site of residual disease. Palliative RT is an established treatment for the management of symptoms of pain, bleeding, or obstruction caused by locally advanced and metastatic bladder cancer. Most data on palliative RT are in the treatment of painful bony metastasis, as well as control of urinary symptoms and hematuria (Coen et al., 2007; Yi, Yoder, Zaner, & Hirsch, 2007). However, little evidence supports the use of RT for pain associated with locally recurrent bladder cancer that is refractory to medical pain management.

Yi et al. (2007) reported the case of an 80-year-old woman with recurrent bladder cancer who had undergone radical cystectomy, total abdominal hysterectomy, bilateral salpingo-oophorectomy, partial vaginectomy, and ileal conduit reconstruction. After five cycles of chemotherapy, the patient had intractable pelvic pain refractory to oral and transdermal pain medications. Palliative pelvic RT to a dose of 50 Gy in 25 fractions was administered with complete resolution of pain symptoms. The patient experienced an improved quality of life as demonstrated by a decrease in pain medication, increased overall activity level, and significant improvement in sleep quality and appetite even prior to completion of the RT.

Patients may be treated with RT for uncommon bladder tumors, which comprise approximately 10% of all bladder tumors and include those with nonurothelial cell types of squamous cell, small cell, and carcinosarcoma (Hoshi et al., 2007; Lester, Hudson, & Barber, 2006; NCCN, 2009; Petrovich et al., 2004). Squamous cell tumors are associated with local regional recurrences as the primary cause of death, have an infrequent incidence of distant metastasis, and have limited responsiveness to combination therapy of surgery with adjuvant radiotherapy with or without chemotherapy with an average of 30% disease-free survival at 52 months (NCCN; Petrovich et al.). Data are limited on the treatment of rare small cell cancers with a combination of polychemotherapy and pelvic radiation; however, literature with small study populations demonstrates a three-year disease-free survival of 30%–70% (Lester et al. ; NCCN; Petrovich et al.). Carcinosarcomas are

very aggressive malignant lesions, and treatment outcomes are extremely poor, even in patients with limited disease to the pelvis who receive aggressive multimodality treatment that includes pelvic irradiation. Only one case report demonstrated a durable CR for 30 months after treatment (Hoshi et al.).

Treatment with alternative forms of RT is infrequent, but includes electron beam, intraoperative RT with or without EBRT, and neutron therapy. All three methods were associated with a potentially higher risk of treatment-related toxicities (some severe) and lack of therapeutic gain. Thus, alternative forms of RT are not recommended in the management of recurrent or metastatic bladder cancer (Petrovich et al., 2004).

Side Effects and Complications

Treatment-related toxicity from RT after bladder preservation is limited to the specific areas targeted. Symptoms are discussed in the context of an intact bladder during treatment. Two-phase radiation regimens that only boost specific areas of bladder to highest doses demonstrated less bowel and bladder toxicity than whole-bladder regimens with an overall 19% reduction in RTOG grade 3–4 toxicity (Mangar et al., 2006; Petrovich et al., 2004). RT to the abdominal/pelvic area produces acute side effects related to bladder irritability resulting from mucositis with decreased bladder capacity, which causes urinary frequency, urgency/urge incontinence, dysuria, and incomplete bladder emptying, all of which resolve within several weeks after completion of therapy. GI symptoms may include diarrhea, abdominal cramping, increased number of bowel movements, and anal irritation (during the last weeks of treatment) and are rarely severe. Bowel obstruction is extremely rare. Depending upon the form of EBRT delivery (e.g., three-dimensional conformal, IMRT, TomoTherapy), volume of field size, and total cumulative dose, there may be mild decreases in white blood cell and platelet counts and increased tiredness and fatigue. In patients treated with RT after limited surgery, approximately 50% of men retained sexual potency, and 70% of women were able to have a normal sexual life with or without mild associated dyspareunia (Kelly & Miaskowski, 1996; Little & Howard, 1998; NCI, 2008).

Late complications, defined as those occurring three months or later after completion of RT, may include interstitial fibrosis and bladder contracture, as well as blood vessel changes within the bladder and bowel. Symptoms may include painless hematuria, blood in the stool, chronic frequency, or dysuria. Although 5%–11% of patients develop a contracted bladder, further workup is warranted because as many as 50% of these patients are found to have local tumor recurrence as the main cause of their symptoms (Petrovich et al., 2004). A higher probability of late complications is compounded by the addition of surgery and/or concurrent chemotherapy to RT (Petrovich et al.).

Nursing Management and Patient Education

Nursing care of patients being treated with RT as part of a multimodality therapy for bladder cancer is multifocal. Symptom management of acute bowel and bladder effects (see Table 5-2) are a primary focus; however, patient education regarding potential late complications and ongoing assessment of psychosocial needs are paramount. Nursing management should include

- Specific medical interventions for altered urinary and bowel elimination
- Assessment of changes in performance status
- Obtaining interval blood chemistries as indicated
- Enhancing coping strategies to deal with anticipated symptoms
- Education regarding the necessity of post-treatment surveillance
- Continuity of care with telephone support.

Providing patients with the appropriate education, counseling, and follow-up care regarding sexual dysfunction will serve to establish and maintain open communication between not only the patient and the nurse, but between the patient and his or her partner. A randomized controlled trial of nurse-led follow-up care in men treated with radiotherapy for bladder cancer demonstrated through self-assessment questionnaires that men were significantly more satisfied with the care of their symptoms and quality of life than men receiving conventional medical care (Faithfull, Corner, Meyer, Huddart, & Dearnaley, 2001). Additionally, Faithfull et al. reported a significant cost benefit, with a 31% reduction in cost with nurse-led care compared to conventional medical care. Nurse-led care focuses on education of identifying behaviors that may contribute to decreased incidence or recurrence of their cancer, such as smoking cessation.

Special considerations also should be given to patients undergoing pelvic radiotherapy who are not candidates for surgery because of coexisting medical conditions or advanced age. A conventional EBRT course of six to seven weeks, five days a week, may result in noncompliance and premature discontinuation of therapy because of physical or psychosocial hardship. In these circumstances, consideration for alternative fractionated treatment schedules is warranted to prevent a less-than-optimal total radiation dose being delivered, which may result in more aggravated symptoms of progressive disease such as pain, gross hematuria, frequency, dysuria, and ureteral obstruction (Petrovich et al., 2004).

Nurses must educate patients regarding the importance of post-treatment testing. NCCN (2009) recommends follow-up that may include cystoscopy, urine cytology, blood chemistries, CT or magnetic resonance imaging scans of the abdomen and pelvis, plain radiographs of chest and kidneys, bone scan, or recommendation for further treatment, including inclusion in a clinical trial.

Nursing Implications of Radiation Therapy

Nurses address not only the physiologic needs of their patients with bladder cancer, but also the psychological needs (see Table 5-3). Direct medical intervention for patients receiving pelvic radiotherapy is only part of the multifaceted care that should be delivered. Patient education is critical for allaying fears and enhancing patients' ability to cope with treatment-related urinary and bowel side effects, late complications, sexual dysfunction, the need for post-treatment testing, possible behavior modification, and the discussion of the importance of clinical trials or additional treatment, if indicated.

Chemotherapy

Chemotherapy as a treatment option for bladder cancer (bladder and upper tracts) can be used in a variety of different regimens and may be used at various stages of the disease. It may be administered as part of a constellation of interventions for patients with superficial tumors, invasive bladder cancer, recurrent bladder cancer, or metastatic disease. Options include intravesical therapy for superficial bladder cancers or systemic therapy for muscle-invasive bladder cancers.

Intravesical Treatment of Carcinoma In Situ

The treatment of choice for carcinoma in situ (CIS) is a six-week induction course of bacillus Calmette-Guérin (BCG) as a single agent or in combination with interferon (Lamm, McGee, & Hale, 2005; Lerner, 2006). Radical cystectomy can be the first treatment of choice for young, otherwise healthy patients with high-grade T1 disease, or for patients with multifocal CIS who cannot tolerate BCG. The European Association of Urology recommended intravesical BCG to treat CIS for the highest rate of CR and the highest long-term disease-free rate (van der Meijden et al., 2005). More recent guidelines do not specifically recommend one agent over another; it is more important that the patient receive intravesical therapy with chemotherapy or BCG, as one agent has not been shown to be better than the other agents (Hall et al., 2007). Also recommended is the use of maintenance therapy after induction therapy to reduce the risk of recurrence and progression (Brassell & Kamat, 2006). If the response is not complete at six months, the treatment of choice is radical cystectomy. Radical cystectomy at the time of diagnosis of CIS, instead of intravesical BCG, provides excellent disease-free survival, but as many as 50% of the patients can be over-treated (Lamm et al., 1998). In patients who are not candidates for cystectomy, a conservative treatment should be considered.

Table 5-3. Standard of Nursing Practice for Patients With Bladder Cancer Receiving Radiation

Nursing Diagnosis	Outcome	Nursing Intervention
Knowledge deficit related to bladder radiation therapy	The patient will be able to verbalize understanding of radiation to the bladder and self-care measures. The patient will immediately notify the healthcare provider of any significant postoperative symptoms.	• Assess patient's understanding of postoperative side effects for which the healthcare team must be notified. • Assess patient's baseline understanding of radiation to the bladder. • Identify and address misconceptions and provide education as to daily treatment regimen. • Provide education as to self-care measures, expected side effects, complications, and significant problems/issues/symptoms to report to health care provider.
Potential for altered urinary elimination secondary to bladder inflammation possibly interfering with voiding	The patient will be able to verbalize understanding of expected inflammation to bladder causing anticipated urinary symptoms, the need for adherence to prescription medication regimens, and an understanding of when to notify healthcare provider if unable to urinate within a specific time frame.	• Review patient's preexisting urinary function and related medical conditions prior to procedure. • Educate patient of importance of adhering to prescribed medication regimens despite current level of urinary symptoms. • Educate patient to ensure proper fluid intake, and to measure intake and output as necessary if discomfort ensues or persists. • Educate patient regarding the importance of avoiding dietary bladder irritants that may aggravate urinary symptoms. • Assess patient's understanding of need to notify healthcare provider and/or seek emergent medical attention if inability to urinate lasts greater than an agreed upon, specified period of time. • If patient is to be sent home with an indwelling catheter or taught intermittent self-catheterization, assess patient's understanding of how to take care of catheter and when to perform self-catheterization. Educate patient of need of keeping urine clear.
Potential for alteration in bowel elimination related to inflammation from bladder irradiation	The patient will verbalize understanding of expected bowel changes and identify significant changes in bowel function requiring the need to contact healthcare provider or seek emergency care.	• Review patient's preexisting bowel function and related medical conditions prior to procedure. • Educate patient of importance of adhering to prescribed medication regimen despite current level of change of bowel function. • Educate patient regarding when to notify healthcare provider for prolonged constipation, diarrhea, pain, presence or an increase in rectal bleeding. • Educate patient regarding importance of proper fluid intake. • Educate patient regarding importance of diet, low residue versus high residue, depending on symptoms.
Risk for sexual dysfunction related to disease or post-treatment sequelae	Patient will verbalize understanding of temporary and potentially permanent erectile dysfunction and/or libido after radiation therapy.	• Address psychogenic and other causes (e.g., stress, marital problems, job responsibilities) and refer as necessary for counseling. • Assess associated physiologic causes of impotence pre-treatment (e.g., diabetes, hypertension, alcohol, tobacco, aging) and educate patient on behavior modification where possible (cessation of smoking, reduce alcohol consumption, control blood sugar level). • Educate patient as to radiation-related erectile dysfunction and expected time frame of dysfunction. • Educate patient (and significant other) as to medical interventions available for use during period of dysfunction.
Psychosocial distress related to disease/radiation side effects	Patient will verbalize concerns and fears over treatment plan and anticipated side effects.	• Assess patient's level of knowledge regarding disease and intended treatment plan. • Assess for evidence of barriers to compliance with treatment. • Assess resources available to patient to include financial, family, relationship status, others as indicated. • Educate patient about disease in relation to treatment plan and anticipated side effects. • Reinforce availability of resources and nursing/medical support throughout the treatment process. • Refer for counseling as appropriate.

Note. Based on information from Kelly & Miaskowski, 1996; National Cancer Institute, 2008. Table courtesy of the Dattoli Cancer Center, Sarasota, FL. Reprinted with permission.

Intravesical Therapy

Intravesical therapy is the use of topical immunotherapy or chemotherapy instilled into the bladder for the treatment of superficial cancers as a local treatment approach. Intravesical therapy for superficial bladder tumors may be used to treat high-risk patients such as those with CIS, T1 disease, large tumors, or multiple bladder tumors (Barocas & Clark, 2008). Intravesical BCG therapy is a useful treatment for CIS, especially for transitional cell tumors (Bernier, 2005). The goal of any intravesical therapy is prevention of recurrent superficial or higher grade or stage tumors. Studies show that intravesical chemotherapy may reduce superficial tumor recurrence by 20% in the short term when compared to TURBT alone, and long-term (5–8 years) recurrence is reduced by 7% (Pawinski et al., 1996). Intravesical chemotherapy can significantly improve the duration of disease-free intervals; although, historically, studies have not demonstrated a clear advantage in terms of progression to invasive disease or distant metastasis, or duration of survival and progression-free survival (Pawinski et al.). Recent studies have suggested that BCG slightly decreases the risk of progression in patients with high-risk tumors (Hendricksen & Witjes, 2007). Some researchers believe that BCG is the agent of choice in the treatment of superficial bladder cancer (Han & Pan, 2006).

Generally, patients receive weekly treatments over a six-week cycle (Boyd, 2003). The first intravesical therapy is with mitomycin C, which is administered within six hours of TURBT for the best outcome (Brassell & Kamat, 2006; Hall et al., 2007; Han & Pan, 2006; Lamm et al., 2005; Sylvester, Oosterlinck, & van der Meijden, 2004). BCG is not used until 14 days after TUR because early use increases the risk of a systemic infection (Boyd). Patients with low-risk disease only require one intravesical treatment to reduce the risk of recurrence, but patients with high-risk disease require adjuvant therapy (Barocas & Clark, 2008). Maintenance treatments may be prescribed after cystoscopic follow-up 12–16 weeks after completion of the first cycle, depending on the stage of the original tumor: High-grade tumors may be treated with maintenance therapy, whereas low-grade tumors followed with cystoscopy with no evidence of recurrence may be followed by cystoscopy and urine cytology alone, only returning to intravesical therapy if the superficial tumors recur (Bernier, 2005).

Intravesical treatments with BCG are diluted with sterile solution in various volumes; as little as 30 ml is adequate for installation (mixed in the pharmacy). This is for instillation into the bladder through a urethral catheter, which is then removed so the solution may dwell for two hours. If a patient cannot void, the catheter is left in place and clamped for two hours, and then the bladder is drained and the catheter removed. If a patient can void, he or she is instructed to retain the instilled medication for two hours. Historically, patients were asked to reposition themselves side-to-side or supine-to-prone every 15–30 minutes, and some facilities and urologists still use this approach (Washburn, 2007). However, other centers no longer do this (McDonald, 2007). Once the two hours have passed, the patient voids. Finally, the patient is instructed to drink a minimum of two glasses of water prior to voiding to help flush the bladder and minimize side effects (Bernier, 2005).

If two treatment cycles of intravesical immunotherapy with first-line agents such as BCG have been ineffective, most urologists recommend switching to a second-line agent such as an alkylating agent (Lamm et al., 2005). If a second-line agent also is not effective in controlling the tumor growth, then a third-line agent, such as an antitumor antibiotic, can be considered. If the intravesical approach is ineffective at prevention of recurrence, a cystectomy may be needed.

Treatment with intravesical instillation of an alkylating agent or antitumor antibiotics is another treatment option. These agents provide topical treatment with relatively little systemic absorption. Side effects from superficial exposure to the chemotherapy agent used are similar to those with BCG (Bernier, 2005). Drugs that may be used to treat superficial, low-grade papillary tumors include thiotepa, mitomycin C, doxorubicin, and epirubicin (Barocas & Clark, 2008; Bernier; McDonald, 2007; Washburn, 2007). Gemcitabine has been used as intravesical therapy for recurrent superficial tumors but with lower disease-free intervals in recently published articles (Maffezzini, Campodonico, Canepa, Capponi, & Fontana, 2007). Agents such as docetaxel for intravesical therapy are in clinical trials (McKiernan et al., 2006). Because CIS alone is not considered an invasive tumor, systemic chemotherapy is not considered the first line of therapy. Aggressive CIS that does not respond to immunotherapy or chemotherapy administered intravesically is treated most often with surgery, as this has the highest potential for rendering the patient disease-free (Joudi & O'Donnell, 2004). Rare cases of upper tract disease in the renal pelvis or ureters with documented low-grade disease or CIS may be treated with BCG from "above" by placement of a percutaneous nephrostomy tube in the renal pelvis. The BCG is diluted and allowed to drip into the kidney through the percutaneous nephrostomy tube using the same schedule of drug delivery as the bladder instillations.

Side effects and potential complications of intravesical immunotherapy with BCG or chemotherapeutic agents can be locally aggravating but managed. Common side effects after instillation include bladder irritation resulting in urinary frequency, urgency, nocturia, and dysuria. These effects, often referred to as *urinary bother*, usually resolve within one to two days but may last until the cycle of weekly treatments is completed. Less frequently, hematuria, fever, malaise, nausea, chills, joint pain, and pruritus develop. These clinical findings are more representative of systemic reaction to the intravesical therapy and should be promptly reported to the healthcare provider. Normal voiding should resume by day three after treatment.

Nursing Care of Patients Receiving Intravesical Treatments

Nursing management of intravesical immunotherapy or chemotherapy includes patient education, administration of the immunotherapeutic or chemotherapy agent, patient care throughout the procedure, management of side effects, and monitoring for complications after administration.

Patient Preparation

Preparation before immunotherapy or chemotherapy bladder instillation requires fluid restriction for up to four hours before the instillation to decrease the need to void for two hours afterward. The patient needs to know that a catheter will be inserted into the bladder before the instillation and that it will be necessary to retain the instilled medication for two hours. After the dwell time, oral fluids are encouraged to flush the bladder and urinary tracts and promote voiding. Patients should be taught that treatments are typically repeated weekly for six to eight weeks and then monthly for varying periods depending on the maintenance schedule. Follow-up monitoring of urine cytology and cystoscopy is required to monitor the bladder and ureters for any recurrent tumor growth.

Side effects such as pain, dysuria, burning, and urinary bother may develop after treatment. Some patients may report that symptoms increase with cumulative doses. Hematuria is a rare side effect, and if present, requires that the weekly dose be held until the hematuria resolves; then, the patient's schedule of therapy is reinitiated. Pain is managed with analgesics. Dysuria or burning while voiding may result from the therapy itself, placement of an indwelling catheter, or residual bladder tumor. Irritative symptoms such as dysuria, frequency, and urgency from the catheter will diminish when the catheter is removed and will improve after two to three days.

Patient Education

Teaching the patient how the BCG or chemotherapy works and what results and side effects to expect is important (see Table 5-4). Reassure the patient that dysuria, frequency, and urgency from catheter placement and intravesical treatment will diminish with increased oral fluid intake. Review prescribed analgesics, antispasmodics, or anticholinergics, and explain how they should be taken. If a fever together with joint pain or extreme fatigue develops after BCG instillation in particular, the healthcare provider should be notified immediately. These signs and symptoms may be an indication of infection, and BCG may need to be discontinued and antibiotics prescribed. Treatment with isoniazid or other medications used to treat tuberculosis may be required if systemic infection is identified. Evaluation of a fever after BCG or intravesical chemotherapy includes a CBC and cultures followed by appropriate antibiotic therapy. Inform the patient and family or caregivers how and when to alert the healthcare provider of complications. Patients who have received intravesical chemotherapy, especially thiotepa or other low-molecular-weight drugs, will need a CBC to monitor the platelet and white blood cell counts (Washburn, 2007).

Table 5-4. Examples of Intravesical Immunotherapy and Chemotherapy Agents			
Agent	Mechanism	Dosage	Side Effects
Immunotherapy (e.g., bacillus Calmette-Guérin [BCG])	Intravesical BCG produces a local or regional granulomatous response and stimulates macrophages that have tumoricidal effects. Interleukin (IL)-2 is produced by activated helper T cells and activates natural killer cells. Patients who responded to BCG treatment had IL-2 in their urine. However, the exact antineoplastic mechanism of BCG is unknown (Micromedex, 2009).	1 vial in 50 ml sterile and preservative-free normal saline. Given intravesically once a week for 6 weeks, then approximately once a month for 6–12 months. To avoid systemic absorption and reduce the risk of serious adverse reactions, one should wait 1–3 weeks after TURBT before starting BCG treatment (McAleer et al., 2007; Micromedex, 2009).	Common: Axillary or cervical lymphadenopathy, bladder irritability, dysuria, hematuria, frequency of urination, influenza-like illness with low fever (38.3°C). Serious: Disseminated systemic infection and sepsis. 60%–80% of patients will experience cystitis and 5% will develop serious infection (McAleer et al., 2007; Micromedex, 2009).
Chemotherapy (e.g., mitomycin C, docetaxel)	Mechanism is thought to be inhibiting DNA synthesis, a degradation of preformed DNA, nuclear lysis and formation of giant cells (Micromedex, 2009).	Instill weekly for 6–8 weeks at dose of 20–60 mg (Jones & Campbell, 2007).	Common: Nausea and vomiting Serious: Myelosuppression (severe), hemolytic uremic syndrome (< 10%), nephrotoxicity (Micromedex, 2009)

Safety

The potential toxicity of intravesical immunotherapy and chemotherapy instillation agents requires that a safe work environment be provided. Most centers require that the nurses who administer immunotherapy have certification in the proper technique. Personal protective equipment (PPE), including face shield, closed front gown, and gloves, is required for personnel administering the agent. The linens must be protected with a plastic-backed absorbent drape. All equipment used in administration is disposed of as hazardous material. This includes the catheter used for administration, the PPE, and all other equipment (Washburn, 2007). For six hours after treatment with BCG, all urine is considered contaminated and the toilet bowl must be disinfected with bleach according the healthcare facility's policies. This often includes adding bleach to the toilet after the patient voids and allowing it to dwell for 15 minutes before flushing to ensure that live BCG is not flushed into the septic or sewer system. Patients are instructed to perform this bleach disinfection in their home toilet, as well. Patients receiving intravesical chemotherapy are encouraged to avoid getting urine on their hands or skin from touching or splashing because it may contain medication; therefore, good hand washing is required. However, bleach should not be used on the skin.

Systemic Chemotherapy

Treatment with chemotherapy usually is recommended for muscle invasive (T2–T4), high-grade, locally advanced recurrent or metastatic bladder cancer (Bernier, 2005). Some cases of invasive disease mixed with CIS may be treated with chemotherapy (Langerak & Dreisbach, 2001). Chemotherapy has five uses in patients with bladder cancer.

Chemotherapy for invasive bladder cancer is used as part of a protocol of a bladder-sparing approach with concomitant EBRT (Hagan et al., 2003). It also can be used preoperatively for more advanced disease in hopes of downstaging before a cystectomy. If the tumor responds, then the patient will progress to surgery with hopes of improved surgical outcomes. Third, chemotherapy can be used as adjuvant therapy after cystectomy, depending on surgical pathologic findings and extent of disease, with the goal of improving cancer-free survival. Also, chemotherapy may be used for recurrent or metastatic bladder cancer with or without surgery (NCCN, 2009). Another use of systemic chemotherapy is to prolong life in patients with widely metastatic disease as a palliative measure to reduce symptoms and possibly halt disease progression. A number of chemotherapy regimens may be utilized for recurrent disease and metastatic disease. Several regimens have emerged as standard and effective therapies for bladder cancer (see Table 5-5). Determining which patients are the best candidates for chemotherapy requires a multidisciplinary team approach. Variables such as patient age; performance status; renal and hepatic function; comorbidities such as hypertension, coronary artery disease, and COPD; potential interaction with other medications such as immunosuppressive agents; and cardiac status should be assessed. Evaluation of risks versus benefit should be determined for each patient. Patients receiving immunotherapy and chemotherapy for bladder cancer are at risk for both systemic and local complications; however, the benefits of therapy may outweigh the potential complications. Patients selecting chemotherapy must understand the potential risks and benefits to make an informed decision.

Side effects (see Appendix) can occur in any system of the body. The most common is bone marrow depression with thrombocytopenia, febrile neutropenia, and anemia. Cisplatin-based therapies may cause nephrotoxicity, ototoxicity, and peripheral nephropathies. Monitoring patients by laboratory test results and assessing for signs and symptoms of infection is important. The potential for nausea and vomiting requires premedication with antiemetics for emesis prophylaxis. Regimens that include chemotherapy agents with a risk of hypersensitivity reactions or anaphylactoid reactions require premedication with dexamethasone, a histamine-2 blocker, and diphenhydramine. Nephrotoxic agents require IV hydration to minimize side effects.

Patient Education

Nurses can help their patients by providing patient education and support. Patients are instructed about the signs and symptoms to report (e.g., extravasation, changes in the skin at the IV site, fever, bleeding, intractable nausea, hearing changes) and how to reach the cancer care team when the clinics are closed. They are instructed in dietary manipulations to maximize hydration, electrolyte replacement, and caloric intake to sustain energy levels while undergoing chemotherapy. Many healthcare centers prepare chemotherapy calendars for patients that outline the days of treatment, premedications, and laboratory schedules. These calendars help to increase compliance with these important elements of care. Often patients are evaluated in the clinic on their weeks off chemotherapy in order to be examined, have side effects and toxicities assessed and managed, and to determine their response to treatment. Documenting response to therapy through radiologic imaging helps the team to decide if chemotherapy should continue, if additional cycles of therapy should be added, or if the regimen should be changed.

Combination Chemotherapy and Radiation for Invasive Bladder Cancer

The goal of bladder cancer RT is to eliminate the tumor and to preserve a functioning bladder without compromising survival. In general, cancer cells do not have DNA

Table 5-5. Common Intravenous Chemotherapeutic Agents for Invasive Bladder Cancer

Regimen	Drugs	Dose	Frequency	Side Effects and Toxicities
CMV	Cisplatin	100 mg/m^2	Day 1	Nausea, vomiting, nephrotoxicity peripheral neuropathy, neurotoxicity
	Methotrexate	30 mg	Day 1, 8	Nephrotoxicity
	Vinblastine	4 mg/m^2	Day 1, 8	Monitor for extravasation. Nephrotoxicity, bone marrow suppression.
MVAC	Methotrexate	30 mg	Day1, 15, 22	Nephrotoxicity
	Vinblastine	3 mg/m^2	Day 2, 15, 22	Neurotoxicity. Monitor for extravasation.
	Doxorubicin	30 mg/m^2	Day 2	Reduce dose with radiation therapy. Cardiac toxicity. Monitor for extravasation. Monitor bilirubin.
	Cisplatin	70 mg/m^2	Day 2	Nephrotoxicity, nausea, peripheral neuropathy.
Gemcitabine and cisplatin	Gemcitabine	1,000 mg/m^2	Day 1, 8, 15	Thrombocytopenia is the dose-limiting toxicity.
	Cisplatin	70 mg/m^2	Day 1	Nephrotoxicity, nausea, peripheral neuropathy.
Paclitaxel and carboplatin	Paclitaxel	200 mg/m^2	Day 1	Allergic reaction
	Carboplatin	AUC 5	Day 1	Myelosuppression, thrombocytopenia, nausea

Note. Based on information from Chu & De Vita, 2006; Langerak & Dreisbach, 2001; National Comprehensive Cancer Network, 2009.

repair mechanisms as effective in repairing the damage from radiation compared with normal cells (Milosevic et al., 2007; Milosevic, Bristow, & Gospodarowicz, 2006). Because of improvements in the delivery of high-precision, image-guided radiation and advances in bladder cancer biology, RT alone or in combination with chemotherapy and surgery could achieve this outcome (Milosevic et al., 2006). Currently, a trimodality regimen of surgery, RT, and chemotherapy is utilized to treat muscle-invasive bladder cancer, in order to cure the cancer and to preserve the bladder as well as to have equivalent survival in appropriately selected patients (Bellmont & Albiol, 2007; Perdona et al., 2007). When chemotherapy is used with RT, cisplatin is the preferred agent, as it has single-agent activity and enhances the activity of RT (Milosevic et al., 2007).

Muscle-Invasive Bladder Cancer (T2, T3, T4)

Definitive RT has been used for muscle-invasive bladder cancer since the early 1900s (Gospodarowicz, Warde, & Bristow, 1999). The ideal outcome is having a preserved, functioning bladder with total eradication of the tumor without compromising survival. EBRT alone has demonstrated short- and long-term responses to invasive bladder cancer, particularly with smaller tumors; patients can be cured of their cancer with normal functioning bladders (Milosevic et al., 2006). However, given the relatively poor local control in invasive disease, RT is not recommended

as sole treatment (Chung et al., 2007). Because patients with more invasive (T2, T3) cancers are at risk for nodal metastases and progression, even though their tumors are localized, they require more aggressive treatments of surgery, radiation, or a trimodality regimen (Stoller, Kane, & Carroll, 2007). Radical RT frequently is used in the curative treatment regimens, either in trimodality therapy in medically fit patients or alone after maximal TURBT in patients who cannot tolerate chemotherapy (Coen et al., 2007). One study demonstrated that concurrent intra-arterial cisplatin and RT resulted in a 90% CR rate in evaluable patients, along with 75% who were able to retain their bladders, infrequent salvage cystectomy, and similar survival (Eapen, Stewart, Collins, & Peterson, 2004).

In a Cochrane analysis by Shelley, Barber, Wilt, and Mason (2001, p. 1), "the mean overall survival (intention-to-treat analysis) at 3 and 5 years were 45% and 36% for surgery, and 28% and 20% for radiotherapy," respectively, which "were significantly in favor of surgery." They commented that the analysis included only three trials, sample sizes were small, and that many participants did not receive the treatment they were randomized to. Many patients receiving RT are older, have advanced disease at presentation, or are high risk for surgery such as cystectomy because of comorbidities (Milosevic et al., 2006). The outcomes of RT in this patient population are predisposed to the worst possible, rather than the optimal.

However, encouraging RT research has been published. Shipley et al. (2002) studied patients with muscle-invasive T2–T4a bladder carcinoma treated with chemo-radiation after rigorous TURBT. They reported that their results were similar to patients undergoing radical cystectomy. Based on the initial tumor response, the trimodality therapy can be safely offered for bladder sparing. However, commitment to and compliance with lifelong bladder surveillance are essential to prevent new or recurrent bladder cancer from being missed (Shipley et al., 2002).

Summary

Treating superficial and invasive bladder cancer requires a multidisciplinary team approach. Nursing expertise in the management of complications that can ensue for various treatments described will ultimately benefit patient outcomes. Advocating for the patient as well as providing guidance regarding potential side effects of surgery, chemotherapy, and radiation is a key component in managing patients with bladder cancer.

The editor would like to acknowledge Sandra Cochran, BSN, RN, CWOCN, as a consultant on the Surgery section of this chapter.

References

Anvari, M., Birch, D.W., Bamehriz, F., Gryfe, R., & Chapman, T. (2004). Robotic-assisted laparoscopic colorectal surgery. *Surgical Laparoscopy, Endoscopy and Percutaneous Techniques, 14*(6), 311–315.

Barocas, D.A., & Clark, P.E. (2008). Bladder cancer. *Current Opinion in Oncology, 20*(3), 307–314.

Baumgartner, G., Wells, N., Chang, S., Cookson, M.S., & Smith, J.A., Jr. (2002). Causes of increased length of stay following radical cystectomy. *Urologic Nursing, 22*(5), 319–326.

Bellmont, J., & Albiol, S. (2007). Invasive bladder cancer: ESMO clinical recommendations for diagnosis, treatment and follow-up. *Annals of Oncology, 18*(Suppl. 2), ii38–ii39.

Bernier, F. (2005). Management of clients with urinary disorders. In J.M. Black & J.H. Hawks (Eds.), *Medical-surgical nursing: Clinical management for positive outcomes* (pp. 857–972). St. Louis, MO: Elsevier Saunders.

Boyd, L.A. (2003). Intravesical bacillus Calmette-Guérin for treating bladder cancer. *Urologic Nursing, 23*(3), 189–199.

Brassell, S.A., & Kamat, A.M. (2006). Contemporary intravesical treatment options for urothelial carcinoma of the bladder. *Journal of the National Comprehensive Cancer Network, 4*(10), 1027–1036.

Chakravarti, A., Winter, K., Wu, C.L., Kaufman, D., Hammond, E., Parliament, M., et al. (2005). Expression of the epidermal growth factor receptor and Her-2 are predictors of favorable outcome and reduced complete response rates, respectively, in patients with muscle-invading bladder cancers treated with concurrent radiation and cisplatin-based chemotherapy: A report from the Radiation Therapy Oncology Group. *International Journal of Radiation Oncology, Biology, Physics, 62*(2), 309–317.

Chambers, A. (2002). Transurethral resection syndrome—it does not have to be a mystery. *AORN Journal, 75*(1), 156–164, 166, 168–170.

Chu, E., & DeVita, V.T., Jr. (2006). *Physicians' cancer chemotherapy drug manual 2006.* Sudbury, MA: Jones and Bartlett.

Chung, P.W.M., Bristow, R.G., Milosevic, M.F., Yi, Q., Jewett, M.A.S., Warde, P.R., et al. (2007). Long-term outcome of radiation-based conservation therapy for invasive bladder cancer. *Urologic Oncology, 25*(4), 303–309.

Coen, J.J., Zietman, A.L., Kaufman, D.S., Heney, N.M., Althausen, A.F., & Shipley, W.U. (2006). Trimodality therapy in the management of muscle-invasive bladder cancer: A selective organ-preserving approach. In S.P. Lerner, M.P. Schoenberg, & C.N. Sternberg (Eds.), *Textbook of bladder cancer* (pp. 569–577). Abingdon, Oxon, UK: Taylor & Francis Group.

Coen, J.J., Zietman, A.L., Kaufman, D.S., & Shipley, W.U. (2007). Benchmarks achieved in the delivery of radiation therapy for muscle-invasive bladder cancer. *Urologic Oncology, 25*(1), 76–84.

Colwell, J.C., Goldberg, M.T., & Carmel, J.E. (2004). *Fecal and urinary diversions: Management principles.* St. Louis, MO: Mosby.

Dreicer, R. (2001). Locally advanced and metastatic bladder cancer. *Current Treatment Options in Oncology, 2*(5), 431–436.

Eapen, L., Stewart, D., Collins, J., & Peterson, R. (2004). Effective bladder sparing therapy with intra-arterial cisplatin and radiotherapy for localized bladder cancer. *Journal of Urology, 172*(4), 1276–1280.

Faithfull, S., Corner, J., Meyer, L., Huddart, R., & Dearnaley, D. (2001). Evaluation of nurse-led follow up for patients undergoing pelvic radiotherapy. *British Journal of Cancer, 85*(12), 1853–1864.

Girard, N.J. (2005). Clients having surgery. In J.M. Black & J.H. Hawks (Eds.), *Medical-surgical nursing: Clinical management for positive outcomes* (7th ed., pp. 263–312). St. Louis, MO: Elsevier Saunders.

Gofrit, O.N., Shapiro, A., Pode, D., Sidi, A., Nativ, O., Leib, Z., et al. (2004). Combined local bladder hyperthermia and intravesical chemotherapy for the treatment of high-grade superficial bladder cancer. *Urology, 63*(3), 466–471.

Gospodarowicz, M.K., Warde, P., & Bristow, R.G. (1999). Radiation therapy in bladder cancer. In R.R. Hall (Ed.), *Clinical management of bladder cancer* (pp. 213–240). New York: Oxford University Press.

Hagan, M.P., Winter, K.A., Kaufman, D.S., Wajsman, Z., Zietman, A.L., Heney, N.M., et al. (2003). RTOG 97-06: Initial report of a phase I–II trial of selective bladder conservation using TURBT, twice-daily accelerated irradiation sensitized with cisplatin, and adjuvant MCV combination chemotherapy. *International Journal of Radiation Oncology, Biology, Physics, 57*(3), 665–672

Hall, M.C., Chang, S.S., Dalbagni, G., Pruthi, R.S., Seigne, J.D., Skinner, E.C., et al. (2007). Guideline for the management of nonmuscle invasive bladder cancer (stages Ta, T1, and Tis): 2007 update. *Journal of Urology, 178*(6), 2314–2330.

Han, R.F., & Pan, J.G. (2006). Can intravesical bacillus Calmette-Guérin reduce recurrence in patients with superficial bladder cancer? A meta-analysis of randomized trials. *Urology, 67*(6), 1216–1223.

Hendricksen, K., & Witjes, J.A. (2007). Treatment of intermediate-risk non–muscle-invasive bladder cancer (NMIBC). *European Urology Supplements, 6*(14), 800–808.

Hoshi, S., Sasaki, M., Muto, A., Suzuki, K., Kobayashi, T., Tukigi, M., et al. (2007). Case of carcinosarcoma of urinary bladder obtained a pathologically complete response by neoadjuvant chemoradiotherapy. *International Journal of Urology, 14*(1), 79–81.

Huncharek, M., Muscat, J., & Geschwind, J.F. (1998). Planned preoperative radiation therapy in muscle invasive bladder cancer: Results of a meta-analysis. *Anticancer Research, 18*(3B), 1931–1934.

Jemal, A., Siegel, R., Ward, E., Hao, Y., Xu, J., Murray, T., et al. (2008). Cancer statistics, 2008. *CA: A Cancer Journal for Clinicians, 58*(2), 71–96.

Jones, J.S., & Campbell, S.C. (2007). Non-muscle-invasive bladder cancer (Ta, T1, and CIS). In P.C. Walsh, A.B. Retik, E.D. Vaughan, & A.J. Wein (Eds.), *Campbell-Walsh Urology* (pp. 2447–2467). Philadelphia: Lippincott Williams & Wilkins.

Joudi, F., & O'Donnell, M. (2004). Second-line intravesical therapy versus cystectomy for bacille Calmette-Guérin (BCG) failures. *Current Opinion in Urology, 14*(5), 271–275.

Kaufman, D.S. (2006). Challenges in the treatment of bladder cancer. *Annals of Oncology, 17*(Suppl. 5), v106–v112.

Kelly, L.P., & Miaskowski, C. (1996). An overview of bladder cancer: Treatment and nursing implications. *Oncology Nursing Forum, 23*(3), 459–468.

Krause, F., Rauch, A., Schrott, K., & Engehausen, D. (2006). Clinical decisions for treatment of different staged bladder cancer based on multitarget fluorescence in situ hybridization assays? *World Journal of Urology, 24*(4), 418–422.

Lamm, D.L., Herr, H.W., Jakse, G., Kuroda, M., Mostofi, F.K., Okajima, E., et al. (1998). Updated concepts and treatment of carcinoma in situ. *Urologic Oncololgy, 4*(4–5), 130–138.

Lamm, D.L., McGee, W.R., & Hale, K. (2005). Bladder cancer: Current optimal intravesical treatment. *Urologic Nursing, 25*(5), 323–332.

Langerak, A.D., & Dreisbach, L. (2001). *Chemotherapy regimens and cancer care.* Georgetown, TX: Landes Bioscience.

Lara, P.C., Rey, A., Santana, C., Afonso, J.L., Diaz, J.M., Gonzalez, G.J., et al. (1998). The role of Ki67 proliferation assessment in predicting local control in bladder cancer patients treated by radical radiation therapy. *Radiotherapy and Oncology, 49*(2), 163–167.

Lerner, S.P. (2006). Treatment of high-risk, non-muscle-invasive bladder cancer. *Nature Clinical Practice Urology, 3*(8), 398–399.

Lester, J.F., Hudson, E., & Barber, J.B. (2006). Bladder preservation in small cell carcinoma of the urinary bladder: An institutional experience and review of the literature. *Clinical Oncology, 18*(8), 608–611.

Little, F.A., & Howard, G.C. (1998). Sexual function following radical radiotherapy for bladder cancer [Abstract 344]. *Radiotherapy and Oncology, 48,* 87.

Maffezzini, M., Campodonico, F., Canepa, G., Capponi, G., & Fontana, V. (2007). Short-schedule intravesical gemcitabine with ablative intent in recurrent Ta-T1, G1-G2, low- or intermediate-risk, transitional cell carcinoma of the bladder. *European Urology, 51*(4), 956–961.

Mangar, S.A., Foo, K., Norman, A., Khoo, V., Shahidi, M., Dearnaley, D.P., et al. (2006). Evaluating the effect of reducing the high dose volume on the toxicity of radiotherapy in the treatment of bladder cancer. *Clinical Oncology, 18*(6), 466–473.

McAleer, S.J., Johnson, C.W., & Johnson, W.J., Jr. (2007). Tuberculosis and parasitic and fungal infection of the genitourinary system. In P.C. Walsh, A.B. Retik, E.D. Vaughan, & A.J. Wein (Eds.), *Campbell-Walsh urology* (pp. 436–459). Philadelphia: Lippincott Williams & Wilkins.

McBain, C.A., & Logue, J.P. (2005). Radiation therapy for muscle-invasive bladder cancer: Treatment planning and delivery in the 21st century. *Seminars in Radiation Oncology, 15*(1), 42–48.

McDonald, C.E. (2007). Intraoperative intravesical epirubicin: Implementing the process. *Urologic Nursing, 27*(3), 210–212.

McKiernan, J., Masson, P., Murphy, A., Goetzl, M., Olsson,C., Petrylak, D., et al. (2006). Phase I trial of intravesical docetaxel in the management of superficial bladder cancer refractory to standard intravesical therapy. *Journal of Clinical Oncology, 24*(19), 3075–3080.

McMahon, C.N., Smith, C.J., & Shabsigh, R. (2006). Treating erectile dysfunction when PDE5 inhibitors fail. *BMJ (Clinical Research Edition), 332*(7541), 589–592.

Menon, M., Tewari, A., Peabody, J.O., Shrivastava, A., Kaul, S., Bhandari, A., et al. (2004). Vattikuti Institute prostatectomy, a technique of robotic radical prostatectomy for management of localized carcinoma of the prostate: Experience of over 1100 cases. *Urologic Clinics of North America, 31*(4), 701–717.

Menon, M., Tewari, A., Shrivastava, A., Shoma, A.M., El-Tabey, N.A., Shaaban, A., et al. (2003). Nerve-sparing robot-assisted radical cystoprostatectomy and urinary diversion. *British Journal of Urology, 92*(3), 232–236.

Messing, E.M. (2007). Urothelial tumors of the bladder. In P.C. Walsh, A.B. Retik, E.D. Vaughan, & A.J. Wein (Eds.), *Campbell-Walsh urology* (pp. 2407–2467). Philadelphia: Lippincott Williams & Wilkins.

Micromedex. (2009). Retrieved February 11, 2009, from http://www.thomsonhc.com/hcs/librarian

Milosevic, M., Gospodarowicz, M., Zietman, A., Abbas, F., Haustermans, K., Moonen, L., et al. (2007). Radiotherapy for bladder cancer. *Urology, 69*(Suppl. 1), 80–92.

Milosevic, M.F., Bristow, R., & Gospodarowicz, M.K. (2006). Optimal radiotherapy for bladder cancer. In S.P. Lerner, M.P. Schoenberg, & C.N. Sternberg (Eds.), *Textbook of bladder cancer* (pp. 552–567). Abingdon, Oxon, UK: Taylor & Francis Group.

Naslund, I., Nilsson, B., & Littbrand, B. (1994). Hyperfractionated radiotherapy of bladder cancer. *Acta Oncologica, 33*(4), 397–402.

National Cancer Institute. (2002). *What you need to know about bladder cancer.* Retrieved April 14, 2007, from http://www.cancer.gov/cancertopics/wyntk/bladder/page11

National Cancer Institute. (2008, May 16). *Bladder cancer (PDQ®): Treatment.* Retrieved February 18, 2009, from http://www.cancer.gov/cancertopics/pdq/treatment/bladder/HealthProfessional/page4

National Comprehensive Cancer Network. (2009). *NCCN Clinical Practice Guidelines in Oncology™: Bladder cancer including upper tract tumors and urothelial carcinoma of the prostate* [v.1.2009]. Retrieved February 11, 2009, from http://www.nccn.org/professionals/physician_gls/PDF/bladder.pdf

Nieh, P.T., & Marshall, F.F. (2007). Surgery in bladder cancer. In A.J. Wein, L.R. Kavoussi, A.C. Novick, A.W. Partin, & C.A. Peters (Eds.), *Campbell-Walsh urology* (9th ed., pp. 2479–2505). St. Louis, MO: Elsevier Saunders.

Overstreet, D., & Sims, T. (2006). Care of the patient undergoing radical cystectomy with a robotic approach. *Urologic Nursing, 26*(2), 117–122.

Pawinski, A., Sylvester, R., Kurth, K.H., Bouffioux, C., van der Meijden, A., & Parmar, M.K., et al. (1996). A combined analysis of European Organization for Research and Treatment of Cancer, and Medical Research Council randomized clinical trials for the prophylactic treatment of stage TaT1 bladder cancer. *Journal of Urology, 156*(6), 1934–1940.

Perdona, S., Autorino, R., Damiano, R., De Sio, M., Morrica, B., Gallo, L., et al. (2007). Bladder-sparing, combined-modality approach for muscle-invasive bladder cancer. *Cancer, 112*(1), 75–83.

Petrovich, Z., Stein, J.P., Jozsef, G., & Formenti, S.C. (2004). Bladder. In C. Perez, L. Brady, E. Halperin, & R. Schmidt-Ullrich (Eds.), *Principles and practice of radiation oncology* (4th ed., pp. 1664–1691). Philadelphia: Lippincott Williams & Wilkins.

Raghavan, D. (2006, June 7). *Bladder, renal, and testicular cancer: Cancer of the bladder.* Retrieved August 28, 2007, from http://www.medscape.com/viewarticle/534553

Rodel, C. (2004). Current status of radiation therapy and combined-modality treatment for bladder cancer. *Strahlentherapie und Onkologie, 180*(11), 701–709.

Shelley, M.D., Barber, J., Wilt, T., & Mason, M.D. (2001). Surgery versus radiotherapy for muscle invasive bladder cancer. *Cochrane*

Database of Systematic Reviews 2001, Issue 4. Art. No.: CD002079. DOI: 10.1002/14651858.CD002079.

Shipley, W.U., Kaufman, D.S.E., Heney, N.M., Lane, S.C., Thakral, H.K., Althausen, A.F., et al. (2002). Selective bladder preservation by combined modality protocol treatment: Long-term outcomes of 190 patients with invasive bladder cancer. *Urology, 60*(1), 62–67.

Shipley, W.U., Kaufman, D.S., Tester, W.J., Pilepich, M.V., & Sandler, H.M. (2003). Overview of bladder cancer trials in the Radiation Therapy Oncology Group. *Cancer, 97*(Suppl. 8), 2115–2119.

Shurpin, K., & DeSimone, M. (1998). Preoperative evaluation. *American Journal of Nurse Practitioners, 2*(2), 7–12.

Steers, W.D., LeBeau, S., Cardella, J., & Fulmer, B. (2004). Establishing a robotics program. *Urologic Clinics of North America, 31*(4), 773–780.

Stoller, M.L., Kane, C.J., & Carroll, P.R. (2007). Bladder cancer. In S.J. McPhee, M.A. Papadakis, & L.M. Tierney Jr. (Eds.), R. Gonzales, & R. Zeiger (Online Eds.), *Current medical diagnosis and treatment.* Retrieved September 8, 2007, from http://www.accessmedicine.com/content.aspx?aID=12409

Sylvester, R.J., Oosterlinck, W., & van der Meijden, A.P. (2004). A single immediate postoperative instillation of chemotherapy decreases the risk of recurrence in patients with stage Ta T1 bladder cancer: Meta-analysis of published results of randomized clinical trials. *Journal of Urology, 171*(6, Pt. 1), 2186–2190.

van der Heijden, A.G., Kiemeney, L.A., Gofrit, O.N., Nativ, O., Sidi, A., Leib, Z., et al. (2004). Preliminary European results of local microwave hyperthermia and chemotherapy treatment in intermediate or high risk superficial transitional cell carcinoma of the bladder. *European Urology, 46*(1), 65–71.

van der Meijden, A.P.M., Sylvester, R., Oosterlinck, W., Solsona, E., Boehle, A., Lobel, B., et al. (2005). EAU guidelines on the diagnosis and treatment of urothelial carcinoma in situ. *European Urology, 48*(3), 363–371.

Washburn, D.J. (2007). Intravesical antineoplastic therapy following transurethral resection of bladder tumors. *Clinical Journal of Oncology Nursing, 11*(4), 553–559.

Yamanouchi Pharmaceutical Co. (2004). *Physician desk reference: Urology prescribing guide.* Tokyo, Japan: Author.

Yi, S.K., Yoder, M., Zaner, K., & Hirsch, A.E. (2007). Palliative radiation therapy of symptomatic recurrent bladder cancer. *Pain Physician, 10*(2), 285–290.

Zhang, Z., Shirakawa, T., Hinata, N., Matsumoto, A., Fujisawa, M., Okada, H., et al. (2003). Combination with CD/5-FC gene therapy enhances killing of human bladder-cancer cells by radiation. *Journal of Gene Medicine, 5*(10), 860–867.

CHAPTER 6

Treatment of Penile Carcinoma

Albert A. Rundio Jr., PhD, DNP, APRN-BC

Introduction

Penile carcinoma is a devastating disease for any man and his partner. It is a rare cancer, occurring annually in only 1% of the male population in the United States and accounting for about 1% of all malignancies (Jemal et al., 2008).

Squamous cell carcinoma is the most common type of penile cancer and is a potentially fatal malignancy, especially when inguinal lymph node metastases are present (Igarashi et al., 1996; Lopes et al., 1996). One of the most common causes of this disease is poor hygiene in uncircumcised men. Other conditions and risk factors include smoking, unprotected sexual activity with multiple partners, human papillomavirus (HPV), and other sexually transmitted diseases such as genital warts (Harish & Ravi, 1995; Hoofnagle, Kandzari, & Lamm, 1996; Misra, Chaturvedi, & Misra, 2004). Risk factors are presented in detail in Chapter 4.

Patients who have been diagnosed with penile carcinoma tend to seek medical treatment later than patients with other types of cancer and present with a wide range of tumor sizes. Treatment often is delayed for more than one year in 15%–50% of patients because of "fear, embarrassment, ignorance of the disease, and personal neglect" (Misra et al., 2004, p. 242). This chapter addresses the surgical treatment of penile cancer along with a discussion on the use of radiation therapy and chemotherapy. The psychosocial and nursing issues associated with this difficult diagnosis also are discussed.

Surgery

Treatment strategies vary and are dependent upon the clinician. Variations in treatment include surgical excision of the lesion, Mohs micrographic surgery (Mohs, Snow, Messing, & Kuglitsch, 1985), laser surgery, subtotal or total penectomy, surgical excision of inguinal lymph nodes, and endoscopic excision of inguinal lymph nodes, as they are usually the first

site of metastasis. Although utilized primarily when a patient refuses conventional treatment therapies, local treatment to the lesion may be accomplished using laser treatments and radiation.

According to Goroll and Mulley (2000), during Mohs micrographic surgery, the initial tumor is excised under local anesthesia. The tissue is examined directly under the microscope to determine if the tumor has been completely excised. Additional sections of the skin and tissue are removed until all of the borders are histologically free of tumor. The five-year survival rate is 80% with subtotal penectomy in the treatment of T1 and T2 penile carcinomas in the absence of inguinal metastases (T1N0 and T2N0) using standard subtotal penectomy (Goroll & Mulley).

The goal of the surgical intervention is to achieve a 2 cm margin free of tumor cells. The residual stump also is serviceable for micturition in the upright position and for sexual functioning (Magoha, 1995). The current practice of having a 2 cm margin of clearance for tumors is not based on evidence-based medicine or on histopathologic evidence but on recurrence rate. Without adequate margins of clearance of at least 2 cm, the incidence of local recurrence is high, approximately 40% (Kroon, Horenblas, & Nieweg, 2005; Loughlin, 2006; Micali, Nasca, Innocenzi, & Schwartz, 2006).

In order to determine the best surgical approach for patients, Agrawal, Pai, Ananthakrishnan, Smile, and Ratnakar (2000) prospectively assessed histologic grade and presence of tumor cell extension beyond the gross tumor in 68 patients. Each patient's gross tumor was removed by partial or total penectomy dependent on the size of the tumor. The specimens were then processed in the pathology laboratory and cut in 5 mm cross-section slices and examined microscopically. Based on the extent of tumor spread, patients with grade 1 and 2 tumors need a 10 mm margin of normal tissue in the surgical specimen, and patients with grade 3 tumors need a 15 mm margin. This surgical approach would reduce the number of total penectomies.

Nursing Assessment and Care of the Surgical Patient

Nursing History

It is essential for the nurse to obtain a thorough history. The patient should be questioned about presenting signs and symptoms and their duration and if circumcision was performed and when. If the patient has not been circumcised, it is important to determine the patient's hygiene habits and history. Obtaining an accurate sexual history is mandatory, and the nurse must ascertain if the patient has been exposed to or has had an HPV infection. The patient should also be asked about smoking history, number of packs per day, and type of tobacco products used. A good psychological history should be obtained that includes history of any past hospitalizations for psychiatric disorders with a specific focus on depression and suicide ideation.

Preoperative Nursing Assessment

Subjective assessment: The patient needs to be assessed subjectively as well as objectively (White, 2001). The subjective assessment should be completed prior to the objective assessment. See Figure 6-1 for questions to direct the interview.

Objective assessment: The objective assessment is performed after the subjective assessment. The nurse must be comfortable with examining male genitalia. The patient also needs to be comfortable with the examining nurse. The patient should be asked if he would prefer that a male nurse, if available, perform the objective assessment. The objective assessment consists of inspection and palpation of the penis, testes, and bilateral inguinal lymph nodes.

The site of the lesion (the shaft of the penis versus the glans penis), the type and extent of the lesion, and the treatment will define the nursing care that is necessary for patients diagnosed with penile carcinoma (Clark, 2004). For example, if a patient decides to have radiation of the lesion rather than surgical excision of the lesion, the nursing care will differ. The nursing assessment includes evaluation of the presenting lesion. The lesion should be measured and clearly described. For example, document if the lesion is papular in nature, indurated, or open and draining. Also document the number and size of any palpable inguinal lymph nodes. It is incumbent for the nurse to assess the patient's psychological status, with attention to anxiety, depression, and suicide ideation with and without a plan.

According to Lasseter (1992) and White (2001), the objective nursing assessment also includes review and evaluation of baseline laboratory, radiologic, electrocardiographic, and pulmonary function tests. These test results will assist the nurse in anticipating the patient's possible response to surgery and in anticipating nursing needs and patient education.

Figure 6-1. Preoperative Subjective Nursing Assessment

- Has the patient been circumcised? If yes, at what age?
- What are the patient's hygiene habits?
- Has the patient had any sexually transmitted diseases? If yes, what types? When did they occur? How were they treated?
- When was the lesion first noted?
- Exactly what location is the lesion located?
- Does the lesion cause pain?
- Has the patient noted any lymph node swelling?
- Has the patient had any fatigue?
- Has the patient noted any recent weight loss? If so, over what time period and how much?
- Does the patient have any allergies?
- What are the patient's current medications, both prescription and over the counter?
- Does the patient have any preexisting medical problems?
- Has the patient had previous surgeries? A positive response should trigger other questions, such as has the patient had any postoperative complications from any surgeries?
- Has the patient had anesthesia in the past? A positive response should trigger other questions, such as what type of anesthesia and any complications from anesthesia?
- The patient needs an emotional assessment with questioning focused on depression, anxiety, and in some cases, suicide ideation with or without a plan.
- The patient also needs an educational assessment. This assessment is best performed if the nurse knows what treatment interventions are planned for the client. Educational needs for surgery will differ than educational needs for radiation treatment without surgical intervention.
- At what literacy level is the patient functioning?
- What cultural norms are apparent in this particular patient?
- What support systems does the patient have?
- Does the patient have any financial issues/problems?
- Have treatment options been explained to the patient? Does he understand these options?
- Is the patient willing to comply with proposed treatment interventions?

Note. Based on information from White, 2001.

Nursing Care

Nursing care is dependent upon the treatment selected by the patient and performed by the physician. Surgical postoperative care will be necessary if either a partial or total penectomy is performed. Care of the patient postoperatively will vary depending on whether a lymph node dissection is performed. The physician who performed the surgical procedure will define routine surgical care for both circumstances.

If the patient undergoes surgical excision of the lesion, or subtotal or total penectomy, nurses should monitor
- Vital signs
- The incision site
- Intake and output.

Nurses also should assess patients for

- Hypotension
- Tachycardia
- Excessive incision drainage
- Redness or swelling around the incision
- Bright red drainage
- Decreased urinary output.

These are potential signs of surgical complications such as infection, sepsis, or bleeding (White, 2001).

The care that is provided to patients diagnosed with any type of cancer needs to be multidisciplinary. This is no different for the patient diagnosed with and treated for penile carcinoma. Generally, care focuses on post-treatment interventions. It is always important to involve patients and their significant others when providing nursing care and teaching. Skin care and healing strategies are going to be needed whether a patient has radiation therapy, surgical excision, or a combination of both treatment modalities. The nurse needs to be aware of the possibility of urethral strictures and urethracutaneous fistula development. If the patient has catheters placed in the perineal area, nursing care includes assessing for urine leakage. Urine leaking on radiated skin can cause additional skin irritation and further problems, which need to be prevented by good skin hygiene (Blanco-Yarosh, 2007). Patients who have undergone a total penectomy will require special tube care. Teaching includes care of the perineal urethrostomy site and the perineal catheter through which urine drains. Teaching will be required for care of the catheter itself as well as perineal care after bowel movements. The goal is to prevent wound contamination and urinary tract infection (Blanco-Yarosh). Frequently, prophylactic antibiotics are administered postoperatively. Nurses will need to monitor antibiotic therapy, the response to such therapy, and any resulting complications.

Radiation and Laser Therapy

Other treatment options include radiation therapy of the lesion, with or without radiation therapy to the regional lymph nodes. An option to treat small, superficial, exophytic lesions in young male patients is radiation therapy with external beam therapy, interstitial implants, or mould techniques (cesium [Cs-137], iridium [Ir-192]) (Azrif et al., 2006; Crook, Grimard, Tsihlias, Morash, & Panzarella, 2002). This can allow for the preservation of sexual function with a high cure rate. In case of relapse, surgery may be necessary (Sanchez-Ortiz & Pettaway, 2003). It must be emphasized that radiation treatment is indicated for small, superficial lesions. Sometimes, it may be utilized for regional lymphadenopathy or in patients for whom surgery is not an option. Certain situations require—and some healthcare providers prefer—a combination of both surgery and radiation. For example, if the tumor is large, radiation is used initially to shrink tumor size so that it is more resect-

able. Meijer, Boon, van Venrooij, and Wijburg (2007) used an Nd:YAG laser to treat 44 patients with carcinoma in situ (CIS), T1, or T2 penile cancer. Phimosis was present in 22 patients, and cancer was found after circumcision in 11 others. Disease relapse occurred in 29 patients and was managed with partial penectomy or repeat laser procedures. Inguinal lymph node metastases were found in 10 patients, with two of them at the time of initial diagnosis with T2 disease. The eight other patients developed nodal metastases at a later time; six of these patients had T2 disease at the time of diagnosis. The mean time from initial diagnosis to the development of nodal metastases was 41 months. Researchers have found that patient survival is more dependent on lymph node status than on the status of the local disease (Mobilio & Ficarra, 2001; Ravi, 1993). They also concluded that wider laser excision at the initial time of therapy is needed and that laser treatments should be limited to three subsequent treatments. Laser therapy is more suitable for patients with CIS and T1 tumors.

Certain healthcare providers utilize a much more conservative approach to treatment. That is, if there is no indication of lymph node metastases once initial therapy has been accomplished (e.g., surgery), the patient is monitored extremely closely for the first indication of regional lymph node metastases. Physical examination is the mainstay of follow-up care. Computed tomography (CT) scanning also can be of benefit.

Abdominal and pelvic CT scans are performed every three to four months for the first year after treatment. Close follow-up is recommended even in patients with low-volume inguinal lymph node metastases because of the potential for cure. Therefore, the importance of prompt identification of nodal metastases cannot be understated (Montie, 1994).

According to Bouchot, Auvigne, Peuvrel, Glemain, and Buzelin (1989), one challenge is the differentiation of inflammatory lymph nodes from those with metastatic involvement because inguinal and pelvic lymphadenectomy has significant associated morbidity. Another challenge is determining which patients without palpable lymph nodes on initial examination are most likely to develop secondary metastatic sites. In addition, Bouchot et al. noted that "patients with tumor localization in the glans or foreskin survived somewhat longer compared to those with localization in the shaft or in the glans and shaft; however, no statistically significant differences were noted" (p. 413). The authors noted that palpable lymph nodes at the initial presentation did not always indicate tumor presence. They reported that 80% of patients who had a negative groin examination for lymphadenopathy had no associated subclinical metastatic nodes (Bouchot et al.). After reviewing other research findings, Bouchot et al. concluded that a superficial lymph node biopsy at the time of the primary surgery is reasonable, as the five-year survival rate for patients with a negative superficial lymph node biopsy has been reported to be 90%. Inguinal lymph node dissection is associated with morbidity. In a study that explored lymph node mapping to determine if dissection was warranted, Spiess et al. (2007) concluded that superficial lymph node dissections should not be replaced.

Lymphadenectomy

Sotelo et al. (2007) reported that bilateral inguinal lymphadenectomy remains the gold standard for treating metastatic penile carcinoma. The authors studied a new technique of endoscopic inguinal lymphadenectomy for penile carcinoma (ELPC) in eight patients with a mean age of 56 years (range = 34 to 75 years). These patients had clinical stages of T2, N0–3, and M0. All of these patients had partial penectomy prior to the procedure and received a four-week course of antibiotics before the procedure. Antibiotics were used before the procedure as a preventive measure against the development of operative site infection and lymphedema that could follow the procedure. The procedure used preoperative Doppler ultrasound mapping of the inguinal regions on the patients who qualified to enroll in the study. Doppler ultrasound mapping was done to delineate the course of the saphenous vein and to map the inguinal lymph nodes. Sotelo et al. reported no postoperative surgical complications, with the exception of lymphoceles that developed in the groin of patients who had previously undergone a saphenous vein ligation procedure. ELPC potentially will be beneficial for patients, but additional research on this procedure is required. The authors reported that more experience and long-term follow-up is required prior to this procedure replacing the standard open dissection of lymph nodes. Tobias-Machado et al. (2007) reported on video endoscopic inguinal lymphadenectomy (VEIL). The authors described a study in which 10 patients underwent this procedure during the period of 2003–2005. Standard inguinal lymphadenectomy was performed on one side and VEIL was performed on the opposite side. The patients were at high risk for the development of bilateral inguinal metastases. No intraoperative complications were reported. A decrease in cutaneous infections was noted in the VEIL procedure side. A trend in decreased overall morbidity also was observed on the VEIL treatment side. A mean follow-up time of 18.7 months revealed no evidence of disease recurrence or disease progression on either side. The authors concluded that VEIL is a safe alternative procedure for those patients with penile carcinoma and nonpalpable lymph nodes.

As the morbidity from lymph node dissection oftentimes can be more severe than the cancer itself, some surgeons are now performing superficial lymph node dissection. If these nodes are negative for metastases, complete lymph node dissection is not performed, thus sparing the patient the morbidity of total lymph node dissection. Lont et al. (2007) examined 308 patients with penile carcinoma. The intent of the study was to identify if the number of inguinal lymph nodes with cancer could predict pelvic lymph node metastases and overall survival. The authors concluded that "patients with only 1 or 2 inguinal lymph nodes involved with no evidence of extracapsular growth and no poorly differentiated tumor within those nodes were at low risk of development of pelvic lymph node involvement" (p. 947). These patients have a good prognosis, and five-year survival rates have been estimated at 90%. Surgical complications included lymphocele, wound infection, skin flap necrosis, lymphedema, deep vein thrombosis, and stroke (Lont et al.).

Nursing Care of the Patient With an Inguinal Lymphadenectomy

Preoperative care includes assessment of the inguinal region. Inguinal areas need to be palpated for the presence of lymphadenopathy. The number of palpable lymph nodes should be noted and reported to the healthcare provider.

Postoperative care includes assessment of the surgical incision sites. Drainage from wound sites needs to be documented. Any excessive bleeding needs to be reported promptly. When dressing changes are performed, the nurse assesses the incision for any signs of wound healing, or infection such as erythema and drainage (especially purulent drainage), which require sending a wound culture and sensitivity to evaluate the infection. Vital signs are monitored, as an elevated temperature is a sign of infection. The patient's complete blood count (CBC) with differential also needs to be monitored, as an elevated WBC count is indicative of infection.

Patient Teaching

Patient teaching is paramount in the provision of nursing care for patients treated for penile carcinoma. Teaching self-care skills, such as perineal care, lower extremity care on the side of inguinal node dissection, and voiding techniques, is essential in the provision of holistic patient care (Clark, 2004).

Chemotherapy

Bermejo et al. (2007) described the use of combination chemotherapy for advanced penile carcinoma with a retrospective review of 59 patients. The patients were treated from 1985 through 2000. Ten patients underwent inguinal lymph node resection after a stable or better response to chemotherapy. Tumor burden involved pelvic and inguinal metastases. Bermejo et al. concluded, "select patients with metastatic penile carcinoma that show disease stabilization or a response to chemotherapy should be considered for surgical consolidation in order to extend survival" (p. 1335). Involvement of the patient in the treatment plan is paramount. The clinician provides the patient with the most current research findings; however, the ultimate decision must be the patient's. When treatment options are considered, it is also vitally important to consider other predisposing factors and patient comorbidities.

When surgical resection cannot be performed immediately in advanced penile carcinoma, combination chemotherapy is used to shrink the tumor prior to surgical resection. Bleomycin, cisplatin, and methotrexate all have single-agent activity in penile cancer with response rates ranging from 15%–21% for cisplatin and 38%–61% for methotrexate (Culkin & Beer, 2003). According to Leijte, Kerst, Bais, Antonini, and Horenblas (2007), the following chemotherapy drugs and drug combinations have been used to treat advanced penile carcinoma.

1. Bleomycin (15 mg IV days 1 and 3, repeated weekly until total maximum dose of 200–300 mg)
2. Bleomycin/vincristine/methotrexate (bleomycin 15 mg IV days 1 and 2, vincristine 1 mg IV day 1, methotrexate 30–50 mg IV day 3, repeated with a one-week interval until maximum of 12 cycles)
3. 5-fluorouracil (5-FU)/cisplatin (5-FU 1,000 mg/m^2 IV days 1–5, cisplatin 100 mg/m^2 IV day 1, repeated with a three-week interval until maximum of five cycles)
4. Bleomycin/cisplatin/methotrexate (bleomycin 15 mg IV days 2–5, cisplatin 20 mg/m^2 IV days 2–5, methotrexate 200 mg/m^2 IV day 1, repeated with a three-week interval until maximum of four cycles)

Adjuvant and neoadjuvant administration of vincristine, bleomycin, and methotrexate for patients with metastatic disease to the lymph nodes produced responses of approximately 42 months, and some patients underwent lymph node dissection (Pizzocaro & Piva, 1988). Neoadjuvant therapy for penile cancer with 5-FU and cisplatin produced unsustained responses (Culkin & Beer, 2003). The toxicity associated with bleomycin, cisplatin, and methotrexate is severe, and the regimen is not used as part of standard therapy (Culkin & Beer; Hakenberg, Nippgen, Froehner, Zastrow, & Wirth, 2006).

Nursing Care of Patients Receiving Chemotherapy

Nursing care centers on the safe administration of chemotherapeutic agents and monitoring patients for side effects and signs of toxicity. Nurses need to monitor laboratory results, especially the CBC with differential count, and renal function tests (blood urea nitrogen, creatinine, and glomerular filtration rate). Patients with decreased white blood cell counts are more prone to infection, and those with decreased platelet counts are at risk for bleeding (Blanco-Yarosh, 2007). Changes in patient blood counts need to be reported promptly. In every setting of chemotherapy administration, it is important to include the patient and family in patient education, as long as the patient provides consent for family involvement.

When administering bleomycin, nurses must take a systems approach in monitoring the patient. Patients must be observed for the development of fever, chills, rigors, headache, nausea, vomiting, stomatitis, and prolonged anorexia, dyspnea, crackles on auscultation, and a nonproductive cough. Patients receiving this medication can develop pneumonitis and pulmonary fibrosis. It is also important for nurses to observe for changes in the skin such as desquamation of hands, feet, and pressure areas. Hardening and discoloration of the palmar and plantar skin may occur. Alopecia often develops in these patients. It is also vitally important that nurses observe patients for hypersensitivity reactions, which can have a delayed onset (*Springhouse Nurse's Drug Guide,* 2008).

Nurses must assess and monitor the patients for peripheral nervous system toxicity when administering vincristine. Therefore, they should assess the patient for numbness and tingling of extremities, loss of deep tendon reflexes, foot drop, and wrist drop. Nurses also need to assess patients' gait, as difficulty in ambulation, ataxia, and slapping gait may be present. Bowel function also must be monitored, as constipation may be an early sign of neurotoxicity, and ileus may develop from autonomic nervous system neurotoxicity (*Springhouse Nurse's Drug Guide,* 2008; Wilkes & Barton-Burke, 2008).

Cisplatin administration requires that nurses monitor serum magnesium, potassium, and other electrolytes, as well as CBCs and renal function lab tests. Hydration before and after treatment as well as a diuretic are administered, and the patient is premedicated with antiemetics to reduce the risk of nausea and vomiting. The patient must be voiding prior to starting the drug infusion. Because hearing loss may occur, it is important to monitor audiometry results, if performed. Peripheral neuropathy also may develop. Nurses also need to be alert for adverse reactions and drug toxicities such as acute renal failure (*Springhouse Nurse's Drug Guide,* 2008; Wilkes & Barton-Burke, 2008).

Methotrexate produces gastrointestinal toxicities such as stomatitis, nausea, and vomiting. Patients need to be taught a prophylactic oral regimen such as using a soft toothbrush and nonabrasive toothpaste and rinsing with saline four times a day. Antiemetics are administered before treatment, and intake and output are closely monitored. Methotrexate is excreted via the kidneys and can cause renal impairment and renal failure. Renal laboratory test values are closely monitored through therapy. Bone marrow depression may develop, so nurses must teach patients the signs and symptoms of infection, bleeding, and anemia, as well as instruct patients to report any evidence of these side effects immediately to their healthcare providers. It is important to monitor the uric acid level, as well as liver function tests, as patients may develop hepatic dysfunction. Nurses should routinely monitor CBCs and need to observe for adverse reactions and drug interactions (*Springhouse Nurse's Drug Guide,* 2008; Wilkes & Barton-Burke, 2008).

When administering 5-FU, it is important to monitor lab values as previously described. Patients may develop leukopenia, thrombocytopenia, stomatitis, diarrhea, gastrointestinal ulceration, bleeding, and hemorrhage. The topical form can induce adverse reactions and systemic effects, including drug toxicity. The nadir (lowest white blood cell count) occurs 9–14 days after the chemotherapy dose. Thus, monitoring CBCs is important during this period (*Springhouse Nurse's Drug Guide,* 2008). See Appendix.

Patient Teaching

Patients and family members need education on cytotoxic therapy and the resultant side effects with an emphasis on prevention and management. Nurses must teach oral hygiene, skin care, infection and immune system precautions, pulmonary hygiene, and perineal care (Clark, 2004). In addition, nurses must inform patients and caregivers regarding safety precautions for neurotoxicities, pulmonary toxicities, and cardiac toxicities because certain chemotherapeutic agents can cause complications such as pulmonary fibrosis and cardiac abnormalities.

The Psychology of Penile Carcinoma

Psychological and Sexual Manifestations

Men frequently delay treatment for carcinoma of the penis because they deny that a problem exists. Psychological manifestations are present both pre- and postoperatively. Patients with very early-stage disease not affecting the glans penis or the shaft of the penis and who may be treated successfully with radiation, cryosurgery, circumcision, and laser therapy often recover uneventfully. One difficulty in trying to assess a patient's psychological state is that sample size is often small because penile carcinoma is not common.

Psychological manifestations may result upon diagnosis and the recommendation of a partial or total penectomy as the preferred treatment option. Patients may feel that they are losing their "manhood," and in a society and culture where masculinity and being sexually active are equated with manhood, such news may be extremely devastating to any patient. Cultural considerations must be addressed, for example, in certain societies and cultures where machismo is the norm for a male. There is no question that partial to total penectomy results in severe disfigurement of the male image. Nurses need to assess the patient for evidence and signs and symptoms of depression and the possibility of suicide ideation with or without a plan. Patients who have suicide ideation promptly need to be referred to an advanced practice nurse with a specialty in psychiatry such as a psychiatric nurse practitioner, or a social worker, psychologist, or psychiatrist.

D'Ancona et al. (1997) examined the quality of life after partial penectomy. The authors specifically addressed the aspects of sexuality, social adjustment, and emotional state. The patients were evaluated through a semistructured interview and four standardized questionnaires. The tools utilized in this research were the Overall Sexual Functioning Questionnaire, the Social Problem Questionnaire, the General Health Questionnaire, and the Hospital Anxiety and Depression Scale. Patients who underwent penectomy were found to be well-adapted to their condition. The authors discovered that the patients' quality of life was maintained. Limitations to this study were the small sample size (14 patients) and use of a convenience sample. The quantity of patients who are diagnosed with penile carcinoma is not a large number, and this contributes to relatively small study sample sizes in certain geographic regions. In industrialized nations such as the United States, penile carcinoma is rare because circumcision, good hygiene, and HPV prevention strategies are common.

Ficarra et al. (2000) evaluated the general state of health and psychological well-being in a group of 155 patients who had surgical interventions for malignant neoplasms. Sixteen of these patients had surgery for squamous cell penile carcinoma. Results from the study group were compared with a group of patients who had retropubic prostatectomy for benign prostatic hypertrophy. Data were collected by face-to-face interviews. The results demonstrated that the general state of health and psychological well-being were more compromised in patients who had surgery for malignant neoplasms when compared to patients who had surgery for benign prostatic hypertrophy. Data in this study demonstrated significant impairment in the general state of health and psychological well-being in patients after partial penectomy ($p = 0.0001$). Pathologic levels of anxiety, as determined by a general health questionnaire and the Hospital Anxiety and Depression Scale, were noted in the partial penectomy group, and sexual function was the most impaired domain for these patients. The results in this study contrast with D'Ancona et al. (1997), who found that patients adapted well to their surgical intervention for penile carcinoma. Partial and total penectomy still remain the gold standard for the treatment of penile carcinoma. Further research in the area of psychological well-being, sexuality, and social adjustment certainly is warranted.

Patients who undergo subtotal or total penectomy may be subject to severe psychological manifestations. Body image is a major concern. Men often judge themselves by the size of their penis. Hence, loss of this organ can be devastating. Sexual counseling, psychological therapy, and family counseling must be offered. Nurses skilled in this area can provide counseling and suggest alternative ways to express intimacy. Despite either partial or full loss of their penis, patients need to be assured of their ability to have an orgasm. Frank discussions on different methods for the patient to provide pleasure to their partner also must be incorporated into the plan of care (Blanco-Yarosh, 2007). Some patients accept their altered body image and are thankful that they are cured of cancer and have been given a "second chance." Others contemplate and even commit suicide. Hem, Loje, Haldorsen, and Ekeberg (2004) concluded that suicide risk in patients with cancer is highest in the first month after diagnosis. Therapy must be tailored to the individual patient and the environment, which is inclusive of their family support system, family structure, work environment, and other factors. Antidepressants and antianxiety medications may be indicated. The selective serotonin reuptake inhibitor class of medication is widely prescribed for depression and also may be used for anxiety. The benzodiazepine class is widely prescribed for anxiety; however, this class of medication has addictive properties.

Psychosocial Nursing Care

Attention to patients' psychological needs is important. Patients need to be continually assessed for anxiety, depression, and suicide ideation. Referral to psychiatry will be based on the nursing assessment and the physician's orders. Nurses are excellent holistic care providers, and patients diagnosed with penile carcinoma need to be treated according to the holistic care philosophy. Nurses need to educate patients with penile carcinoma regarding care of the surgical wound, sexual counseling and education, self-examination (especially assessment for lymphadenopathy), and any medications that the physician may prescribe. Nurses need to explain the importance of and necessity for follow-up care of patients who are treated for penile carcinoma.

Summary

Penile carcinoma can be a devastating illness. Early diagnosis and treatment are essential to long-term survival from this disease.

References

Agrawal, A., Pai, D., Ananthakrishnan, N., Smile, S.R., & Ratnakar, C. (2000). The histological extent of the local spread of carcinoma of the penis and its therapeutic implications. *BJU International, 85*(3), 299–301.

Azrif, M., Logue, J.P., Swindell, R., Cowan, R.A., Wylie, J.P., & Livsey, J.E. (2006). External-beam radiotherapy in T1-2 N0 penile carcinoma. *Clinical Oncology, 18*(4), 320–325.

Bermejo, C., Busby, J.E., Spiess, P.E., Heller, L., Pagliaro, L.C., & Pettaway, C.A. (2007). Neoadjuvant chemotherapy followed by aggressive surgical consolidation for metastatic penile squamous cell carcinoma. *Journal of Urology, 177*(4), 1335–1338.

Blanco-Yarosh, M. (2007). Penile cancer: An overview. *Urologic Nursing, 27*(4), 286–290.

Bouchot, O., Auvigne, J., Peuvrel, P., Glemain, P., & Buzelin, J.M. (1989). Management of regional lymph nodes in carcinoma of the penis. *European Urology, 16*(6), 410–415.

Clark, J. (2004). Genitourinary cancers. In C.G. Verricchio (Ed.), *A cancer source book for nurses* (8th ed., pp. 277–294). Sudbury, MA: Jones and Bartlett.

Crook, J., Grimard, L., Tsihlias, J., Morash, C., & Panzarella, T. (2002). Interstitial brachytherapy for penile cancer: An alternative to amputation. *Journal of Urology, 167*(2, Pt. 1), 506–511.

Culkin, D.J., & Beer, T.M. (2003). Advanced penile carcinoma. *Journal of Urology, 170*(2, Pt. 1), 359–365.

D'Ancona, C.A., Botega, N.J., DeMoraes, C., Lavoura, N.S., Jr., Santos, J.K., & Rodrigues Netto, N., Jr. (1997). Quality of life after partial penectomy for penile carcinoma. *Urology, 50*(4), 593–596.

Ficarra, V., Righetti, R., D'Amico, A., Pilloni, S., Balzarro, M., Schiavone, D., et al. (2000). General state of health and psychological well-being in patients after surgery for urological malignant neoplasms. *Urologia Internationalis, 65*(3), 130–134.

Goroll, A.H., & Mulley, A.G., Jr. (2000). *Primary care medicine: Office evaluation and management of the adult patient.* Philadelphia: Lippincott Williams & Wilkins.

Hakenberg, O.W., Nippgen, J.B.W., Froehner, M., Zastrow, S., & Wirth, M.P. (2006). Cisplatin, methotrexate and bleomycin for treating advanced penile cancer. *BJU International, 98*(6), 1225–1227.

Harish, K., & Ravi, R. (1995). The role of tobacco in penile carcinoma. *British Journal of Urology, 75*(3), 375–377.

Hem, E., Loje, J.H., Haldorsen, T., & Ekeberg, O. (2004). Suicide risk in cancer patients from 1960 to 1999. *Journal of Clinical Oncology, 22*(20), 4209–4216.

Hoofnagle, R.F., Jr., Kandzari, S., & Lamm, D.L. (1996). Deoxyribonucleic acid flow cytometry of squamous cell carcinoma of the penis. *West Virginia Medical Journal, 92*(5), 271–273.

Igarashi, H., Oishi, Y., Kishimoto, K., Yanada, S., Kondo, N., & Hasegawa, N. (1996). A case of penile cancer treated with combination of chemotherapy, radiation and radical operation. *Hinyokika Kiyo—Acta Urological Japonica, 42*(6), 465–467.

Jemal, A., Siegel, R., Ward, E., Hao, Y., Xu, J., Murray, T., et al. (2008). Cancer statistics, 2008. *CA: A Cancer Journal for Clinicians, 58*(2), 71–96.

Kroon, B.K., Horenblas, S., & Nieweg, D.E. (2005). Contemporary management of penile squamous cell carcinoma. *Journal of Surgical Oncology, 89*(1), 43–50.

Lasseter, S.J. (1992). Cancer of the penis: Perioperative interventions. *AORN Journal, 56*(1), 19–30.

Leijte, J., Kerst, J., Bais, E., Antonini, N., & Horenblas, S. (2007). Neoadjuvant chemotherapy in advanced penile carcinoma. *European Urology, 52*(2), 488–494.

Lont, A.P., Kroon, B.K., Gallee, M.P.W., van Tinteren, H., Moonen, M.F., & Horenblas, S. (2007). Pelvic lymph node dissection for penile carcinoma: Extent of inguinal lymph node involvement as an indicator for pelvic lymph node involvement and survival. *Journal of Urology, 177*(3), 947–952.

Lopes, A., Hidalgo, G.S., Kowalski, L.P., Torloni, H., Rossi, B.M., & Fonseca, F.P. (1996). Prognostic factors in carcinoma of the penis: Multivariate analysis of 145 patients treated with amputation and lymphadenectomy. *Journal of Urology, 156*(5), 1637–1642.

Loughlin, K.R. (2006). Surgical atlas. Surgical management of penile carcinoma: The inguinal nodes. *BJU International, 97*(5), 1125–1134.

Magoha, G.A. (1995). Management of carcinoma of the penis: A review. *East African Medical Journal, 72*(9), 547–550.

Meijer, R.P., Boon, T.A., van Venrooij, G., & Wijburg, C. (2007). Long-term follow-up after laser therapy for penile carcinoma. *Urology, 69*(4), 759–762.

Micali, G., Nasca, M.R., Innocenzi, D., & Schwartz, R.A. (2006). Penile cancer. *Journal of the American Academy of Dermatology, 54*(3), 369–391.

Misra, S., Chaturvedi, A., & Misra, C. (2004). Penile carcinoma: A challenge for the developing world. *Lancet Oncology, 5*(4), 240–247.

Mobilio, G., & Ficarra, V. (2001). Genital treatment of penile carcinoma. *Current Opinion in Urology, 11*(3), 299–304.

Mohs, F.E., Snow, S.N., Messing, E.M., & Kuglitsch, M.E. (1985). Microscopically controlled surgery in the treatment of carcinoma of the penis. *Journal of Urology, 133*(6), 961–966.

Montie, J.E. (1994). Follow-up after penectomy for penile cancer. *Urologic Clinics of North America, 21*(4), 725–727.

Pizzocaro, G., & Piva, L. (1988). Adjuvant and neoadjuvant vincristine, bleomycin, and methotrexate for inguinal metastases from squamous cell carcinoma of the penis. *Acta Oncologica, 27*(6b), 823–824.

Ravi, R. (1993). Correlation between the extent of nodal involvement and survival following groin dissection for carcinoma of the penis. *British Journal of Urology, 72*(5, Pt. 2), 817–819.

Sanchez-Ortiz, R.F., & Pettaway, C.A. (2003). Natural history, management, and surveillance of recurrent squamous cell penile carcinoma: A risk-based approach. *Urology Clinics of North America, 30*(4), 853–867.

Sotelo, R., Sanchez-Salas, R., Carmona, O., Garcia, A., Mariano, M., Neiva, G., et al. (2007). Endoscopic lymphadenectomy for penile carcinoma. *Journal of Endourology, 21*(4), 364–367.

Spiess, P.E., Izawa, J.I., Besset, R., Kedar, D., Busby, J.E., Wong, F., et al. (2007). Preoperative lymphoscintigraphy and dynamic sentinel node biopsy for staging penile cancer: Results with pathological correlation. *Journal of Urology, 177*(6), 2157–2161.

Springhouse nurse's drug guide (9th ed.). (2008). Philadelphia: Lippincott Williams & Wilkins.

Tobias-Machado, M., Tavares, A., Ornellas, A.A., Molina, W.R., Jr., Juliano, R.V., & Wroclawski, E.R. (2007). Video endoscopic inguinal lymphadenectomy: A new minimally invasive procedure for radical management of inguinal nodes in patients with penile squamous cell carcinoma. *Journal of Urology, 177*(3), 953–957.

White, L. (2001). *Foundations of nursing: Caring for the whole person*. Albany, NY: Delmar.

Wilkes, G.M., & Barton-Burke, M. (2008). *Oncology nursing drug handbook 2008*. Sudbury, MA: Jones and Bartlett.

CHAPTER 7

Treatment of Renal Cell Carcinoma

Laura S. Wood, RN, MSN, OCN®

Introduction

Treatment of renal cell carcinoma (RCC) has changed significantly over the past 10 years. Changes include advances in surgical techniques and the U.S. Food and Drug Administration (FDA) approval of new systemic therapies for patients with advanced disease. Since 1992, immunotherapy has been the main systemic therapy for clear cell renal cancer. The FDA approved interleukin (IL)-2 after it demonstrated a 14% objective response rate (Fyfe et al., 1995). Knowledge gained about the biology of RCC has led to an understanding of the histologic subtypes and the von-Hippel Lindau (VHL) protein. Both have an impact on the pathogenesis of renal cancer. In conditions of abnormal VHL function or increased tumor hypoxia, the VHL protein does not bind to hypoxia-inducible factor-1α (HIF-1α), leading to an accumulation of HIF-1α and activation of hypoxia-inducible genes. These genes include vascular endothelial growth factor (VEGF), platelet-derived growth factor-beta (PDGF-β), transforming growth factor-alpha (TGF-α), and erythropoietin (EPO). Loss of VHL gene function allows for increased secretion of VEGF, PDGF, TGF-α, and EPO, leading to increased renal tumor vascularization (Cohen & McGovern, 2005; Kim & Kaelin, 2004).

Extensive efforts to identify the proangiogenic pathways involved in renal cancer resulted in the development and approval of several targeted therapies that interfere with downstream signaling responsible for vascular development and tumor progression in RCC. VEGF, PDGF, ras kinase, and the mammalian target of rapamycin (mTOR) are key pathways in RCC pathogenesis. Drugs that target these pathways include sorafenib (Nexavar®, Bayer Healthcare Pharmaceuticals and Onyx Pharmaceuticals), which was approved for the treatment of advanced RCC in December 2005, followed by sunitinib (Sutent®, Pfizer Inc.) in January 2006, temsirolimus (Torisel®, Wyeth Pharmaceuticals) in May 2007, and everolimus (Afinitor®, Novartis Pharmaceuticals) in March 2009.

Prognostic Criteria

Prognostic factors associated with favorable, intermediate, or poor risk have been identified for untreated patients with renal cancer (see Figure 7-1) and were validated and expanded (see Figure 7-2) (Mekhail et al., 2005; Motzer, Bacik, Murphy, Russo, & Mazumdar, 2002). Some criteria evaluated were Karnofsky performance status, time from diagnosis to treatment with interferon (IFN) alfa, and hemoglobin, lactate dehydrogenase, and corrected serum calcium levels. These factors also were identified for patients who have received prior cytokine therapy (see Figure 7-3) (Motzer et al., 2004). Median survival rates differ for each risk group, and stratification using these prognostic factors has been beneficial in determining the effectiveness of new therapies in renal cancer. These may provide clinicians with additional useful information for guiding them toward treatment decisions specific to a particular patient.

Figure 7-1. Prognostic Factors and Median Survival in Untreated Renal Cancer

Prognostic Factors
- Karnofsky performance status is less than 80%.
- Time from diagnosis to treatment with interferon alfa is less than 12 months.
- Hemoglobin is less than the lower limit of normal.
- Lactate dehydrogenase is greater than 1.5 times the upper limit of normal.
- Corrected serum calcium is greater than 10 mg/dl.

Risk Groups	Number of Prognostic Factors	Median Overall Survival
Favorable	0	29.6 months
Intermediate	1 or 2	13.8 months
Poor	Greater than 2	4.9 months

Note. Based on information from Motzer et al., 2002.

Figure 7-2. Expanded Prognostic Factors and Median Survival in Untreated Renal Cancer

Prognostic Factors

- Time from diagnosis to treatment with interferon alfa is less than 12 months.
- Hemoglobin is less than the lower limit of normal.
- Lactate dehydrogenase is greater than 1.5 times the upper limit of normal.
- Corrected serum calcium is greater than 10 mg/dl.
- Prior radiation therapy
- Presence of hepatic, lung, or retroperitoneal nodal metastasis

Risk Groups	Number of Prognostic Factors	Median Overall Survival
Favorable	0 or 1	29 months
Intermediate	2	14.4 months
Poor	Greater than 2	7.3 months

Note. Based on information from Mekhail et al., 2005.

Figure 7-3. Prognostic Factors and Median Survival in Previously Treated Renal Cancer

Prognostic Factors

- Karnofsky performance status is less than 80%.
- Corrected serum calcium is greater than 10 mg/dl.
- Hemoglobin is less than or equal to 13 g/dl for men or less than or equal to 11.5 for women.

Risk Groups	Number of Prognostic Factors	Median Overall Survival
Favorable	0	22 months
Intermediate	1	11.9 months
Poor	2 or 3	5.4 months

Note. Based on information from Motzer et al., 2004.

Surgery

Patients with localized or metastatic RCC may benefit from surgical intervention. The type and timing of surgery varies significantly based on location of the primary tumor, extent of local tissue invasion, vascular involvement, and presence of metastatic disease. Excision of the primary renal mass may be curative for patients with localized disease, and cytoreductive nephrectomy should be considered for patients who present with synchronous metastatic disease. Treatment options for the primary renal mass are listed in Figure 7-4. Surveillance strategies following definitive surgery for localized disease incorporate various characteristics, including tumor, node, and metastasis staging; Eastern Cooperative Oncology Group

performance status; the natural history of RCC; nuclear grade; and histology (Chin, Lam, Figlin, & Belldegrun, 2006; Kattan, Reuter, Motzer, Katz, & Russo, 2001; Leibovich et al., 2003). Follow-up care for these patients includes physical examination, laboratory tests, and radiographic procedures. More frequent monitoring is recommended for patients at high risk for recurrence, specifically those patients with renal vein involvement and tumors that invade beyond the Gerota fascia (National Comprehensive Cancer Network, 2009; Russo, 2006).

The laparoscopic approach to radical or partial nephrectomy provides benefits that include decreased postoperative pain, shortened hospital stay, quicker convalescence, and improved cosmesis (Gill et al., 2007; Ogan, Cadeddu, & Stifelman, 2003). Surgical approach is based on tumor location (Gill, 2003).

Surgery can be performed from a retroperitoneal approach or a transperitoneal approach. The transperitoneal approach is used for anterior, anterolateral, lateral, and upper-pole apical tumors and allows control of the renal artery and vein before dissection of the kidney (Gill, 2003). The retroperitoneal approach is used for posterior or posterolaterally located tumors and allows control of the renal artery and vein. Partial nephrectomy initially was indicated for small, peripheral, superficial, exophytic tumors, and may be appropriate in carefully selected patients with more complex tumors (Gill). This approach also is indicated for more complex tumors in the setting of a single kidney or when a radical nephrectomy will result in dialysis to maintain renal function. With the detection of renal masses at an earlier stage, partial nephrectomy or nephron-sparing surgery has evolved as an effective alternative to radical nephrectomy (Russo, 2000). Early renal functional and oncologic outcomes were similar between the laparoscopic and open partial nephrectomy procedures in a large multicenter study of 1,800 patients (Gill et al., 2007).

Treatment for patients who present with synchronous metastatic disease should be a collaborative decision involving both a medical oncologist and urologist. Consideration

Figure 7-4. Treatment Options for the Primary Renal Mass

Procedure

- Partial nephrectomy
- Radical nephrectomy
- Ablative partial nephrectomy
- Radiofrequency ablation
- Cryoablation

Surgical Approach

- Open thoracoabdominal approach (Chevron incision)
- Laparoscopic
  - "Hands-free"
  - "Hand-assisted"

Note. Based on information from Wood & Calabrese, 2005.

regarding the potential for surgical removal of the primary renal mass, the timing of surgery, and systemic therapy is a critical part of treatment planning. Some patients will benefit from having surgery first, whereas others should have systemic therapy followed by consideration of surgery. Cytoreductive nephrectomy followed by IFN demonstrated a survival benefit compared to interferon alone in two randomized studies (Flanigan et al., 2001; Mickisch et al., 2001). Surgical morbidity and mortality was acceptable and allowed almost all patients to begin postoperative treatment within three weeks (Flanigan et al., 2004). Cytoreductive nephrectomy should not be performed in all patients because of potential complications and preexisting comorbid conditions. Selection criteria include a good performance status, a resectable primary tumor representing the majority of the tumor burden, no evidence of rapidly progressing extrarenal disease, and no prohibitive medical comorbidities (Rini & Campbell, 2007).

Nursing care includes patient education, assessment, and management of side effects. Patient education begins during the preoperative period and continues through discharge planning (see Figure 7-5). Postoperative nursing care (see Figure 7-6) includes ensuring adequate pain control and monitoring for potential surgical complications, which can be classified as intraoperative or postoperative (Galli, Munver, Sawczuk, & Kochis, 2005; Gill et al., 2007).

Radiation Therapy

Radiation therapy is used in the treatment and palliation of metastatic RCC. External beam radiation is used to treat metastatic bone lesions to prevent pathologic fracture and as palliative treatment for pain caused by the development of lytic lesions. Brain metastasis can be managed with corticosteroids, whole brain radiotherapy, or stereotactic radiosurgery in select situations (Flanigan & Orris, 2006). Treatment decisions in-

---

Figure 7-6. Nursing Care: Postoperative Care

Intraoperative Complications
- Injury to adjacent organs, major vessels, ureter, or pleura
- Urinary leak
- Hemorrhage

Postoperative Complications
- Urinary leak
- Hematuria
- Renal failure
- Infection
- Thromboembolic events
- Alterations in incision structure

Postoperative Nursing Assessment and Care
- Pain management
- Minimize nausea and vomiting
- Pulmonary hygiene
- Phlebitis and deep vein thrombosis prophylaxis, including use of sequential compression stockings
- Oral hygiene
- Incision care
- Assessment for bowel sounds
- Nutritional assessment
- Progressive ambulation
- Discharge planning and patient education
  - Incision care
  - Monitor incision for erythema or drainage
  - Monitor for fever or chills
- Instruct patient to call doctor's office for development of fever, chills, cough, shortness of breath, drainage or bleeding from incision, hematuria, or worsening of pain.

Note. Based on information from Galli et al., 2005; Gill et al., 2007.

---

clude consideration regarding (Vogelbaum & Suh, 2006)
- Status of the patient's systemic disease
- Tumor type
- Karnofsky performance status
- Neurologic status
- Number and locations of lesions
- Presence of leptomeningeal disease.

Advances in treatment modalities allow clinicians to achieve superior levels of tumor control within the brain (Vogelbaum & Suh, 2006). Surgical resection is appropriate when gross total resection with minimal neurologic injury is possible based on tumor location and patient characteristics. Gamma knife radiosurgery provides a high dose of radiation to a localized brain tumor volume in a single session. Lesions that are well demarcated on CT or magnetic resonance images are usually amenable to stereotactic radiosurgery (Sheehan, Sun, Kondziolka, Flickinger, & Lunsford, 2003). Whole brain radiotherapy is indicated when patients have brain metastasis not amenable to surgical or radiosurgical intervention. Patients who receive whole brain radiotherapy in addition to stereotactic radiosurgery may have an improved clinical outcome (Brown, Brown,

---

Figure 7-5. Nursing Care: Patient Education

Preoperative
- Overview of preoperative, surgical, and immediate postoperative experience
- Dietary restrictions
- Bowel preparation regimen
- Day of surgery appointment information

Postoperative
- Pulmonary hygiene
- Phlebitis and deep vein thrombosis prophylaxis
- Strategies for effective pain management
- Progressive ambulation
- Incision care and assessment
- Discharge planning and follow-up appointments

Note. Based on information from Galli et al., 2005; Kidney Cancer Association, 2007.

Pollock, Gorman, & Foote, 2002). Whole brain radiotherapy following complete surgical resection remains controversial, as most patients die from systemic disease progression (Patchell et al., 1998; Vogelbaum & Suh). Early detection of brain metastasis, aggressive treatment of systemic disease, and the use of radiosurgery or whole brain radiotherapy can offer patients an extended survival (Brown et al.; Sheehan et al.).

Nursing care, including patient education and management of side effects, assists patients to complete radiation therapy as planned while minimizing severe side effects and maximizing quality of life (see Figure 7-7). It is important to be aware of acute, delayed, and potentially chronic side effects associated with specific types of radiation therapy and the location of treatment (see Figure 7-8) (Armstrong & McCaffrey, 2006; Maher, 2005; McQuestion, 2006; Shih, Miaskowski, Dodd, Stotts, & MacPhail, 2003). Side effects are dependent on the location and organ being treated, fractionation, treatment volume, and total dose of radiation (Sadler et al., 2003; Williams, Chen, Rubin, Finkelstein, & Okunieff, 2003).

Systemic Therapy

Immunotherapy

RCC demonstrates immunogenicity that is the basis for therapeutic strategies, including IL-2 and IFN (Uzzo et al.,

---

Figure 7-8. Side Effects of Radiation Therapy

Acute Side Effects
- Develop within hours or days of treatment
- Occur because proliferating cells are more radiosensitive than quiescent cells

Subacute Side Effects
- Develop several weeks to months following completion of treatment
- Result from recurrent cellular insult and inability of cells to completely repair radiation-induced damage

Late Side Effects
- Develop several months following completion of treatment
- Result from perpetual cascade of cytokine expression causing progressive cellular damage and tissue destruction

Note. Based on information from Maher et al., 2005; Williams et al., 2003.

2003). High-dose IV IL-2 provides a durable response for patients who achieve a complete response to initial therapy, but no survival benefit when compared to low-dose IV or subcutaneously administered IL-2 (Fisher, Rosenberg, & Fyfe, 2000; Yang et al., 2003). Side effects depend on the drug, route of administration, and dose administered.

Interleukin-2

High-dose IL-2 (aldesleukin) was approved for the treatment of metastatic renal cancer in 1992. Intravenous administration of 600,000–720,000 IU/kg is administered as follows (Chiron Corporation, 2000).
- As an inpatient regimen every eight hours
- As a 15-minute infusion
- For up to 14 doses
- Over five days as clinically tolerated
- Followed by a nine-day rest period

A second identical cycle of treatment is given following five to nine days of rest depending on the patient's tolerance of side effects and adequate organ function. This two-cycle regimen can be repeated every 6–12 weeks in stable or responding patients as clinically appropriate. Long-term follow-up demonstrated a 54-month median response duration for all objective responders (Fisher et al., 2000).

IL-2 has been administered subcutaneously on an outpatient basis using various doses, as monotherapy, or in combination with IFN, chemotherapy, or more recently in combination with targeted therapeutic agents (Atzpodien et al., 2004; McDermott et al., 2005; Sleifer et al., 1992). Comparison of IL-2 administered as a high-dose IV, low-dose IV, or subcutaneous regimen demonstrated a superior response rate for the high-dose IV group (21%) compared to low-dose IV (11%) and subcutaneous IL-2 (10%). However, there was no significant

---

Figure 7-7. Nursing Care for Patients Who Are Receiving Radiation Therapy

Patient Education
- Treatment plan and simulation process
- Use of masks, frames, blocks, or immobilization devices
- Total dose and fractionation of radiation
- Skin care during and following completion of treatment
- Nutrition guidelines
- Side effect management based on structures or organs in the radiation field
- Emphasis on maintaining adequate fluid and caloric intake

Nursing Care
- Assessment of integumentary system, gastrointestinal system, urinary function, nutritional and hydration status, and cognitive function
- Initiate strategies to manage side effects
- Evaluation of interventions

Skin Care
- Maintaining skin integrity
- Cleanliness and hygiene
- Comfort
- Pain control
- Protection from trauma
- Prevention and management of infections
- Promotion of a healing environment

Note. Based on information from Maher, 2005; McQuestion, 2006.

difference in survival for any of the groups (e.g., high-dose versus low-dose p = 0.04) (Yang et al., 2003).

Interferon

IFN is widely used in the treatment of advanced renal cancer as IFN alfa-2a (Roferon®, Hoffmann-La Roche) and IFN alfa-2b (Intron A®, Schering-Plough). In renal cancer, IFN is administered subcutaneously utilizing a variety of regimens with different doses and frequency. The most common regimen involves dose escalation to a final dose of 9 million units (MU) three times weekly. Treatment begins with IFN 3 MU in week 1, 6 MU in week 2, escalating to 9 MU in week 3, and beyond if tolerated. The median time to progression in patients treated with IFN as first-line therapy results in an average of 4.7 months, with an overall survival of 13 months (Motzer et al., 2002). Survival stratified according to Memorial Sloan-Kettering Cancer Center (MSKCC) risk factors resulted in a median overall survival of 30 months for "favorable-risk," 14 months for "intermediate-risk," and 5 months for "poor-risk" group (Motzer et al., 2002). IFN was used as the comparative arm in the front-line comparison studies of sunitinib and sorafenib.

Side Effects of Immunotherapy

IL-2 and IFN are associated with a cascade of side effects that are unique to immunotherapy and are dose-dependent in their severity (Mavroukakis, Muehlbauer, White, & Schwartzentruber, 2001; Mekhail, Wood, & Bukowski, 2000; Reiger, 2001). Side effects have been classified as "constitutional" or flu-like symptoms including fever, chills or rigors, fatigue, and anorexia. Acetaminophen and indomethacin are used to treat fever, whereas meperidine and hydromorphone are used to treat chills or rigors. Cardiovascular symptoms are particularly dependent on dose, with more severe symptoms often becoming dose limiting for patients receiving high-dose IL-2 therapy. Cardiopulmonary side effects include hypotension, pulmonary edema, capillary leak syndrome, atrial fibrillation, and hypoxia. Neurologic side effects include mental confusion or agitation, fatigue, and impaired cognitive function. Clinical pathways offer practical tools for anticipating and managing side effects associated with administration of IL-2 (Mavroukakis et al.; Tyre & Quan, 2007). Patients may experience more severe side effects, especially impaired renal function, and be less tolerant of IL-2 during subsequent cycles of treatment (Marroquin, White, Steinberg, Rosenberg, & Schwartzentruber, 2000). This may be the result of cytokine production, including tumor necrosis factor-alpha and administration of nephrotoxic drugs during IL-2 therapy. Low-dose dopamine may improve renal perfusion during IL-2 therapy, and renal function may return to baseline following interruption or completion of therapy (Marroquin et al.; Reiger).

Targeted Therapies in Renal Cancer

Advances over the past 10 years in understanding the molecular biology of renal cell carcinoma have led to the recent approval of three targeted therapies for advanced renal cancer. VEGF, PDGF (see Figure 7-9), and mTOR play a crucial role in tumor angiogenesis, cell growth, and cell survival (see Figure 7-10). An understanding of their role in the pathogenesis of RCC has led to the rational development of recently approved therapeutic strategies (see Figures 7-11 and 7-12), and many additional agents currently are being investigated in various stages of clinical trials in renal cancer. VEGFR-2 is believed to be the major receptor mediating the angiogenic effects of VEGF in RCC (Ferrara, Gerber, & LeCouter, 2003). VEGF expression results from inactivation of the VHL tumor suppressor gene and leads to increased VEGF transcription, overexpression of VEGF protein, and increased angiogenesis (Linehan, Walther, & Zbar, 2003; Rini & Small, 2005). Inactivation of the VHL gene is observed in the majority of clear cell renal tumors and is a critical component of renal cancer tumor angiogenesis (Rini & Small).

Sorafenib

Sorafenib is a small-molecule tyrosine kinase inhibitor of Raf, VEGFR, and platelet-derived growth factor receptor (PDGFR) that was approved as treatment for advanced RCC in December 2005. Approval was based on a phase III, randomized, placebo-controlled trial of 903 patients with clear cell renal cancer who failed initial therapy (Escudier

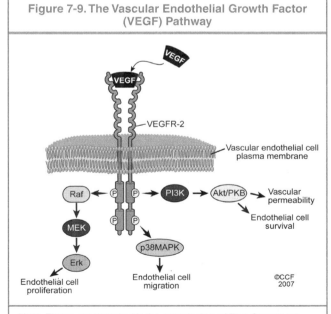

Figure 7-9. The Vascular Endothelial Growth Factor (VEGF) Pathway

Note. Figure reprinted with the permission of The Cleveland Clinic Center for Medical Art and Photography, © 2008. All rights reserved.

Figure 7-10. The Mammalian Target of Rapamycin (mTOR) Pathway

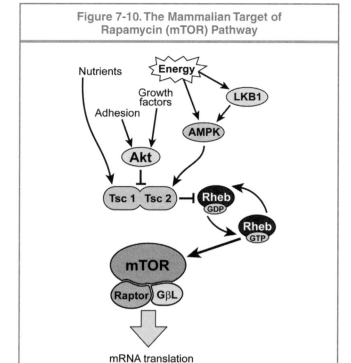

©CCF 2007

dose should be administered one hour before or two hours after meals because food intake affects drug absorption (Onyx Pharmaceuticals, 2007). Dose modification for side effects includes an initial dose reduction to 400 mg once daily with a subsequent dose reduction to 400 mg every other day (Onyx Pharmaceuticals).

The most common side effects (≥ 15% all grades) associated with sorafenib include diarrhea, skin rash and desquamation, fatigue, hand-foot skin reaction, alopecia, nausea, pruritus, hypertension, anorexia, and vomiting (Onyx Pharmaceuticals, 2007). Patient education and nursing care (see Figure 7-13) include timely notification of side effect development to healthcare providers, which allows for early intervention and management, thus maximizing the potential to avoid treatment interruption and dose modification (Wood, 2006). Hypertension can be managed with the initiation or escalation of antihypertensive therapies, with severe or uncontrolled hypertension requiring dose interruption or dose reduction. Diarrhea generally can be managed effectively with standard antidiarrheal agents and dietary modifications (e.g., rice and bananas). The hand-foot skin reaction associated with sorafenib may initially present as paresthesias of fingers, palms, or soles of the feet, and may develop thickened calluses, areas of hyperkeratosis, and acral erythema, which can be painful and lead to disruptions in the patient's ability to tolerate activity (Robert et al., 2005; Wood & Manchen, 2007). Treatment with colloidal oatmeal lotion may be helpful in the treatment of skin toxicities associated with sorafenib (Alexandrescu, Vaillant, & Dasanu, 2006).

et al., 2007). This study demonstrated a median progression-free survival of 5.5 months in the sorafenib group and 2.8 months in the placebo group at the first interim analysis (p < 0.01) (Escudier et al.). Partial responses were observed in 10% of patients randomized to sorafenib and 2% of patients randomized to placebo (Escudier et al.). Based on the statistically significant progression-free survival benefit for patients randomized to sorafenib at the interim analysis, crossover was permitted from placebo to sorafenib with ongoing analysis of all patients. A final analysis of overall survival demonstrated a median survival of 17.8 months for patients receiving sorafenib and 15.9 months for patients in the placebo group who did not cross over (Bukowski et al., 2007; Escudier et al.). Sorafenib was compared to IFN in the frontline setting in a phase II randomized trial of 189 patients with advanced clear cell renal cancer and demonstrated no difference in progression-free survival for sorafenib versus IFN with 5.7 months versus 5.6 months, respectively (Szcylik et al., 2007).

Sorafenib is formulated as a 200 mg tablet administered at a dose of 400 mg twice daily on a continuous basis. Each

Figure 7-11. Vascular Endothelial Growth Factor (VEGF) Agents in Renal Cell Carcinoma

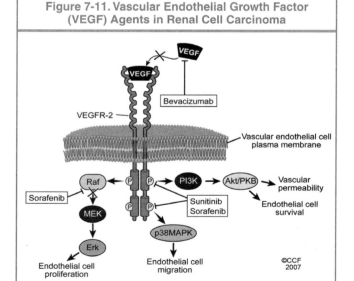

©CCF 2007

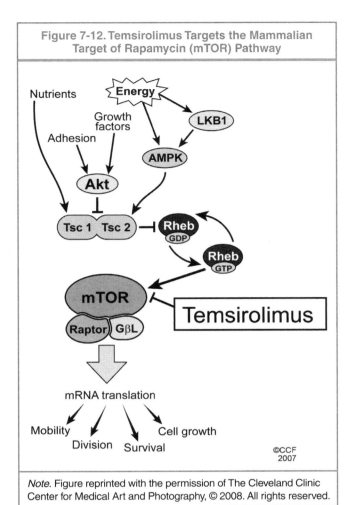

Figure 7-12. Temsirolimus Targets the Mammalian Target of Rapamycin (mTOR) Pathway

©CCF 2007

Sunitinib Malate

Sunitinib malate is a small-molecule tyrosine kinase inhibitor of VEGFR (types 1–3) and PDGFR (alpha and beta) that was approved for advanced RCC in January 2006. Approval initially was based on two multicenter phase II studies of 168 patients with cytokine-refractory renal cancer. The combined median time to progression was 8.4 months, with a median overall survival of 22.3 months (Rosenberg et al., 2007). Sunitinib has been compared to IFN in the front-line setting in a phase III randomized trial of 750 patients with advanced clear cell renal cancer that demonstrated a significant improvement in progression-free survival for sunitinib (11 months) versus IFN (5 months) (p < 0.001) (Motzer et al., 2007).

Sunitinib is formulated in a capsule containing 50 mg, 25 mg, and 12.5 mg strengths. It is administered once daily (irrespective of food intake) for 28 days followed by a 14-day rest (Pfizer Inc., 2007). Dose modification for side effects includes an initial dose reduction to 37.5 mg daily, with a subsequent dose reduction to 25 mg daily, if needed.

Common side effects of sunitinib (≥ 20% all grades) include fatigue, diarrhea, nausea, mucositis/stomatitis, altered taste, anorexia, hypertension, bleeding, vomiting, dyspepsia, rash, abdominal pain, hand-foot syndrome, and asthenia (Pfizer Inc., 2007). Laboratory abnormalities (≥ 50% all grades) include leukopenia, neutropenia, anemia, elevated creatinine, thrombocytopenia, lymphopenia, elevated aspartate aminotransferase, and elevated lipase. Hypothyroidism may occur because of treatment with sunitinib. Patients should have thyroid tests performed at baseline and should be monitored periodically throughout therapy (Rini et al., 2007). Although no specific guidelines have been published recommending the monitoring of thyroid function tests, it is reasonable to check the TSH, T_3, and T4/FTI at baseline and every 12 weeks (Dr. B.I. Rini, personal communication, June 30, 2008). Hypertension may require the initiation of therapy or adjustment of a patient's antihypertensive medication regimen, using caution to monitor for hypotension during the 14-day off-drug period. Mucositis observed with sunitinib is most frequently a *functional mucositis*, which interferes with oral intake. Treatment for functional mucositis may require treatment interruption, IV hydration, and dose modification for severe cases. With functional mucositis, oral inspection reveals no lesion in the mouth but the patient complains of oral discomfort or pain. The use of viscous xylocaine or lidocaine may provide symptomatic relief, with antifungal therapies seldom required (Wood, 2006). Diarrhea can most often be effectively managed with the use of loperamide (Imodium®, McNeil-PPC), diphenoxylate hydrochloride with atropine sulfate (Lomotil®, Pfizer Inc.), or other antidiarrheal agents, in addition to dietary modifications commonly used for the management of diarrhea. The hand-foot syndrome associated with sunitinib may involve both the palms of the hands and soles of the feet, with the potential to become painful and interfere with activities of daily living. Nausea and vomiting can be controlled with standard antinausea medication and supportive care, including IV hydration, if clinically indicated. Nursing care and patient education are critical for patients to receive maximal benefit of therapy with tolerable side effects.

Temsirolimus

The signaling pathway composed of insulin-like growth factor receptor, phosphatidylinositol 3-kinase (also known as PI3K), protein kinase B (also known as Akt/PKB), and mTOR is crucial for cell growth and survival (Dutcher, 2004). Temsirolimus was approved in May 2007 for the treatment of advanced RCC based on a phase III trial of 626 patients with advanced renal cancer with three or more criteria of poor prognosis using the MSKCC poor-prognosis criteria modified to include more than one site of metastatic disease (Hudes et al., 2007). Patients were randomized to receive temsirolimus 25 mg as a weekly IV infusion, IFN alfa 3 MU escalating to 18 MU subcutaneously three times a week, or a combination of temsirolimus 15 mg IV weekly with IFN alfa 6 MU subcutaneously three times a week. The median progression-free survival was better for temsirolimus (5.5 months) compared to IFN alfa (3.1 months) p < 0.001 (Hudes et al.). An increase in median overall survival for temsirolimus (10.9 months) compared to IFN alfa (7.3 months) was statistically significant (p = 0.008) (Hudes et al.).

Temsirolimus is administered as a weekly IV infusion of 25 mg peripherally or via an IV access device for patients with poor venous access. Dose reduction for toxicities should be considered, with an initial dose reduction to 20 mg followed by an additional reduction to 15 mg, if clinically indicated. Temsirolimus is supplied with a diluent, and should be added to 250 ml of 0.9% normal saline. Additional preparation instructions are provided in the package insert (Wyeth Pharmaceuticals, 2007). The solution should be protected from light and infused within six hours of preparation. Patients should receive prophylactic IV diphenhydramine 25 mg or 50 mg (or similar antihistamine) approximately 30 minutes before the start of each dose because of the potential for hypersensitivity reaction (Wyeth Pharmaceuticals). Temsirolimus should be infused over a 30-minute period, with the initial infusion of 60 minutes followed by subsequent infusions of 30 minutes for patients who do not experience hypersensitivity reactions. Treatment should be held for patients with an absolute neutrophil count less than 1,000/mm³, platelet count less than 75,000/mm³, or other severe side effects (Wyeth Pharmaceuticals).

The most common side effects (≥ 25% in all grades) observed with temsirolimus include asthenia, rash, nausea, facial or peripheral edema, mucositis, pain, dyspnea, cough, and diarrhea (Wyeth Pharmaceuticals, 2007). Common laboratory abnormalities (≥ 40% all grades) include anemia, hyperglycemia, elevated cholesterol, elevated triglycerides, elevated alkaline phosphatase, elevated creatinine, lymphopenia, hypophosphatemia, and thrombocytopenia (Wyeth Pharmaceuticals).

Nursing care includes patient education regarding the potential for hypersensitivity reaction during the first or subsequent infusions and emphasizing early notification of a healthcare provider with the patient's onset of dyspnea, cough, rash, or hives. Hypersensitivity reactions can be easily managed using standard institutional guidelines for hypersensitivity reactions. Almost all patients will be able to complete the infusion following interruption of the infusion, administration of steroids or other supportive medications, and a slower infusion rate. Standard management strategies for treatment of rash and associated pruritus should allow patients to continue treatment on schedule. Severe rash with or without pruritus may require short-course steroid therapy, dosing interruption, and consideration of dose modification. Standard management of nausea, mucositis, diarrhea, and other clinical side effects will allow most patients to receive treatment without interruptions or dose reductions. Medications to treat elevated blood sugar, cholesterol, or triglycerides should be considered, and treatment may need to be interrupted for elevations in serum creatinine. Treatment with temsirolimus should continue until disease progression or the onset of an unacceptable toxicity.

Figure 7-13. Nursing Care for Patients Who Are Receiving Targeted Therapies

Patient Education
- Treatment plan and drug administration
  - Route and frequency of drug administration
- Sorafenib
  - Twice a day 1 hour before or 2 hours after meals
  - Continuous dosing
- Sunitinib
  - Once a day, irrespective of meals
  - Daily for 28 days followed by 14-day rest period
- Temsirolimus
  - IV administration
  - Once weekly
- Appointment schedule
- Supportive strategies for management of gastrointestinal side effects
  - Nausea
  - Vomiting
  - Diarrhea
  - Constipation
- Supportive strategies for management of dermatologic side effects
  - Hand-foot skin reaction
  - Callus formation
  - Rash
  - Pain

Nursing Care
- Assess compliance with drug administration for oral therapies.
- Monitor for hypersensitivity reaction during temsirolimus infusions.
- Assess presence and severity of nausea, vomiting, and diarrhea.
- Evaluate effectiveness of antiemetics and antidiarrheal agents.
- Assess hydration and nutritional status.
- Administer IV hydration if appropriate.
- Initiate dietary consult if appropriate.
- Assess for possible dermatologic side effects.
- Evaluate compliance with skincare regimen.
- Evaluate management strategies and modify as needed.
- Assess blood pressure, and review patient blood pressure diary, if appropriate.
- Notify physician if hypertension develops or worsens.
- Monitor laboratory results, and notify physician of abnormalities.

Effective patient education and nursing care will allow patients to receive maximal benefit from therapy (see Figure 7-13).

Everolimus

On March 31, 2009, the FDA approved everolimus, an oral mTOR inhibitor, for the treatment of patients with advanced renal cell carcinoma after failure of treatment with sunitinib or sorafenib. This was based on an international, multicenter, randomized, double-blind trial comparing everolimus and placebo in patients with metastatic renal cell carcinoma whose disease had progressed despite prior treatment with sunitinib (Kay et al., 2009; Novartis Pharmaceuticals, 2009).

Summary

Significant advances have been made in the treatment of advanced RCC. Unanswered questions remain regarding the management of metastatic renal cancer and the benefits of adjuvant therapy for those patients at risk of recurrence. The potential for biomarkers to identify patients who will benefit most from cytokine therapy continues to be investigated. Questions remain regarding the evaluation of response to therapy, the definition of clinical benefit, and the optimal timing of discontinuing targeted therapy in patients with slowly progressive disease (Bukowski & Wood, 2007). Maximizing side effect management and quality of life will continue to guide clinical practice as combination and sequential strategies emerge and new agents are approved for use in the treatment of RCC.

References

Alexandrescu, D.T., Vaillant, J.G., & Dasanu, C.A. (2006). Effect of treatment with a colloidal oatmeal lotion on the acneform eruption induced by epidermal growth factor receptor and multiple tyrosine-kinase inhibitors. *Clinical and Experimental Dermatology, 32*(1), 71–74.

Armstrong, J.A., & McCaffrey, R. (2006). The effects of mucositis on quality of life in patients with head and neck cancer. *Clinical Journal of Oncology Nursing, 10*(1), 53–56.

Atzpodien, J., Kirchner, H., Jonas, U., Bergmann, L., Schott, H., Heynemann, H., et al. (2004). Interleukin-2 and interferon alfa 2-a-based immunochemotherapy in advanced renal cell carcinoma: A prospectively randomized trial of the German cooperative renal carcinoma chemoimmunotherapy group (DGCIN). *Journal of Clinical Oncology, 22*(7), 1188–1194.

Brown, P.D., Brown, D.A., Pollock, B.E., Gorman, D.A., & Foote, R.L. (2002). Stereotactic radiosurgery for patients with "radioresistant" brain metastases. *Neurosurgery, 51*(3), 656–667.

Bukowski, R.M., Eisen, T., Sczylik, C., Stadler, W.M., Simantov, R., Shan, M., et al. (2007). Final results of the randomized phase III trial of sorafenib in advance renal cell carcinoma: Survival and biomarker analysis. *Journal of Clinical Oncology, 25*(18S, Pt. I), Abstract 5023.

Bukowski, R.M., & Wood, L.S. (2007). Renal cell carcinoma: State-of-the-art diagnosis and treatment. *Clinical Oncology News Special Edition, 2*(2), 1–12.

Chin, A.I., Lam, J.S., Figlin, R.A., & Belldegrun, A.S. (2006). Surveillance strategies for renal cell carcinoma patients following nephrectomy. *Reviews in Urology, 8*(1), 1–7.

Chiron Corporation. (2000). Proleukin [Package insert]. Emeryville, CA: Author.

Cohen, H.T., & McGovern, F.J. (2005). Renal-cell carcinoma. *New England Journal of Medicine, 353*(23), 2477–2490.

Dutcher, J.P. (2004). Mammalian target of rapamycin (mTOR) inhibitors. *Current Oncology Reports, 6*(18, Pt. 2), 111–115.

Escudier, B., Eisen, T., Stadler, W.M., Szczylik, C., Oudard, S., Siebels, M., et al. (2007). Sorafenib in advanced clear-cell renal-cell carcinoma. *New England Journal of Medicine, 356*(2), 125–134.

Ferrara, N., Gerber, H.P., & LeCouter, J. (2003). The biology of VEGF and its receptors. *Nature Medicine, 9*(6), 669–676.

Fisher, R.I., Rosenberg, S.A., & Fyfe, G. (2000). Long-term survival update for high-dose recombinant interleukin-2 in patients with renal cell carcinoma. *Cancer Journal From Scientific American, 6*(Suppl. 1), S55–S57.

Flanigan, R.C., Mickisch, G., Sylvester, R., Tangen, C., Van Poppel, H., & Crawford, E.D. (2004). Cytoreductive nephrectomy in patients with metastatic renal cancer: A combined analysis. *Journal of Urology, 171*(18), 1071–1076.

Flanigan, R.C., & Orris, B.G. (2006). Management of metastatic renal cell carcinoma. In N.J. Vogelzang, P.T. Scardino, W.U. Shipley, F.M.J. Debruyne, & W.M. Linehan (Eds.), *Comprehensive textbook of genitourinary oncology* (3rd ed., pp. 767–780). Philadelphia: Lippincott Williams & Wilkins.

Flanigan, R.C., Salmon, S.E., Blumenstein, B.A., Bearman, S.I., Roy, V., McGrath, P.C., et al. (2001). Nephrectomy followed by interferon alfa-2b compared with interferon alfa-2b alone for metastatic renal cell cancer. *New England Journal of Medicine, 345*(23), 1655–1699.

Fyfe, G., Fisher, R.I., Rosenberg, S.A., Sznol, M., Parkinson, D.R., & Louie, A.C. (1995). Results of treatment of 255 patients with metastatic renal cell carcinoma who received high-dose recombinant interleukin-2 therapy. *Journal of Clinical Oncology, 13*(3), 688–696.

Galli, B., Munver, R., Sawczuk, I., & Kochis, E. (2005). Laparoscopic radical nephrectomy in renal cell carcinoma. *Urologic Nursing, 25*(2), 83–86, 133.

Gill, I.S. (2003). Minimally invasive nephron-sparing surgery. *Urologic Clinics of North America, 30*(3), 551–579.

Gill, I.S., Kavoussi, L.R., Lane, B.R., Blute, M.L., Babineau, D., Colombo, J.R., et al. (2007). Comparison of 1,800 laparoscopic and open partial nephrectomies for single renal tumors. *Journal of Urology, 178*(1), 41–46.

Hudes, G., Carducci, M., Tomczak, P., Dutcher, J., Figlin, R., Kapoor, A., et al. (2007). Temsirolimus, interferon alfa, or both for advanced renal-cell carcinoma. *New England Journal of Medicine, 356*(22), 2271–2281.

Kay, A., Motzer, R., Figlin, R., Escudier, B., Oudard, S., Porta, C., et al. (2009). Updated data from a phase III randomized trial of everolimus (RAD001) versus PBO in metastatic renal cell carcinoma (mRCC) [Abstract]. *2009 Genitourinary Cancers Symposium.* Alexandria, VA: American Society of Clinical Oncology.

Kattan, M.W., Reuter, V., Motzer, R.J., Katz, J., & Russo, P. (2001). A post-operative prognostic nomogram for renal cell carcinoma. *Journal of Urology, 166*(1), 63–67.

Kidney Cancer Association. (2007). *We have kidney cancer: A practical guide for patients and families.* Evanston, IL: Author.

Kim, W.Y., & Kaelin, W.G. (2004). The role of VHL gene mutation in human cancer. *Journal of Clinical Oncology, 22*(24), 4991–5004.

Leibovich, B.C., Blute, M.L., Cheville, J.C., Lohse, C.M., Frank, I., Kwon, E.D., et al. (2003). Prediction of progression after radical nephrectomy for patients with clear cell renal cell carcinoma: A stratification tool for prospective clinical trials. *Cancer, 97*(7), 1663–1671.

Linehan, W.M., Walther, M.M., & Zbar, B. (2003). The genetic basis of cancer of the kidney. *Journal of Urology, 170*(6, Pt. 1), 2163–2172.

Maher, K.E. (2005). Radiation therapy: Toxicities and management. In C.H. Yarbro, M.H. Frogge, & M. Goodman (Eds.), *Cancer nursing: Principles and practice* (6th ed., pp. 283–314). Sudbury, MA: Jones and Bartlett.

Marroquin, C.E., White, D.E., Steinberg, S.M., Rosenberg, S.A., & Schwartzentruber, D.J. (2000). Decreased tolerance to interleukin-2 with repeated courses of therapy in patients with metastatic melanoma or renal cell cancer. *Journal of Immunotherapy, 23*(3), 387–392.

Mavroukakis, S.A., Muehlbauer, P.M., White, R.L., Jr., & Schwartzentruber, D.J. (2001). Clinical pathways for managing patients receiving interleukin 2. *Clinical Journal of Oncology Nursing, 5*(5), 207–217.

McDermott, D.F., Regan, M.M., Clark, J.I., Flaherty, L.E., Weiss, G.R., Logan, T.F., et al. (2005). Randomized phase III trial of high-dose interluekin-2 versus subcutaneous interleukin-2 and interferon in patients with metastatic renal cell carcinoma. *Journal of Clinical Oncology, 23*(2), 133–141.

McQuestion, M. (2006). Evidence-based skin care management in radiation therapy. *Seminars in Oncology Nursing, 22*(3), 163–173.

Mekhail, T., Wood, L., & Bukowski, R. (2000). Interleukin-2 in cancer therapy: Uses and optimum management of adverse effects. *BioDrugs, 14*(5), 299–318.

Mekhail, T.M., Abou-Jawde, R.M., Boumerhi, G., Malhi, S., Wood, L., Elson, P., et al. (2005). Validation and extension of the Memorial Sloan-Kettering prognostic factors model for survival in patients with previously untreated metastatic renal cell carcinoma. *Journal of Clinical Oncology, 23*(4), 832–841.

Mickisch, G.H., Garin, A., van Poppel, H., de Prijck, L., Sylvester, R., & European Organisation for Research and Treatment of Cancer Genitourinary Group. (2001). Radical nephrectomy plus interferon-alfa-based immunotherapy compared with interferon alfa alone in metastatic renal-cell carcinoma: A randomized trial. *Lancet, 358*(4286), 966–970.

Motzer, R.J., Bacik, J., Murphy, B.A., Russo, P., & Mazumdar, M. (2002). Interferon-alfa as a comparative treatment for clinical trials of new therapies against advanced renal cell carcinoma. *Journal of Clinical Oncology, 20*(1), 289–296.

Motzer, R.J., Bacik, J., Schwartz, L.H., Reuter, V., Russo, P., Marion, S., et al. (2004). Prognostic factors for survival in previously treated patients with metastatic renal cell carcinoma. *Journal of Clinical Oncology, 22*(3), 454–463.

Motzer, R.J., Hutson, T.E., Tomczak, P., Michaelson, D., Bukowski, R.M., Rixie, O., et al. (2007). Sunitinib versus interferon alfa in metastatic renal-cell carcinoma. *New England Journal of Medicine, 356*(2), 115–124.

National Comprehensive Cancer Network. (2009). *NCCN Clinical Practice Guidelines in Oncology™: Kidney cancer* [v.1.2009]. Retrieved January 9, 2009, from http://www.nccn.org/professionals/physician_gls/PDF/kidney.pdf

Novartis Pharmaceuticals. (2009). Afinitor [Package insert]. East Hanover, NJ: Author

Ogan, K., Cadeddu, J.A., & Stifelman, M.D. (2003). Laparoscopic radical nephrectomy: Oncologic efficacy. *Urologic Clinics of North America, 30*(3), 543–550.

Onyx Pharmaceuticals. (2007). Nexavar [Package insert]. Emeryville, CA: Onyx and Bayer Pharmaceuticals.

Patchell, R.A., Tibbs, P.A., Regine, W.F., Dempsey, R.J., Mohiuddin, M., Kryscio, R.J., et al. (1998). Postoperative radiotherapy in the treatment of single metastases to the brain: A randomized trial. *JAMA, 280*(17), 1485–1489.

Pfizer Inc. (2007). Sunitinib malate (Sutent) [Package insert]. New York: Author.

Reiger, P.T. (2001). Interleukin-2: A paradigm for developing nursing strategies for patient management. *A Continuing Education Program for Nurses by Pro-Ed Communications*, pp. 1–26.

Rini, B.I., & Campbell, S.C. (2007). The evolving role of surgery for advanced renal cell carcinoma in the era of molecular targeted therapy. *Journal of Urology, 177*(6), 1978–1984.

Rini, B.I., & Small, E.J. (2005). Biology and clinical development of vascular endothelial growth factor-targeted therapy in renal cell carcinoma. *Journal of Clinical Oncology, 23*(5), 1028–1043.

Rini, B.I., Tamaskar, I., Shaheen, R., Salas, R., Garcia, J., Wood, L., et al. (2007). Hypothyroidism in patients with metastatic renal cell carcinoma treated with sunitinib. *Journal of the National Cancer Institute, 99*(1), 81–83.

Robert, C., Soria, J.C., Spatz, A., LeCesne, A., Malka, D., Pautier, P., et al. (2005). Cutaneous side-effects of kinase inhibitors and blocking antibodies. *Lancet Oncology, 6*(7), 491–500.

Rosenberg, J.E., Motzer, R.J., Michaelson, M.D., Redman, B.G., Hudes, G.R., Bukowski, R.M., et al. (2007). Sunitinib therapy for patients (pts) with metastatic renal cell carcinoma (mRCC): Updated results of two phase II trials and prognostic factor analysis for survival. *Journal of Clinical Oncology, 25*(18S, Pt. I), Abstract 5095.

Russo, P. (2000). Renal cell carcinoma: Presentation, staging, and surgical treatment. *Seminars in Oncology, 27*(2), 160–176.

Russo, P. (2006). Open radical nephrectomy for localized renal cell carcinoma. In N.J. Vogelzang, P.T. Scardino, W.U. Shipley, F.M.J. Debruyne, & W.M. Linehan (Eds.), *Comprehensive textbook of genitourinary oncology* (3rd ed., pp. 725–730). Philadelphia: Lippincott Williams & Wilkins.

Sadler, G.R., Stoudt, A., Fullerton, J.T., Oberle-Edwards, L.K., Nguyen, Q., & Epstein, J.B. (2003). Managing the oral sequelae of cancer therapy. *Medical-Surgical Nursing, 12*(1), 28–36.

Sheehan, J.P., Sun, M.H., Kondziolka, D., Flickinger, J., & Lunsford, L.D. (2003). Radiosurgery in patients with renal cell carcinoma metastasis to the brain: Long-term outcomes and prognostic factors influencing survival and local tumor control. *Journal of Neurosurgery, 98*(2), 342–349.

Shih, A., Miaskowski, C., Dodd, M.J., Stotts, N.A., & MacPhail, L. (2003). Mechanisms for radiation-induced oral mucositis and the consequences. *Cancer Nursing, 26*(3), 222–229.

Sleifer, D.T., Janssen, R.A.J., Buter, J., deVries, E.G.E., Willemse, P.H.B., & Mulder, N.H. (1992). Phase II study of subcutaneous interleukin-2 in unselected patients with advanced renal cell cancer on an outpatient basis. *Journal of Clinical Oncology, 10*(7), 1119–1123.

Szcylik, C., Demkow, T., Staehler, M., Rolland, F., Negrier, S., Hutson, T.E., et al. (2007). Randomized phase II trial of first-line treatment with sorafenib versus interferon in patients with advanced renal cell carcinoma: Final results. *Journal of Clinical Oncology, 25*(18S, Pt. I), Abstract 5025.

Tyre, C.C., & Quan, W. (2007). Nursing care of patients receiving high-dose, continuous-infusion interleukin-2 with pulse dose and famotidine. *Clinical Journal of Oncology Nursing, 11*(4), 513–519.

Uzzo, R.G., Cairns, P., Al-Saleem, T., Hudes, G., Haas, N., Greenberg, R.E., et al. (2003). The basic biology and immunobiology of renal cell carcinoma: Considerations for the clinician. *Urologic Clinics of North America, 30*(3), 423–436.

Vogelbaum, M.A., & Suh, J.H. (2006). Resectable brain metastases. *Journal of Clinical Oncology, 24*(8), 1289–1294.

Williams, J., Chen, Y., Rubin, P., Finkelstein, J., & Okunieff, P. (2003). The biological basis of a comprehensive grading system for the adverse effects of cancer treatment. *Seminars in Radiation Oncology, 13*(3), 182–188.

Wood, L.S. (2006). Managing the side effects of sorafenib and sunitinib. *Community Oncology, 3*(9), 558–562.

Wood, L.S., & Calabrese, D. (2005). Bladder and renal cancers. In C.H. Yarbro, M.H. Frogge, & M. Goodman (Eds.), *Cancer nursing: Principles and practice* (6th ed., pp. 1005–1021). Sudbury, MA: Jones and Bartlett.

Wood, L.S., & Manchen, B. (2007). Sorafenib: A promising new targeted therapy for renal cell carcinoma. *Clinical Journal of Oncology Nursing, 11*(5), 649–658.

Wyeth Pharmaceuticals. (2007). Temsirolimus [Package insert]. Philadelphia: Author.

Yang, J.C., Sherry, R.M., Steinberg, S.M., Tapalian, S.L., Schwartzentruber, D.J., Hwu, P., et al. (2003). Randomized study of high-dose and low-dose interleukin-2 in patients with metastatic renal cancer. *Journal of Clinical Oncology, 21*(16), 3127–3132.

CHAPTER 8

Treatment of Testicular Cancer

Tara S. Baney, RN, MS, AOCN®, Jennifer Cash, ARNP, MS, OCN®,
and Barbara H. Zoltick, MSN, CRNP, CURN

Introduction

The treatment of testicular cancer is dependent upon the histologic makeup of the tumor, stage, serum tumor marker levels, and sites of metastasis if present. If a testicular mass is noted, most patients will undergo a radical orchiectomy for both diagnosis and treatment. Once the histologic makeup of the tumor is determined this will guide whether further surgery, radiation, or chemotherapy is indicated.

Surgery

Surgery has long been the gold standard for the treatment of testicular cancer. Prior to the advent of cisplatin-based chemotherapy regimens, surgery provided the only chance of cure for this disease. Because of the predictable spread of testicular cancer, surgical removal of metastatic disease either before or after chemotherapy is highly successful. Surgical resection is relevant for nonseminomatous and advanced seminomatous disease and will be addressed separately.

Radical Orchiectomy

Radical inguinal orchiectomy is performed to obtain a tissue diagnosis and as treatment for the primary lesion. The inguinal approach with high ligation of the spermatic cords is the accepted surgical procedure (Bosl, Bajorin, Sheinfeld Motzer, & Chiganti, 2005). During this procedure, the nerve and vascular components are doubly clamped and divided. In order to make the surgical removal of the gonadal vessel easier at the time of retroperitoneal lymph node dissection (RPLND), the stumps left behind after removal of the testicle are placed in the retroperitoneal cavity. Finally, because of the risk of spillage, the affected testis and spermatic cord are removed in one piece (called *en bloc*). Bleeding is controlled prior to wound closure. Fine needle biopsies or orchiectomy via trans-scrotal approach are contraindicated. Violation of

the scrotal sac may result in the "development of alternate lymphatic pathways to the pelvic and inguinal nodal basins" (Bosl et al., 2005, p. 1270).

Organ-Sparing Testicular Surgery

Most testicular tumors are unilateral. Bilateral testis tumors are rare and occur in approximately 2%–3% of all cases. They may develop synchronously or sequentially (Heidenreich, 2004). Bilateral inguinal orchiectomy is the gold-standard surgical procedure for bilateral tumors. However, organ-sparing surgery has been explored to preserve fertility and testosterone production and to address the psychosocial issues related to castration (Heidenreich). The tumor must be smaller than 2 cm in diameter and enough normal testicular tissue must be preserved to allow for the synthesis of testosterone in order to employ an organ-sparing procedure (Heidenreich). Additionally, preoperative levels of luteinizing hormone, testosterone, and semen analysis must be normal to proceed with organ-preservation surgery (Heidenreich).

Most testicular tumors have a pseudocapsule, which walls the tumor off from normal tissue so that the surrounding tissue can be scraped away. First, the tumor is enucleated, and then additional frozen sections are obtained from the surrounding tissue. Tumor bed biopsies are performed prior to wound closure to determine if the entire tumor has been removed. During the procedure the testicle is cooled down to reduce blood flow and metabolic activity to preserve remaining tissues. This process is called *cold ischemia* (Heidenreich, 2004).

Research has demonstrated that 85%–92% of patients who underwent organ-preserving surgery have adequate androgen levels postoperatively (Heidenreich, 2004). After an organ-sparing procedure, radiation therapy (RT) to the affected testicle may be administered. Patients undergoing organ-sparing surgery require close follow-up with serial testicular ultrasounds to monitor for recurrence. The first ultrasound usually occurs four to six weeks postoperatively and then at two-month intervals for the first year (Heidenreich et al., 2001; Yossepowitch & Baniel, 2004). On imaging, developing scar tissue is seen in four to six weeks or at the time of the first trans-scrotal ultrasound. After the first test, ultrasound is performed every two months for one year and then twice a year thereafter to monitor for recurrence. If the patient received radiation, physical examination of the testes is adequate to detect recurrence (Heidenreich).

Nursing Care

A radical inguinal orchiectomy or organ-sparing surgery is generally an outpatient procedure. The nursing care focuses on educating the patient about the procedure and postoperative care. The patient will have an incision in the inguinal area on the side of the tumor. The dressing will need to be changed daily and the wound inspected for signs of infection and bleeding. A small amount of serosanguineous drainage may be present on the first day, but any other drainage should be reported to the physician. Pain is managed with a mild opioid such as oxycodone with acetaminophen and cold compress applications (Gray, 2005). While wearing a scrotal support, the patient should ambulate several times a day to reduce the risk of pneumonia and thromboembolism (Gray).

Alteration in body image caused by the loss of a testicle or testicles is common. The loss of one or both of the testicles may have a negative psychological impact. Because of this alteration in body image, patients should receive information about the risks and benefits of the placement of a testicular prosthesis (Chapple & McPherson, 2004). Patients should have ample time to consider the issues of appearance, self-image, comfort, possible short-term complications, and long-term safety (Chapple & McPherson). Men should be referred for counseling if body image alterations persist. Last, men should understand that the removal of one testicle will not have an effect on fertility or sexual function.

Lymphatic Drainage System

The initial site of metastatic disease is the retroperitoneum. This occurs because of the lymphatic drainage pathway from the testis, along the gonadal vessel, and into the spermatic cord. From the spermatic vessels, some of the lymphatics cross ventrally over the ureter, whereas others follow the spermatic vessels up to the inferior vena cava.

The areas of metastasis in the retroperitoneum are called *landing zones* (Bosl et al., 2005). The primary landing zones for a right-sided tumor are the interaortocaval nodes inferior to the renal vessels, as well as the ipsilateral paracaval, preaortic, and the right common iliac nodes. The primary landing zones for a left-sided tumor are the para-aortic nodes inferior to the left renal vessels, as well as the ipsilateral para-aortic, preaortic, and left common iliac nodes (Donohue, Zachary, & Maynard, 1982; Stephenson & Sheinfeld, 2004). Metastatic disease is not commonly found within the common iliac,

external iliac, or inguinal lymph nodes, and usually is caused by large-volume disease with retrograde spread. Previous surgeries such as herniography or vasectomy can predispose a patient to metastatic disease in the inguinal or pelvic nodes because of the changes in the lymphatic drainage pathways. Contralateral retroperitoneal disease is associated with a right testicular tumor or large-volume tumors on either side (Bosl et al., 2005). In advanced disease, metastasis beyond the retroperitoneum also may be seen. Because of the upward drainage of the lymphatic pathway from the retroperitoneum into the cisterna chyli, metastasis also may be found in the retrocrural nodes. Posterior mediastinal and left supraclavicular metastasis occurs via the thoracic duct.

Retroperitoneal Lymph Node Dissection

Early-stage testicular cancer generally is treated surgically utilizing RPLND. Advanced disease requires the combination of chemotherapy and surgical management, or a postchemotherapy RPLND for cure or control of disease. The first reports of RPLND were between 1904 and 1914 in France, Italy, and England. Half of the patients were survivors of their disease, therefore suggesting a benefit from RPLND (Donohue, 2003).

Primary Retroperitoneal Lymph Node Dissection

In early-stage disease, RPLND is a curative procedure with recurrence in the surgical field occurring less than 1% (de Wit & Fizazi, 2006). Therefore, patients with stage IA and IB generally are recommended to have a primary RPLND. Patients also may be candidates for observation/surveillance if there is no vascular invasion or if an embryonal component is not found on pathologic examination of the primary tumor. Observation/surveillance patients must comply with monthly follow-up (Stephenson & Sheinfeld, 2004). The advantage of observation/surveillance is that patients without metastatic disease will not undergo unnecessary treatment, and those who develop metastatic disease will undergo cisplatin-based chemotherapy (Foster & Bihrle, 2002). The disadvantages of observation/surveillance are the psychological stress of monthly follow-up and the possibility of needing chemotherapy if disease appears.

The rationale for completing RPLND versus observation/surveillance in patients who do not have evidence of disease on radiologic examination is that 15%–40% of patients are reported to be clinically under-staged (Bosl et al., 2005). Of the patients thought to be stage I preoperatively, 30%–50% will have retroperitoneal disease found during surgery (de Wit & Fizazi, 2006). Patients with stage IIA disease are candidates for either a primary retroperitoneal dissection or two cycles of chemotherapy (National Comprehensive Cancer Network [NCCN], 2009). However, if tumor markers alpha-fetoprotein

(AFP) and beta human chorionic gonadotropin (HCG) are normal, usually RPLND is the definitive therapy of choice. The administration of chemotherapy after a primary RPLND for clinical stage IA or IB disease will depend on whether disease is found in the retroperitoneal lymph nodes, along with the size and number of lymph nodes (pathologic stage).

The surgical management of testicular cancer has evolved. Originally, the standard area of dissection or template for RPLND was the bilateral infrahilar dissection through either a thoracoabdominal or transabdominal approach. This included the resection of the precaval, retrocaval, paracaval, interaortocaval, retroaortic, preaortic, para-aortic, and the common iliac lymph nodes bilaterally. The gonadal vessel, gonadal vein, and surrounding fibroadipose tissue near the junction with the inferior vena cava (right-sided tumor) or left renal vein (left-sided tumor) also were excised to decrease risk of recurrence (Bosl et al., 2005). To decrease the frequency of retrograde ejaculation, a nerve-sparing unilateral template may be performed. However, if nodes are involved with cancer (grossly or on frozen section), a bilateral template should be utilized, and complete resection of disease should not be compromised in order to reduce the risk of retrograde ejaculation (Stephenson & Sheinfeld, 2004).

A right-sided testis tumor modified nerve-sparing template includes the removal of the right paracaval, precaval, and interaortocaval areas after the sympathetic nerve fibers, which control emission and ejaculatory function, are identified, dissected, and preserved. All of the lymphatic tissue is removed in an en bloc resection, not in a "plucking" the lymph node manner (Foster & Bihrle, 2002). This is important to ensure the removal of the involved lymph nodes so that intraperitoneal seeding does not occur. For a left-sided tumor, the nerve fibers responsible for emission and ejaculation are identified, dissected, and preserved first, then en bloc resection for the left para-aortic and preaortic nodes is completed (Foster & Bihrle). When nerve-sparing techniques are utilized, preservation of ejaculation occurs in 51%–95% of patients (Stephenson & Sheinfeld, 2004).

Clinical stage II disease involves metastasis to the retroperitoneum. The two methods of treatment for stage II disease are RPLND or cisplatin-based chemotherapy. Both treatment methods have an approximate cure rate of 95%. Both approaches have a 30% chance of requiring the other form of treatment in addition to the primary treatment (i.e., chemotherapy then RPLND or RPLND then chemotherapy) (Bosl et al., 2005). Optimum candidates for a primary RPLND for stage II disease are those who have normal postorchiectomy tumor markers, no tumor-related back pain, unifocal disease that is 3 cm in diameter or less, and disease confined to the region below the renal vessels and above the aortic bifurcation (Bosl & Motzer, 1997). Patients who do not meet these criteria most likely have unresectable disease and should receive primary chemotherapy (Stephenson & Sheinfeld, 2004).

A primary RPLND for stage II disease can be completed if ipsilateral solitary nodes are less than 3 cm, have normal serum tumor markers, and are below the renal hilum and within the landing zones (Bosl et al., 2005; Stephenson & Sheinfeld, 2004). Patients who have stage II disease but have bulky retroperitoneal disease, disease-related back pain, elevated serum tumor markers, or supradiaphragmatic disease will require chemotherapy followed by RPLND (Bosl et al., 2005; Stephenson & Sheinfeld). The primary RPLND has far less morbidity than a postchemotherapy RPLND (PC-RPLND) for stage II disease. Patients who undergo RPLND as primary treatment may have a full bilateral RPLND to ensure complete resection, but a modified nerve-sparing procedure may be completed dependent upon location and size of disease (Bosl et al., 2005). In most clinical stage II patients, a nerve-sparing procedure can be completed, but it should not be at the expense of an incomplete dissection. Patients undergoing chemotherapy for clinical stage II disease and requiring a PC-RPLND for residual tumor will have a higher probability of loss of emission and ejaculatory function (Bosl et al., 2005).

Laparoscopic Retroperitoneal Lymph Node Dissection

Several studies have evaluated the use of laparoscopic RPLND for clinical stage I disease (Abdel-Aziz et al., 2006; Bhayani, Allaf, & Kavoussi, 2004; Correa, Politis, Rodriguez, & Pow-Sang, 2007; Neyer et al., 2007). Laparoscopic RPLNDs have a very steep learning curve, but if performed by an experienced surgeon, the morbidity, surgical blood loss, and length of hospital stay may be shorter than with standard RPLND (Janetschek, Hobisch, Peschel, & Bartsch, 2000). The concerns regarding laparoscopic RPLND are related to the template or standard area of dissection. The retroaortic and retrocaval nodes were not removed in several of the series, nor were the interaortocaval nodes for left-sided tumors and the para-aortic nodes for right-sided tumors (Finelli, 2008). The modification of the templates for laparoscopic RPLND places the patient at great risk for recurrence. This procedure should not be performed routinely and should be considered only in an investigational setting (Bosl et al., 2005; NCCN, 2009).

Post-Chemotherapy Retroperitoneal Lymph Node Dissection

Patients who have large-volume metastatic disease will undergo chemotherapy as primary therapy because the cure rate for surgery alone is lower (less than 50%) (Foster & Bihrle, 2002). Patients who have normalized tumor markers but have persistent radiographic disease will undergo PC-RPLND. This is necessary for three reasons: First, a determination of the histologic makeup of the residual disease is needed to determine if more chemotherapy is required. Second, if the residual disease is teratoma, surgical resection is the only effective treatment. If teratoma is not resected, it will continue to grow because of its resistance to chemotherapy and will invade other organs. Finally, if a small amount of cancer remains, surgical resection may be the only other treatment necessary (Stephenson & Sheinfeld, 2004).

PC-RPLND has a higher morbidity rate than a primary RPLND (8% versus 18%) (Sheinfeld, Bartsch, & Bosl, 2007). The factors that contribute to the technical difficulty include tumor bulk, location relative to the major vessels, and the desmoplastic (pervasive growth of dense fibrous tissue around the tumor) reaction that can occur after a tumor is treated with chemotherapy (Stephenson & Sheinfeld, 2004). Complications may include ileus, bleomycin-related pulmonary issues, high risk of retrograde ejaculation, and inclusion of a nephrectomy caused by injury of renal vessels.

The goal of any RPLND is the complete resection of disease. In some cases, removal of other organs such as the kidney may be necessary to ensure complete resection and long-term control. For instance, if the tumor is encasing the renal vessel, the kidney will need to be removed (Stephenson, Tal, & Sheinfeld, 2006). Other procedures such as liver resection, bowel resection, or thoracotomy with resection may be necessary for a complete resection of residual disease.

Salvage or Desperation Retroperitoneal Lymph Node Dissection

Although germ cell tumors (GCTs) have a 70%–80% overall survival rate even with advanced disease upon presentation, a small subset of patients do not do well despite standard therapy. This subset can be categorized into four groups. The first group is those who have received second-line or salvage/high-dose chemotherapy. Often surgery is performed because of an incomplete response to chemotherapy. These patients have a lower rate of complete resection and higher rate (50%) of viable cancer remaining in the residual tumor (Stephenson & Sheinfeld, 2004), but because of the lack of benefit of additional chemotherapy, surgical resection may be the only treatment of benefit. Secondly, there are patients who have undergone chemotherapy and continue to have persistently elevated tumor markers, which indicate disease that is refractory to chemotherapy. Previously, these patients were thought to be unresectable. In a select group of patients undergoing RPLND because of elevated markers, the "desperation RPLND," approximately 20%–47% were reported to not have progression of disease (Eastham, Wilson, Russell, Ahlering, & Skinner, 1994; Murphy et al., 1993; Stephenson & Sheinfeld; Wood et al., 1992). In one study evaluating patients who underwent salvage RPLND for disseminated disease from relapse after salvage chemotherapy, 21% remained disease-free with no other treatment at 46-month follow-up (Murphy et al.).

Another study showed that 37% patients with platinum-resistant disease and with persistent radiographic and serologic disease were alive and disease-free at 74 months after salvage surgery (Eastham et al.). Patients in this group who have elevated AFP versus HCG and retroperitoneal disease instead of visceral metastasis have a more favorable prognosis (Wood et al.). The third group includes those patients with unresectable tumors because of a high relapse rate and poor overall survival rate of 21% (Donohue, Leviovitch, Foster, Baniel, & Tognoni, 1998). The final patient group includes those who have already had an RPLND and chemotherapy. These are classified as redo PC-RPLNDs. This subset emphasizes the importance of a complete resection. The overall survival for this group is 55% versus 84% at five years with a primary PC-RPLND (McKiernan et al., 2003).

Surgical Findings

The histologic findings of a resected mass after PC-RPLND reveal that 59% are fibrosis, 31% show teratoma, and 10% are a persistent germ cell cancer. After salvage chemotherapy, the histologic findings are notably different: 50% are persistent GTCs, 40% are teratomas, and only 10% are fibrosis (Stephenson & Sheinfeld, 2004). Based on these data, PC-RPLND is warranted in patients with normalized markers but persistent disease on radiographic studies, as 90% of the residual tissue will be either persistent disease or teratoma. Patients found to have viable GCT upon PC-RPLND most likely will have partially drug-resistant disease that will progress if not resected. Teratoma is not chemosensitive, and if not resected, it may grow, obstruct, and invade vital organs, or may undergo malignant transformation into a sarcoma or carcinoma (Sheinfeld et al., 2007). Despite the higher morbidity associated with PC-RPLND, the chance of finding tissue other than fibrosis supports its necessity.

Although development of models to predict the patients who have necrosis or fibrosis and who would not need to undergo PC-RPLND has been attempted, to date, these models have not had enough reliability to exclude patients from postchemotherapy surgery (Bosl et al., 2005). Patients who are found to have necrosis or teratoma have a good long-term prognosis, whereas those with residual disease will need to undergo more chemotherapy and have a 66% long-term disease-free prognosis (Foster & Bihrle, 2002).

Post-Chemotherapy Retroperitoneal Lymph Node Dissection for Seminoma

Although seminomas are a type of GCT, they behave differently and require a different treatment strategy then nonseminomatous tumors. Most seminomas (80%) present as clinical stage I disease (Zack, 2005). Patients with stage I, IIA, and IIB disease are treated with RT to the retroperitoneum. For stage IIC, III, and IV disease, chemotherapy is warranted. The management following chemotherapy is controversial. Seminomas rarely have teratomatous components, and often the residual mass is found to be fibrosis (Stephenson & Sheinfeld, 2004). Surgery can be very complicated because of the desmoplastic reaction that occurs when seminomas are exposed to chemotherapeutic agents, thereby increasing the morbidity associated with PC-RPLND for a seminomatous tumor (Stephenson & Sheinfeld). In the past, research was unable to identify factors that could possibly predict the presence of viable seminoma after chemotherapy (Herr et al., 1997). Recent research has concluded that fluorodeoxyglucose positron-emission tomography (FDG-PET) is an accurate tool to assess patients with residual masses for viable disease (Becherer et al., 2005; De Santis et al., 2004). In patients with negative FDG-PET scans, observation is a justifiable course for patients with postchemotherapy seminoma (De Santis et al.).

Nursing Care

Preoperative Workup

A thorough assessment of each patient should include a medical and surgical history, psychosocial history, and medications (including chemotherapy). Preoperative testing, including laboratory blood work, x-rays, and pulmonary function tests (PFTs), may be indicated. Routine laboratory studies include complete blood count (CBC) with differential, liver function test, comprehensive metabolic profile, prothrombin time, partial thromboplastin time and international normalized ratio, tumor markers, and urinalysis. If patients have received chemotherapy recently, their white blood cell count should be more than 3,500 k/mm^3 and the platelet count must be more than 100,000 k/mm^3 in order to proceed with surgery. An abdomen and pelvis CT scan should be completed within the month prior to surgery to provide an updated assessment of the retroperitoneum. A chest x-ray should be performed to rule out metastatic disease (Bosl et al., 2005). If new abnormalities are seen, a chest CT should be completed. If PC-RPLND is being considered, a magnetic resonance imaging (MRI) angiogram may be warranted to evaluate disease related to the major vessels. Patients who received bleomycin as part of their chemotherapy regimen also should undergo a preoperative PFT. An electrocardiogram is warranted to assess cardiac function prior to surgery. A complete and thorough preoperative workup will help to determine potential postoperative complications. Interventions then can be instituted to reduce the risk of complications postoperatively (Donat, 1999).

Although the majority of GCTs occur in younger males, patients must be screened for medical problems that could complicate surgery or the postoperative period (Donat, 1999). These include medical problems such as asthma, diabetes, hypertension, and heart disease. Assessing patients' coping skills is important because testicular cancer can have a profound effect on fertility, and men may feel their disease is a threat to their manhood. Patient education must include information on the incidence of retrograde ejaculation associated with

RPLND. Sperm banking options should be discussed with all patients prior to chemotherapy or surgery. Patients should be referred to social services and psychiatry if they are having difficulty coping with their diagnosis.

Preoperative Education

Because the age of patients with testicular cancer can range from adolescence to adulthood, patient education must be tailored to the appropriate age group (Stevenson & McNeill, 2004). Information regarding preoperative preparations is imperative. With most extensive abdominal surgeries, bowel preparation is necessary. Depending on the complexity of the surgical procedure, bowel preparation may include a clear liquid diet, laxatives, and enemas. Prior to surgery, patients need to hydrate with at least two to three quarts of fluid per day. Avoidance of nonsteroidal anti-inflammatory drugs such as aspirin, ibuprofen, or naproxen for 10 days prior to surgery is important to reduce the risk of intraoperative and postoperative bleeding (Stevenson & McNeill). Anticoagulation therapies such as warfarin, clopidogrel, ticlopidine, heparin, and low-molecular-weight heparin also must be stopped prior to surgery. With the increasing use of herbal remedies, patients should know to stop all herbal remedies and high doses of vitamins (other than a multivitamin) at least 10 days prior to surgery. Many herbal remedies and high doses of vitamins have anticoagulation properties. Smoking cessation assistance should be offered to patients who smoke, as smoking can increase the risk of postoperative complications such as pneumonia and impaired wound healing.

Postoperative Care

The length of stay will depend on the surgical procedure completed (primary RPLND versus PC-RPLND) and is generally four to seven days (Chang et al., 2002). The surgical procedure may require 3 hours for a primary RPLND to more than 10 hours for PC-RPLND. Monitoring of respiratory, cardiovascular, gastrointestinal (GI), bleeding, infection, and pain status are all crucial postoperatively. Knowledge regarding patients' preoperative chemotherapy regimens is critical in the planning of postoperative nursing care and patient education.

Respiratory

Pulmonary hygiene has a direct effect on patients' postoperative recovery. Because of the large abdominal incision, pain can impede respiratory function. The use of incentive spirometry and coughing and deep breathing exercises must be taught preoperatively and initiated immediately postoperatively (Stevenson & McNeill, 2004). Ambulation is valuable in the prevention of pulmonary complications. If breathing exercises and use of the incentive spirometry are difficult, a consultation for chest physiotherapy may be helpful (Stevenson & McNeill). Good pain management will enhance pulmonary hygiene and ambulation (Gray, 2005).

Patients who had bleomycin as part of their chemotherapy regimen are at greater risk for pulmonary complications. Because of the exposure to bleomycin, these patients may have pulmonary fibrosis secondary to collagen deposits within their lungs (Grande, Peao, de Sa, & Aguas, 1998). Pulmonary fibrosis may increase the risk of developing pulmonary edema (Sheinfeld et al., 2007). Because of the decreased lung interstitium caused by fibrosis, there is a reduction in interstitial edema and therefore an increase in alveolar edema (Grande et al.). Surgery and anesthesia time, amount of blood transfused, blood loss, fluid status, type of fluid given, and preoperative forced vital capacity (FVC) are all predictors of the development of postoperative pulmonary complications (Donat & Levy, 1998). Supplemental oxygen therapy must be used with caution in patients who previously have been treated with bleomycin because of the susceptibility of the alveoli to damage (Malhotra, Schwartz, & Schwartzstein, 2007). The amount of time that a patient is on oxygen and the flow rate should be limited as much as possible. Patients may even be maintained at lower oxygen saturation levels as monitored by pulse oximetry to diminish the amount of supplemental oxygen therapy administered and thus reduce the risk of pulmonary toxicity (Lasky & Ortiz, 2007; Malhotra et al.).

Fluid Volume

Patients require meticulous fluid management perioperatively and postoperatively. Often, colloids rather than crystalloids provide better fluid resuscitation in patients who have received bleomycin. Daily weights, daily comprehensive metabolic profile, and monitoring of urine output and accurate fluid intake should be continually assessed postoperatively. Patients may be at risk for fluid volume overload if they received cisplatin or ifosfamide therapy, as these agents are nephrotoxic. The patient will have an indwelling urinary bladder catheter in place for the first few postoperative days to ensure accurate urinary output calculations. Renal function is monitored with daily laboratory studies including blood urea nitrogen (BUN), creatinine, and an electrolyte panel (Fischbach & Dunning, 2006).

Cardiovascular

All patients undergoing surgery are at risk for venous thromboembolism. The use of sequential compression boots for the first two to three days will assist in circulation of the lower extremities. Ambulation beginning postoperative day one and performed three to four times a day also will help to restore circulation. The large abdominal incision requires that good pain control occur to facilitate ambulation. The use of low-molecular-weight heparin in the postoperative course is controversial because of the risk of bleeding (Stevenson & McNeill, 2004). Patients often will be tachycardic but normotensive for the first few days postoperatively because of the manipulation of the sympathetic nerve bundles during the resection (Hickey, 2003; Steele & Richie, 2007). Tachycardia will resolve with time and rarely needs medical or pharmacologic intervention.

Gastrointestinal

Surgical complexity and length of procedure has an impact on the return of bowel function (Stevenson & McNeill, 2004). A nasogastric (NG) tube may be placed in the operating room and remain in place for 24–48 hours after surgery. During the time the NG tube is in place, the patient will receive nothing by mouth (NPO) and usually for 24 hours after its removal. Ongoing GI assessments are needed to evaluate the patient for signs and symptoms of an ileus, which include nausea, vomiting, decreased bowel sounds, abdominal distention, and absence of flatus. The patient will begin with a clear liquid diet upon bowel function return and progress to a regular diet as tolerated. Ambulation assists in the return of intestinal motility. Once patients are tolerating a regular diet, taking a stool softener and drinking at least two quarts of fluid per day will decrease the risk of constipation (Stevenson & McNeill).

The disruption of the lymphatics during the surgery places patients at risk for developing chylous ascites (2%–3%) (Sheinfeld et al., 2007). Chyle is a milky white fluid with a fat content of 4–40 g/dl and protein greater than 30 g/dl (Sheinfeld et al.). Patients who undergo vena caval, suprahilar, or hepatic resection are at greater risk for developing this complication (Baniel, Foster, Rowland, Bihrle, & Donohue, 1995; Link, Amin, & Kavoussi, 2006). Signs and symptoms of a chylous leak include ileus, an abdomen fluid wave, pleural effusions, and milky white fluid leaking from the incision. A paracentesis should be performed to obtain fluid for evaluation. Decompressing the abdomen will enhance the patient's comfort. Dietary management including medium-chain triglycerides (MCTs), and a diet with 5 g/day fat for approximately three months will resolve the leak in 50% of the cases (Leibovitch, Mor, Golomb, & Ramon, 2002; Link et al.). MCTs are shorter than long-chain fatty acids and are absorbed directly into the portal venous circulation, bypassing the bowel and retroperitoneal lymphatics and decreasing chyle flow (Ablan, Littooy, & Freeark, 1990). If the leak does not respond to conservative dietary measures, total parenteral nutrition and possibly the use of octreotide may be implemented. Patients who do not respond to these medical interventions may require surgical repair or peritoneovenous shunting (Leibovitch et al.; Link et al.).

Infection and Bleeding

Vital signs should be assessed every 4 hours for the first 48 hours postoperatively. Atelectasis is usually the cause of a fever in the immediate postoperative period, and aggressive pulmonary hygiene should be instituted. Other sources such as wound infection or urinary tract infection also should be considered for fever etiology. A CBC with differential should be performed each day to monitor white blood cell count for infection and platelet count for bleeding. Patients who have undergone chemotherapy prior to surgery may require granulocyte–colony-stimulating factors (G-CSFs) if their neutrophil count is low. G-CSF increases the number of circulating neutrophils and decreases the risk of infection postoperatively (Polovich, White, & Kelleher, 2005). Hemoglobin and hematocrit results also are useful in monitoring for bleeding postoperatively.

Pain Management

Recovery from an RPLND depends on good pain control for the large abdominal incision that extends from the xyphoid process to the pubic symphysis. If a laparoscopic RPLND is performed, the pain will be caused by the carbon dioxide insufflation during the procedure and will be a referred pain into the shoulder. Patient-controlled analgesia (PCA) is the best method of pain control for the majority of patients while NPO. Oral pain medications should be implemented once the patient is no longer NPO. PCA allows the patient to administer the medication prior to activities that cause pain such as ambulating and pulmonary hygiene exercises. Other nonopioid medications such as ketorolac may be utilized to decrease the use of opioids, which slow the return of bowel function (Cepeda et al., 2005; Ferraz et al., 1995). Contraindications for use of ketorolac are renal insufficiency as evidenced by an elevated creatinine level (normal varies from institution to institution) and risk of GI bleeding (Turkoski, Lance, & Bonfiglio, 2007).

Discharge and Follow-Up

Discharge instructions are essential. They need to include self-care measures, follow-up appointment schedule, and when to call the surgeon and other healthcare providers. Symptoms such as fever greater than 38.3°C (101°F), shortness of breath, calf pain, abdominal pain, nausea, vomiting, bleeding, wound dehiscence, lack of bowel movement in three days, or signs of infection should be reported to the surgeon immediately. Patients should continue to ambulate at home to decrease the risk of pneumonia and thromboembolic events and to stimulate bowel function. Patients will still require a mild analgesic such as oxycodone with acetaminophen so that activity is possible. They also should be taking a stool softener and drinking additional fluids, if opioids are being used, to counteract the side effect of constipation.

The first scheduled follow-up with the surgeon will occur a month after surgery to assess the surgical site and tumor markers and to discuss a follow-up plan. At each follow-up visit, psychosocial assessments should occur to ensure that the patient and partner are coping with treatment-related side effects such as retrograde ejaculation and infertility (Gray, 2005). Referrals to counselors, a fertility specialist, and support groups should be offered as necessary.

Summary of Surgery

Over the past several decades, the survival rates for testicular cancer have increased because of the advent of cisplatin-based chemotherapy and perfection of the technique for RPLND both before and after chemotherapy. Previously, many of these patients would not have undergone these complicated procedures because of the high morbidity. However, with new techniques and the modification of the standard surgical template, the risk of complications has been reduced, thus allowing more patients a chance for increased survival.

Radiation Therapy

Treatment of testicular cancer with RT is guided by a number of factors, including the pathology of seminoma versus nonseminoma, stage after orchiectomy, serum tumor markers, involvement of infradiaphragmatic and subdiaphragmatic lymph node regions, and the extent of metastatic spread (Morton & Thomas, 2004; NCCN, 2009). The two most common staging systems for testicular cancer used today are the Union Internationale Contre le Cancer (Sobin & Whittekind, 1997) and the American Joint Committee on Cancer (2002) Staging and End-Results Reporting. These provide a classification system that incorporates metastatic germ cell malignancies into the tumor, node, metastasis (TNM) system outlined by the International Germ Cell Cancer Collaborative Group (IGCCCG, 1997). The role of RT in the management of nonseminomatous testicular cancer is limited to palliation for brain metastasis. Therefore, this discussion of the use of RT in the treatment of testicular cancer will be confined to the treatment of seminomas (NCCN).

Testicular Intraepithelial Neoplasia

Testicular intraepithelial neoplasm (TIN) is considered the equivalent of carcinoma in situ of the testis and is recognized as a common precursor of testicular germ cell neoplasms (Classen, Dieckmann, Loy, & Bamberg, 1998; Dieckmann, Classen, & Loy, 2003). When cancer is identified in a single testis or bilateral TIN, local RT is the treatment of choice. Delivery of low-dose RT at 18–20 gray (Gy) has been the standard dosing regimen in Germany (Classen et al., 1998; Classen, Souchon, Hehr, & Bamberg, 2001). However, because of reported androgen deficiency requiring testosterone supplementation in nearly one-quarter of patients, dosing regimens of 16 Gy and 18 Gy also have been utilized with sporadic failures noted (Classen et al., 2003; Dieckmann et al.).

Treatment of Local Disease (Stage I)

Stage I testicular seminoma is a highly radiosensitive GCT with cure rates in excess of 95% (Morton & Thomas, 2004;

Neill, Warde, & Fleshner, 2007; Stein et al., 1998; Willan & McGowan, 1985; Zagars, Ballo, Lee, & Strom, 2004). The standard of care for patients with newly diagnosed stage I seminoma is radical inguinal orchiectomy with high ligation of the spermatic cord, followed by optional surveillance versus single-dose carboplatin adjuvant therapy or postoperative megavoltage irradiation of the para-aortic/paracaval lymph nodes, with consideration given to also irradiating the ipsilateral pelvic nodes (i.e., dog-leg treatment field) or mediastinum (rare), dependent upon staging outcomes and risk of microscopic retroperitoneal disease (Morton & Thomas; NCCN, 2009; Raghavan, 2006).

Patients who do not receive adjuvant RT after orchiectomy have a 15%–20% relapse rate associated with surveillance alone, with a median time to relapse of 12 months but upwards of 5 years (Morton & Thomas, 2004; NCCN, 2009). However, 2009 NCCN guidelines now recommend single-dose carboplatin as an alternative treatment to radiation therapy for stages IA and IB disease because of less toxicity and equal outcomes of prevention of disease recurrence. Radiotherapy utilizing 20–40 Gy (10–20 fractions over 2–4 weeks) is directed to para-aortic lymph nodes or dog-leg fields approximately 3–4 weeks after orchiectomy, with similar relapse rates as surveillance 12–18 months following orchiectomy. The European Organisation for the Research and Treatment of Cancer Trial 30942, a randomized trial of 625 patients using 30 Gy versus 20 Gy in the adjuvant treatment of stage I seminoma, reported that lower treatment doses of 20 Gy (versus standard 30 Gy) had less than a 3% difference in mortality. However, a reduction in moderate to severe lethargy (5% versus 20%) and inability to carry out normal work activities (28% versus 46%) four weeks after starting therapy was reported (Jones et al., 2005). Additionally, the omission of pelvic fields in post-orchiectomy patients reduces acute treatment-related hematologic and GI side effects, fatigue, and gonadal toxicity with an average of a 2% difference in pelvic relapse rates (Fossa et al., 1999; Morton & Thomas). Patients with stage IS are treated to a dose of 25–30 Gy to infradiaphragmatic area, including para-aortic lymph nodes with or without ipsilateral ileo inguinal nodes (NCCN). Patients considered not to be good candidates for RT would include those with stage IA or IB disease with a horseshoe or pelvic kidney, those who have inflammatory bowel disease, or those who have undergone prior RT (NCCN).

Treatment of Regional Disease (Stage II/III)

Considerations in treating stage IIA (tumors measuring less than 2 cm) or IIB (tumors measuring 2–5 cm) seminoma are based on bulk of retroperitoneal disease, with irradiation volume and dose modified accordingly (Morton & Thomas, 2004; NCCN, 2009). Recommended dosing regimens for IIA disease are standard infradiaphragmatic radiation fields to include para-aortic and ipsilateral lymph nodes to 35–40 Gy, and

treatment field widths appropriately widened to encompass IIB disease as demonstrated on CT scan or lymphography, with a margin of 2 cm (Morton & Thomas; NCCN). Currently, neither the NCCN guidelines nor Morton and Thomas recommend prophylactic mediastinal lymph node irradiation, as this does not significantly improve outcome by preventing relapse, which is already rare. Smalley, Earle, Evans, and Richardson (1990) reported possible poor tolerance to salvage chemotherapy and subsequent increased cardiopulmonary toxicity associated with prophylactic mediastinal radiotherapy. In the rare circumstances where mediastinal and supraclavicular irradiation are warranted for progression of disease after chemotherapy, 25 Gy is delivered to those sites with margins of 1–1.5 cm (Morton & Thomas). Relapse rates remain low (approximately 8%–10% for IIA and 15%–20% for IIB) in patients receiving appropriate adjuvant RT, according to Morton and Thomas and the European Germ Cell Cancer Consensus Group (Schmoll et al., 2004). According to the National Cancer Institute (NCI, 2009) and NCCN (2009), stage IIC or III seminoma is potentially curable, despite the persistence of residual disease at the completion of primary cisplatin-based chemotherapy. Patients with bulky stage IIC/III disease (tumors larger than 5 cm) typically undergo primary chemotherapy. Upon completion of initial chemotherapy, patients identified with residual/recurrent disease of 3–5 cm or greater (as evidenced by PET scan no less than six weeks after completion of chemotherapy or CT scans if indicated), with or without supradiaphragmatic disease, may warrant RT and surgical excision. If RT is indicated for residual disease, the same treatment fields are utilized as with stage IIB patients, with abdominal fields made larger to encompass known volume of disease, and doses are administered at 36 Gy or greater (Morton & Thomas; NCCN; Schmoll et al.; Smalley et al.). Treatment-related concerns for these patients are potential nephrotoxicity if a large mass overlies one or more kidneys, and cardiopulmonary sequelae secondary to mediastinal irradiation for an enlarging mass (Morton & Thomas; Raghavan, 2006; Smalley et al.). Cure rates for patients with combination therapy of infradiaphragmatic and mediastinal irradiation range from 70%–80% or greater and are slightly lower for those patients receiving infradiaphragmatic irradiation only (Morton & Thomas; Raghavan; Smalley et al.).

Treatment of Metastatic and Relapsed Disease

RT is considered for patients with metastasis or relapse to the whole brain (or single lesions), lungs, liver, and bone, as well as for epidural spinal cord compression, supraclavicular neck masses, and inguinal disease with or without spermatic cord involvement and direct invasion into the surrounding tissue (Bokemeyer et al., 1997; Daugaard, Karas, & Sommer, 2006; Friedman, Sheetz, Levine, Everett, & Hong, 1986; Lee & Calcaterra, 1998; Raghavan, 2006). Aggressive multimodal therapy of surgery, cisplatin-based chemotherapy, and RT may all be utilized with survival rates of 25%–50% and greater. According to NCI (2009), development of a metastasis in a contralateral testicle after undergoing curative therapy ranges from 2%–5% over a 25-year period.

Side Effects and Complications

For patients receiving definitive radiotherapy to lymph node chains in para-aortic and ipsilateral inguinal lymph nodes, expected side effects include fatigue, bone marrow suppression (in larger treatment fields), and GI symptoms of dyspepsia and diarrhea (Hawkins & Miaskowski, 1996; McCullagh & Lewis, 2005; NCI, 2009). Severity of side effects is directly related to the size of treatment fields and total dose delivered (Morton & Thomas, 2004). No major complications were seen when total doses were less than 25 Gy; however, radiation doses greater than 25 Gy demonstrated a 2% chance of major GI complication (e.g., intestinal obstruction, peptic ulcer, hemorrhagic gastritis), and with doses at 40 Gy or greater, a 6% incidence of complications was noted (Morton & Thomas). Radiation scatter to the contralateral testicle during treatment may contribute to temporary or permanent oligospermia (reduced sperm) or azoospermia (no sperm production). However, at least 50% of men have some degree of impairment in spermatogenesis after surgery and prior to radiotherapy (Hawkins & Miaskowski; Morton & Thomas). Testicular retraction and shielding is commonly utilized to decrease the effects of radiation scatter. Cardiopulmonary toxicity is associated with mediastinal irradiation and may be increased further when combined with chemotherapies (Morton & Thomas; NCI).

Patients treated with RT are at an increased risk for development of a second primary malignancy, especially solid tumors within high-dose treatment fields with a latency period of a decade or more (Efstathiou & Logothetis, 2006; Morton & Thomas, 2004; NCI, 2009; van Leeuwen et al., 1993). van Leeuwen et al. reported the first large follow-up patient series of second cancer risk after testicular cancer treatment, with the mean 15-year actuarial risk of all types of second malignancies at 9.8%, more specifically, GI (relative risk 2.6–3.7-fold), contralateral testicular cancer (relative risk 35.7-fold), and leukemia (relative risk 5.1-fold) among 1,909 patients treated in the Netherlands from 1971 to 1985. Other studies have reported similar findings of second malignancies elsewhere including pancreas, stomach, colorectal, prostate, bladder, kidney, lung, pleura, and sarcomas with an incidence of 16%–22.6% at 25 and 30 years after treatment (Efstathiou & Logothetis; McCullagh & Lewis, 2005; Morton & Thomas; NCI).

Patient Education

Patient education for patients with testicular cancer who are undergoing radiotherapy should include
- Education of the disease process
- Management of acute symptoms throughout the treatment course
- Long-term effects after therapy
- Follow-up guidelines.

Men diagnosed with testicular cancer typically are treated rapidly to prevent further complications, and adequate education of sequelae may be missed. Concerns and anxieties related to possible alterations in relationships, sexual performance, and fertility are paramount and need to be addressed appropriately (Hawkins & Miaskowski, 1996; McCullagh & Lewis, 2005).

Because supportive care needs are multifactorial, the initial identification and assessment of knowledge of fertility issues needs to be addressed prior to initiation of RT. Fear of impotency, sterility, and permanent sexual dysfunction are very real concerns related to sexuality and body image (Hawkins & Miaskowski, 1996). Discussion of coping with subsequent appearance-altering treatment (e.g., orchiectomy), loss of libido, and the possible need for erectile dysfunction aids are critical components of education not only for patients but also their significant others. Information regarding fertility preservation measures such as sperm banking or cryopreservation of sperm are options for men desiring to father children, although spontaneous baseline semen quality commonly returns within two years after treatment (Brown, 2004; Morton & Thomas, 2004; Ohl & Sonksen, 1996). Referrals to appropriate clinicians may be warranted, including a sexual counselor, assistive reproductive technology specialist, psychologist, and psychiatrist. The additional cost of sperm banking and erectile dysfunction aids may have a financial impact on the patient, and referral to a social worker for obtaining appropriate resources may be indicated.

The most common acute RT-related symptoms that require management are GI in nature and include nausea, dyspepsia, and diarrhea. Patient education focuses on dietary and prescriptive interventions to decrease the severity, with symptoms well managed with oral antiemetics, antidiarrheals, and histamine-2 blockers, or a proton pump inhibitor (Brown, 2004; Hawkins & Miaskowski, 1996). Potential bone marrow suppression for patients with larger treatment fields for more advanced cancers will need routine blood work to assess level of dysfunction, with referral for intervention as indicated. Because most patients have undergone multiple treatment therapies of radiation, surgery, and chemotherapy, education should focus on fatigue management, signs and symptoms of infection and bleeding (which is rare), and the importance of prompt healthcare provider notification.

Post-treatment follow-up guidelines developed by NCCN (2009) include history and physical, chest x-ray, and serum tumor markers of AFP, beta-HCG, and lactate dehydrogenase (LDH) every three to four months for at least the first year following treatment, with abdominal and pelvic CTs annually or at alternative visits dependent upon stage. PET scans also may be performed as indicated.

Nursing Implications

Providing appropriate information in a timely fashion to patients undergoing continued therapy for a newly diagnosed testicular cancer is critical. Testicular cancer, for the most part, is a disease of younger men. Development of education strategies that focus on relationships, desire to father children, sexuality, and body image should be incorporated into management of acute treatment-related symptoms throughout the course of therapy. Patient fears, concerns, and misconceptions of cancer physically affecting their sexual partner and children must be discussed thoroughly. Nurses are in a unique position to help patients and their families with not only the physiologic aspects of their disease and treatment but the psychological and emotional sequelae with appropriate referrals to community resources.

Chemotherapy

Since the development of cisplatin-based combination chemotherapy, testicular cancer has been considered a "model for a curable neoplasm" (Einhorn, 1990, p. 1777). Most metastatic cancers eventually result in fatality, but the majority of patients treated for testicular cancer, including more than 80% of those with metastatic disease, can be rendered disease-free with appropriate therapy. The goal for these patients is never just palliation, but cure (Einhorn, 1990; Masters & Koberle, 2003). Sensitive tumor markers, a logical series of management trials, and a sophisticated system for prognostic evaluation of gonadal and extragonadal testicular cancer makes possible the selection of treatments most appropriate for achieving cure while avoiding overtreatment and unnecessary toxicity (Horwich, Shipley, & Huddart, 2006; Kopp et al., 2006). These factors, coupled with an improved understanding of the biology of testicular cancer and the continued understanding and development of chemotherapeutic agents, have resulted in cure rates that have not been achieved in other cancers (Kopp et al.). Most patients with testicular cancer are young at diagnosis and will likely live many years as cancer survivors. As more is known about the potential short- and long-term effects of treatment, it is vital to minimize exposure to potential long-term toxic effects of chemotherapy without jeopardizing effectiveness (Jones & Vasey, 2003).

Background

Cisplatin is the foundation of testicular cancer chemotherapeutic treatment. Cisplatin kills cancer cells by binding to and damaging the cells' DNA. Studies indicate that testicular cancer cells are two to four times more sensitive to cisplatin than most other cancer cell types because they lack a particular type of DNA repair mechanism, and thus have a reduced capacity to undo genetic damage caused by cisplatin (Masters & Koberle, 2003). Testicular tumors also are deficient in other aspects of DNA repair, thereby increasing the predisposition for apoptosis (Masters & Koberle).

The identification of cisplatin as an effective agent in the treatment of testicular cancer began in the 1970s. Prior to cisplatin, dactinomycin, as a single agent or combined with methotrexate and chlorambucil, was the standard. Less than 15% of patients with metastatic disease had a durable complete response (Einhorn, 1990). In the 1970s, vinblastine plus bleomycin resulted in more encouraging responses (Einhorn, 1990). However, the era of curative therapy was heralded with a study by Einhorn and Donohue (1977), in which 50 patients with metastatic testicular cancer were treated. Cisplatin was given in combination with vinblastine and bleomycin. This three-drug combination, known as PVB, was chosen as it was thought to fit the four criteria for a model of a potentially successful chemotherapeutic regimen:

- Each agent had single-agent activity.
- Each agent had a different mechanism of action.
- Each agent had a different dose-limiting toxicity.
- There was preclinical evidence of synergism (Einhorn, 1990).

The PVB combination resulted in a complete response rate of 75% (Benedetto, 1999; Einhorn, 1990).

Despite the significant improvement in response rates, a number of patients remained who did not achieve a complete response and some who relapsed, resulting in a search for second-line and salvage therapies. In the late 1970s, the investigational agent etoposide (VP-16) was studied. It appeared to be an active single agent that would act synergistically with bleomycin and exhibited a greater response rate than vinblastine without adding to neurotoxicity (Benedetto, 1999; Williams, Einhorn, Greco, Oldham, & Fletcher, 1980).

Early in the 1980s, a clinical trial by the Southeastern Cancer Study Group compared the combination of bleomycin, etoposide, and cisplatin (BEP) to PVB. The study demonstrated therapeutic equivalency with slightly improved outcomes in patients with high-volume tumors treated on the BEP arm (Benedetto, 1999; Williams, Birch, et al., 1987). Eliminating vinblastine resulted in substantially less neurotoxicity as well. This established BEP as the new standard (Benedetto; Williams, Birch, et al., 1987). BEP remains the standard for first-line chemotherapy (NCCN, 2009). However, in patients with good prognosis but compromised pulmonary function, bleomycin may be eliminated because of the risk of bleomycin-induced pulmonary toxicity. In these patients, four cycles of EP (BEP without bleomycin) is equivalent to three of BEP and can be utilized without compromising potential for cure (Jankilevich, 2004; Kopp et al., 2006). A standard cycle of BEP consists of etoposide and cisplatin daily for five days with bleomycin once weekly, every 21 days (see Table 8-1). A study by de Wit et al. (2001) found that a three-day delivery schedule utilizing the same total weekly dose was as

Table 8-1. First-Line Chemotherapy for Testicular Cancer		
Drug	**Dose**	**Frequency**
BEP × 3 or 4 cycles		
Cisplatin	20 mg/m²	Days 1–5, every 21 days
Etoposide	100 mg/m²	Days 1–5, every 21 days
Bleomycin	30 u	Weekly days 1, 8, and 15, or days 2, 9, and 16
EP × 4 cycles		
Cisplatin	20 mg/m²	Days 1–5, every 21 days
Etoposide	100 mg/m²	Days 1–5, every 21 days

Note. Based on information from National Comprehensive Cancer Network, 2009.

effective as a five-day schedule and had no significant increase in toxicities. Three- and five-day regimens are now used in Europe. In the United States, the five-day regimen remains the standard (de Wit et al., 2001; NCCN).

It is important to note that when treating patients with testicular cancer, dose intensity is crucial in achieving an optimal response and that neither the dose of the drugs, the number of cycles, or intervals between cycles should be modified in the absence of severe adverse events (Kopp et al., 2006). It is essential that the standard chemotherapy protocols be administered using the well-defined guidelines in cancer center settings with staff who are experienced and familiar with the treatments (Jones & Vasey, 2003). Patients treated in large tertiary medical centers have been found to have better outcomes than those treated at smaller centers (Collette et al., 1999; Horwich et al., 2006).

Treatment by Stage

Successful disease treatment with chemotherapy, as well as with surgery and radiation, is based on prognostic indicators. Primary site, pathologic findings, radiographic imaging evaluation, and LDH and serum tumor markers determine the extent of disease at diagnosis. This establishes stage, prognosis, and treatment options. In metastatic disease, patients are divided into three risk groups: good, intermediate, and poor prognosis. Historically, several systems have been used for prognostic classification. To enhance the ability to make appropriate risk-based treatment decisions and to aid in standardizing definitions for clinical trials, IGCCCG developed a simple prognostic factor-based staging classification that has become the standard (IGCCCG, 1997; Poirier & Rawl, 2000).

For some disease stages and classifications, there are treatment options. The NCCN Categories of Consensus ranks treatment recommendations based on varying levels of evidence: Category 1 indicates consensus based on uniform evidence; category 2A is consensus based on lower-level evidence; category 2B is nonuniform evidence; and category C is major disagreement that the recommendation is appropriate (see Figure 8-1) (NCCN, 2009).

Stage and Risk Classification

Early-Stage Disease

Approximately two-thirds of patients with testicular cancer are diagnosed with stage I or IIA/B disease. Despite successful outcomes, the management of stage I disease confined to the testis is a controversial topic in urologic oncology (de Wit & Fizazi, 2006; Poirier & Rawl, 2000). As these patients, most of whom are young, can live for many years, it is necessary to weigh the potential for cure and risk of recurrence with the

---

Figure 8-1. National Comprehensive Cancer Network (NCCN) Categories of Consensus

Category 1: The recommendation is based on high-level evidence (e.g. randomized controlled trials) and there is uniform NCCN consensus.

Category 2A: The recommendation is based on lower-level evidence and there is uniform NCCN consensus.

Category 2B: The recommendation is based on lower-level evidence and there is nonuniform NCCN consensus (but no major disagreement).

Category 3: The recommendation is based on any level of evidence but reflects major disagreement.

All recommendations are category 2A unless otherwise noted.

Note. From *The NCCN Clinical Practice Guidelines in Oncology™ Testicular Cancer* (V.1.2007). © National Comprehensive Cancer Network, Inc. Available at http://www.nccn.org. Accessed July 30, 2007. To view the most recent and complete version of the NCCN Guidelines, go online to www.nccn.org.

These guidelines are a work in progress that will be refined as often as new significant data becomes available.

The NCCN Guidelines are a statement of consensus of its authors regarding their views of currently accepted approaches to treatment. Any clinician seeking to apply or consult any NCCN guideline is expected to use independent medical judgment in the context of individual clinical circumstances to determine any patients care or treatment. The National Comprehensive Cancer Network makes no warranties of any kind whatsoever regarding their content, use, or application and disclaims any responsibility for their application or use in any way.

These guidelines are copyrighted by the National Comprehensive Cancer Network. All rights reserved. These guidelines and illustrations herein may not be reproduced in any form for any purpose without the express written permission of the NCCN.

potential long-term toxicities resulting from over-treatment. The monetary cost of long-term disease surveillance also should be a factor (Christoph, Weikert, Miller, & Schrader, 2005; de Wit & Fizazi).

Clinical Stage I Seminoma

Clinical stage I seminoma has a cure rate of nearly 100%. However, because of undetectable retroperitoneal micrometastases, 15%–20% of patients will relapse. Seminoma is exquisitely radiosensitive, post-orchiectomy adjuvant RT has been the standard treatment for decades. However, radiation can cause both acute and long-term toxicities. With a better understanding of relapse patterns, high-quality imaging tools, and effective salvage chemotherapy in the event of relapse, a carefully followed protocol of surveillance has been found to be a safe alternative to adjuvant RT, thus avoiding over-treatment in the 80%–85% of patients who have been cured by orchiectomy alone (Choo et al., 2005; Neill et al., 2007). The disadvantage of post-orchiectomy surveillance alone is that relapses can occur after three or four years, requiring additional long-term radiologic follow-up with CT scans of the abdomen and pelvis approximately every three to four months for three years, every six months through year seven, then annually until year ten (de Wit & Fizazi, 2006; NCCN, 2009).

Amid the increasing interest in late effects of cancer treatment and more long-term follow-up information on cancer survivors, researchers have been searching for treatment modalities with fewer adverse effects, both acute and long term. With results of 15-year follow-up studies becoming available, unexpectedly high rates of morbidity and mortality from RT have been disclosed, including impaired fertility, peptic ulcers, cardiovascular morbidity, and secondary solid tumor cancers. This has created an interest in single-dose/single-agent chemotherapy with carboplatin as an alternative to adjuvant radiation, in the hope of finding an equally effective treatment with fewer long-term sequelae (Christoph et al., 2005; de Wit & Fizazi, 2006).

A study of 1,477 patients by Oliver et al. (2005) found that patients who received carboplatin had similar outcomes to those who received radiation; however, they relapsed more frequently in the retroperitoneum than those who received radiotherapy, but mediastinal, supraclavicular, and pelvic-node relapse was more common after radiation. One patient in the radiation group ultimately died of seminoma. No disease- or treatment-related deaths occurred in the carboplatin group. The radiotherapy arm versus the carboplatin arm, however, had 10 versus 2 second GCTs in the contralateral testis, and four versus three non–germ-cell metachronous cancers, respectively (Oliver et al., 2005). Because late recurrences can occur after 5–10 years, patient follow-up continued. In 2008, follow-up data revealed that although there was a 94.7% five-year relapse-free rate in the carboplatin arm versus 96% in the radiotherapy arm, the difference in the rate of new GCTs

was 2 versus 15 on the carboplatin and radiotherapy arms, respectively. Thus it was determined that carboplatin was less toxic and equivalent in efficacy to radiotherapy in preventing disease recurrence in this population (Oliver, Mead, Fogarty, Stenning, & MRC TE19 and EORTC 30982 Trial Collaborators, 2008). The 2009 NCCN guidelines now include single agent carboplatin, radiotherapy, and surveillance in selected patients as category 1 treatments for stage IA and IB seminoma (NCCN, 2009). It should be noted that the majority of patients who experience a recurrence can be still be cured with salvage chemotherapy.

The role of carboplatin in the treatment armamentarium for stage I seminoma still remains unclear. Further studies are needed to make an evidence-based determination of the benefits of single-dose adjuvant carboplatin versus adjuvant radiation. NCCN currently classifies single-agent carboplatin for stage I testicular cancer as a category 3 treatment.

Clinical Stage II Seminoma

Surveillance is not an option for patients with stage II seminoma. Standard treatment for stage IIA, nodal mass less than 2 cm, and stage IIB, nodal mass 2–5 cm, is radiotherapy. In patients who are not candidates for radiotherapy, three cycles of standard-dose BEP or four cycles of EP are appropriate. Single-agent carboplatin should never be considered in stage II disease because of the higher risk of recurrence and the absence of any evidence of advantage over RT (Kopp et al., 2006).

Clinical Stage I Nonseminoma

In clinical stage I nonseminoma with normal markers after orchiectomy and negative radiographic studies, men have about a 25%–30% chance of having occult metastases. Stage I nonseminoma is divided into low risk and high risk based on prognostic factors, in particular, the presence or absence of lymphovascular invasion. Risk of relapse without vascular invasion is in the range of 14%–22%. The presence of vascular invasion increases that risk to almost 50%. In an effort to minimize unnecessary treatment, surveillance is the option of choice for compliant patients at low risk (Benedetto, 1999; Oosterhof & Verlind, 2004).

High-risk patients have three options: (a) surveillance, (b) RPLND, or (c) adjuvant chemotherapy utilizing two cycles of BEP. Chemotherapy reduces the risk of recurrence in high-risk men to about 2% (Oosterhof & Verlind, 2004). The choice of treatment is dependent on the risk factors and the individual's preference and willingness to comply with close surveillance. Physician and institutional preferences also affect the treatment choice. In case of relapse, 98%–100% of patients will still be cured with chemotherapy. Subsequent surgery will be required in approximately 30% of patients (Oosterhof & Verlind). Approximately 50% of patients, without further treatment, will not recur and may be exposed to unnecessary treatment if they choose chemotherapy (de Wit & Fizazi).

However, surveillance demands compliance on the part of the patient and experience on the part of the physician. With accumulating evidence concerning the risk of long-term side effects of both chemotherapy and radiation (de Wit & Fizazi), patients must receive counseling on the risks and benefits of each treatment option.

For patients with clinical stage IS and persistently elevated markers without radiographic evidence of disease, the recommendation is standard chemotherapy with three cycles of BEP or four cycles of EP. RPLND is not an option, as these patients have an increased risk of harboring undetectable disseminated disease (NCCN, 2009).

Clinical Stage II Nonseminoma

Clinical stage II nonseminoma is classified as IIA and IIB similar to seminoma, but treatment for IIA disease is stratified by tumor marker levels. Patients with normalized markers following orchiectomy have the option of standard primary chemotherapy followed by RPLND or surveillance. Alternatively, patients can have RPLND first, followed by adjuvant chemotherapy with two cycles of BEP, or surveillance. Patients who choose surveillance following RPLND have the same chance for cure as those who choose adjuvant chemotherapy (Kondagunta & Motzer, 2007; Kopp et al., 2006; NCCN, 2009; Williams, Stablien, et al., 1987). The difference is that postoperative chemotherapy requires only two rather than three or four cycles, and those who ultimately would not recur on surveillance are spared exposure to potential chemotherapy-associated toxicities. As the overall cure rate is 98% and the relapse rate is relatively low, choosing the best modality of treatment for an individual can be difficult for the patient as well as the oncologist. However, clinical stage IIA patients with persistently elevated markers should receive three cycles of BEP or four cycles of EP followed by RPLND if residual disease persists after chemotherapy (Kopp et al.; NCCN; Poirier & Rawl, 2000).

Treatment for stage IIB disease depends on both tumor markers and findings on radiology imaging scans. If markers are normal and disease is minimal and limited to lymphatics, patients can undergo RPLND followed by adjuvant chemotherapy as in stage IIA disease. Otherwise, they could have standard primary chemotherapy followed by RPLND or surveillance. If disease is found outside the lymphatics, initial RPLND is not an option, and patients should receive primary chemotherapy (NCCN, 2009).

Advanced Disease

Patients with advanced disease, clinical stages IIC/D and III, will require standard chemotherapy. These patients have extensive or bulky retroperitoneal, supradiaphragmatic nodal, or visceral metastasis. Adjunct surgery for residual disease often is needed after chemotherapy to render patients disease-free (Bosl et al., 2005). Despite metastatic disease, as many as 80% of these men will be cured with chemotherapy alone

or followed by surgery. However, outcomes vary according to several prognostic factors. The IGCCCG classification system divides patients with metastatic disease into three risk categories: (a) good, (b) intermediate, and (c) poor prognosis. The categories are based on site of primary tumor, presence or absence of nonpulmonary visceral metastasis, LDH, and tumor markers. The classification helps to clarify treatment recommendations and predict outcomes (Jones & Vasey, 2003; Kopp et al., 2006). The treatment recommendations for each prognostic class are similar for both seminoma and nonseminoma, with the exception that a poor prognostic classification does not exist for seminoma (see Table 8-2).

Good Prognosis

Distinguishing good prognosis from intermediate and poor prognosis testicular cancer is important prior to starting chemotherapy. Patients with metastatic testicular cancer who are classified as having good prognosis have an overall five-year survival of 86% for seminoma and 92% for nonseminoma (IGCCCG, 1997). A major goal for these patients is to minimize treatment and thus minimize treatment-related toxicity, while maximizing long-term survival and potential for cure. Studies comparing three cycles of BEP versus four cycles of EP in this population have found them to be equivalent (Culine et al., 2003; Jones & Vasey, 2003; Kopp et al., 2006; Vaughn, 2007). These are category 1 first-line treatments according to the NCCN guidelines (2009). Much research has been conducted to determine if bleomycin can be omitted from the regimen altogether. The overwhelming consensus is that bleomycin, in the absence of significant risk factors, should not be omitted when three cycles are given (de Wit et al., 1997; Loehrer, Johnson, Elson, Einhorn, & Trump, 1995; Vaughn). The decision to utilize or eliminate bleomycin should be based on careful consideration of risks and benefits. In patients with a history of smoking, underlying pulmonary disease, renal insufficiency, or more than 40 years of age, four cycles of EP may be preferred to avoid exposure to bleomycin and possible bleomycin-induced lung toxicity. Also, healthcare professionals should consider the risk in patients with underlying peripheral neuropathy or hearing deficits in whom an additional cycle of cisplatin exposure, which is required when omitting bleomycin, may result in further complications (Vaughn).

Intermediate and Poor Prognosis

Approximately 75% of patients with intermediate prognosis and 45% of those with poor prognosis disease will be cured with standard therapy (Kondagunta & Motzer, 2006). In patients with poor prognosis, clinical trials should be considered whenever possible. Complicated multidrug regimens have been investigated in an effort to improve outcomes. The combination of etoposide, ifosfamide, and cisplatin (VIP) resulted in similar survival compared to BEP but was found to be more toxic. For patients with intermediate and poor

Table 8-2. International Germ Cell Consensus Classification Prognostic Factor-Based Staging System for Metastatic Germ Cell Tumor

Risk Status	Seminoma	Nonseminoma
Good prognosis	Any primary site and No nonpulmonary visceral metastases and Normal AFP and HCG, any LDH	Testicular/retroperitoneal primary and No nonpulmonary visceral metastases and Good markers: AFP < 1,000 ng/ml and HCG < 5,000 iu/L and LDH < 1.5 × upper limit of normal
Intermediate prognosis	Any primary site and Nonpulmonary visceral metastases and Normal AFP, any HCG, any LDH	Testicular/retroperitoneal primary and No nonpulmonary visceral metastases and Intermediate markers: any of AFP ≥ 1,000 ≤ 10,000 ng/ml or HCG ≥ 5,000 and ≤ 50,000 iu/L or LDH ≥ 1.5 and ≤ 10 × upper limit of normal
Poor prognosis	No patient classified as poor prognosis	Mediastinal primary or Nonpulmonary visceral metastases or Poor markers: any of AFP >10,000 ng/ml or HCG > 50,000 iu/L or LDH > 10 × upper limit of normal

AFP—alpha-fetoprotein; HCG—human chorionic gonadotropin; LDH—lactate dehydrogenase

Note. From "International Germ Cell Consensus Classification: A Prognostic Factor-Based Staging System for Metastatic Germ Cell Cancers," by International Germ Cell Cancer Collaborative Group, 1997, *Journal of Clinical Oncology, 15*(2), p. 600. Copyright 1997 by American Society of Clinical Oncology. Adapted with permission.

prognosis seminoma and nonseminoma, four cycles of BEP is category 1 treatment and remains the standard. However, VIP can be used as an alternative treatment for poor prognosis patients with compromised pulmonary function when bleomycin is contraindicated. Although clinical investigations for improved regimens are ongoing, four cycles of BEP will remain the standard until randomized phase III trials exhibit superior outcomes (Kondagunta & Motzer, 2006).

Following chemotherapy, approximately one-third of men will have residual disease on radiographic imaging. In seminoma, FDG-PET has been found to be a beneficial adjunct to MRI and CT techniques in detecting residual viable GCTs after chemotherapy (Putra et al., 2004). Generally, in seminoma, masses measuring less than 3 cm do not require resection; otherwise, the definition of significant disease remains controversial (Dodd & Kelly, 2001).

In nonseminoma, if markers are normalized but significant residual disease is detected on radiographic imaging, surgical resection is required whenever possible (Bosl et al., 2005; NCCN, 2009). Approximately 45%–50% of resected tumors will be necrotic and 35%–45% will be teratoma. If pathology reveals necrotic tissue or mature teratoma, only standard surveillance is required. The presence of residual viable tumor, which will be found in approximately 10% of specimens, will require two additional cycles of BEP. Elevated serum markers after chemotherapy generally imply unresected viable disease, and salvage chemotherapy usually is indicated (Bosl et al., 2005; NCCN).

Relapsed or Refractory Disease

Approximately 20%–30% of patients with advanced testicular cancer will relapse or fail to achieve a complete response after chemotherapy (Bosl et al., 2005; Dodd & Kelly, 2001). However, testicular cancer is one of very few malignancies that can still be cured with second-line chemotherapy. Both conventional-dose salvage therapy and high-dose therapy (HDT) with stem cell rescue have a role in treating patients with relapsed and resistant seminoma and nonseminoma. Long-term remission rates of up to 50% can be achieved using standard-dose cisplatin-based chemotherapy (Kopp et al., 2006). Prognostic factors associated with outcomes of candidates for salvage therapy include the location of the primary tumor, the level of tumor markers, and the duration of remission. Patients with good prognosis disease should receive conventional salvage chemotherapy to avoid potentially increased toxicity associated with HDT (see Table 8-3). Men with poor prognosis, those who fail to achieve a complete response with first-line therapy, and those with a mediastinal primary have less than a 10% chance of cure. These patients should be offered HDT or clinical trials using dose-intense chemotherapy (Bosl et al., 2005; Kondagunta & Motzer, 2006; Kopp et al.).

Conventional salvage therapy combinations for patients with relapsed or refractory disease were developed utilizing ifosfamide and paclitaxel, as each was found to have single-agent activity in patients with refractory testicular cancer (Kondagunta & Motzer, 2006). Salvage chemotherapy regimens include VIP; vinblastine, ifosfamide, and cisplatin (VeIP); and paclitaxel, ifosfamide, and cisplatin (TIP) (Kopp et al., 2006). All three regimens include administration of the chemoprotective agent mesna to prevent ifosfamide-induced hemorrhagic cystitis (Kondagunta & Motzer, 2006; Loehrer et al., 1995; NCCN, 2009). No

evidence has shown one regimen to have an advantage over the others (Kopp et al.).

The use of HDT in testicular cancer made sense to early investigators. As testicular cancer is an exquisitely chemosensitive disease, it was thought that using HDT with rescue had the potential to overcome chemotherapy resistance to standard drug doses. HDT is now the accepted third-line treatment and is a category 2A treatment for patients with disease that is refractory to conventional salvage therapy. HDT is also category 2B second-line therapy for patients with prognostic factors that indicate they have a poor likelihood of achieving a complete response to the standard cisplatin-based salvage chemotherapy (NCCN, 2009).

HDT, with carboplatin and etoposide and autologous bone marrow transplantation (BMT), was first investigated at Indiana University in 1986 as a last attempt to cure refractory disease (Einhorn, 2002). Early studies of high-dose chemotherapy followed by autologous BMT found significant morbidity and mortality in this heavily pretreated population, with a long-term survival rate of 15%–20%. Peripheral hematopoietic stem cells replaced bone marrow cells in the mid-1990s, as they were found to engraft more rapidly, allowing for a second cycle of high-dose chemotherapy within fewer days than was possible with marrow transplants (Einhorn, 2002). This, coupled with better patient selection and improved supportive care, has resulted in treatment-related mortality of less than 2% and long-term, disease-free survival rates that approach 12%–52%, with acceptable toxicity (Bhatia et al., 2000). Predictors of poor response using carboplatin combination HDT chemotherapy include high HCG levels, a mediastinal primary site, and insensitivity to cisplatin (NCCN, 2009).

HDT consists of two cycles of high-dose carboplatin 700 mg/m^2 plus etoposide 750 mg/m^2 IV five, four, and three days before stem cell infusion. The stem cells are harvested after marrow stimulation with G-CSF. If patients respond, a second course of HDT is given after granulocytes and platelets recover. Patients with residual disease following HDT may be candidates for surgical resection (Einhorn et al., 2007).

Patients who relapse or do not respond to HDT are generally not curable (Kopp et al., 2006). Some agents that are useful for palliation are oral etoposide, gemcitabine, paclitaxel, and oxaliplatin, but these usually result in only partial responses in 10%–20% of patients (Kondagunta & Motzer, 2006). Because these patients are heavily pretreated, toxicities often result in the need for frequent dose modifications, treatment delays, and early terminations (Kollmannsberger, Nichols, & Bokemeyer, 2006). Recent phase II studies have found gemcitabine and oxaliplatin to be of some benefit and have manageable toxicities. Based on these studies, the 2009 NCCN guidelines have included two regimens utilizing these agents as palliative second-line salvage therapy: gemcitabine 1,000 mg/m^2 or 1,250 mg/m^2 IV, administered on days 1 and 8, with oxaliplatin 130 mg/m^2 on day 1 every 21 days (NCCN, 2009).

Table 8-3. Salvage Chemotherapy Regimens for Resistant and Relapsed Testicular Cancer

Drug	Dose	Frequency
VeIP × 4 cycles		
Vinblastine	0.11 mg/kg	Days 1 and 2, every 21 days
Ifosfamide	1.2 g/m²	Days 1–5, every 21 days
Mesna	400 mg/m²	Every 8 hours, days 1–5*
Cisplatin	20 mg/m²	Days 1–5, every 21 days
VIP × 4 cycles		
Etoposide	75 mg/m²	Days 1–5, every 21 days
Ifosfamide	1.2 g/m²	Days 1–5, every 21 days
Mesna	400 mg/m²	Every 8 hours, days 1–5*
Cisplatin	20 mg/m²	Days 1–5, every 21 days
TIP × 4 cycles		
Paclitaxel	250 mg/m²	Day 1 over 24 hours
Ifosfamide	1.5 g/m²	Days 2–5
Mesna	500 mg/m²	Before, at 4 hours, and at 8 hours after ifosfamide*
Cisplatin	25 mg/m²	Days 2–5

*Schedule of mesna administration is not standardized.

Note. Based on information from Kondagunta et al., 2005; Loehrer et al., 1995; National Comprehensive Cancer Newtork, 2009; Schuchter et al., 2002.

Novel molecular targets also are being explored in refractory testicular cancer. Early studies suggest that vascular endothelial growth factor (VEGF) may have a role in metastatic disease, and VEGF inhibitors are undergoing evaluation (Kollmannsberger et al., 2006). Jones and Vasey (2003) remind us that in this small population of patients who are unlikely to be cured, it may occasionally be appropriate to consider quality of life rather than striving for likely unattainable cures with aggressive therapy.

Follow-Up

Following treatment, patients who have negative markers and are free of any evidence of disease on radiologic imaging move to a program of close surveillance with regularly scheduled physical examinations, chest x-rays, CT scans, and phlebotomy for tumor markers (NCCN, 2009; Vaughn, Gignac, & Meadows, 2002). Randomized data are scant and there is no evidence-based consensus concerning frequency or intensity of follow-up. Current recommendations are based on the pattern and probability of recurrence using stage, histology, and primary therapy as criteria. Several institutions, in particular NCCN, have outlined guidelines regarding follow-up protocols that are most effective in identifying relapsed disease (Kondagunta, Sheinfeld, & Motzer, 2003), but no evidence-based guidelines for the appropriate follow-up investigations are yet available. Optimal imaging requirements and frequency of surveillance visits need to be further investigated (Gospodarowicz, 2008; Kondagunta et al., 2003).

Acute and Long-Term Toxicity and Supportive Care

Despite its success in curing patients with testicular cancer, chemotherapy can and does cause significant toxicity both in the acute setting and years after treatment. The focus on health-related quality of life, both during and after chemotherapy, has been increasing in this population (Fossa et al., 2003). Much information is available on prevention and treatment of the acute toxicities, but we are just beginning to learn about the long-term effects of chemotherapy in these mostly young patients.

Over the past 20 years, significant gains have been made in supportive care. Drugs including G-CSFs to reduce neutropenia, erythropoietins to reduce anemia, and various new antiemetics have allowed higher maximum tolerated doses of chemotherapeutic agents (Camp-Sorrell, 2000) resulting in expected cures for testicular cancer. More attention and research is being directed toward reducing and preventing side effects, both acute and long-term, with interventions such as counseling and education to enhance self-care and assist with behavior modification (Camp-Sorrell; Nail, 2004). Nurses play a key role in education and management in both the inpatient and outpatient settings.

Acute Toxicity and Management

Acute toxicity, side effects that occur during and shortly after treatment, range from minor and transient to permanent or life threatening. Almost all organ systems can be affected by chemotherapy for testicular cancer (see Table 8-4). It is important to remember that side effects that may be of little consequence to some individuals can be devastating to others.

Myelosuppression

By interfering with rapidly dividing cells, chemotherapy affects bone marrow stem cells, decreasing the ability to replace leukocytes, erythrocytes, and platelets. Myelosuppression is

Table 8-4. Acute Toxicities From Chemotherapy and Supportive Drugs	
System	**Toxicity**
Myelosuppression	• Anemia • Neutropenia • Thrombocytopenia
Gastrointestinal	• Constipation • Gastric reflux • Hiccups • Mucositis, thrush, and herpes simplex • Nausea and vomiting
Neurologic and otologic	• Hearing loss • Peripheral neuropathy • Tinnitus
Nephrologic and urologic	• Hematuria • Kidney dysfunction, elevated creatinine, decreased glomerular filtration rate • Potassium and magnesium wasting
Pulmonary	• Pneumonitis
Dermatologic	• Acne • Alopecia • Hyperpigmentation • Nail changes • Pruritus • Rash
Quality of life	• Cognitive impairment • Depression • Fatigue • Flu-like symptoms
Sexuality	• Erectile dysfunction • Infertility • Loss of libido

Note. Based on information from Beck, 2004; Bosl et al., 2005; Camp-Sorrell, 2000; Coyne & Leslie, 2004; Goodman, 2000; Massey et al., 2004; Vardy et al., 2006; Wilkes, 2001, 2004.

common in all regimens used in testicular cancer. Etoposide used in BEP and EP, and ifosfamide, vinblastine, and paclitaxel used in TIP, VIP, and VeIP are all myelosuppressive agents (Goodman, 2000; Wilkes, 2001). Neutropenia, anemia, and thrombocytopenia are all possible; however, neutropenia is more common. Blood counts usually reach nadir 10–14 days after treatment and gradually recover in 21–28 days (Wujcik, 2004). A CBC with differential should be checked prior to each treatment and more frequently if indicated.

The G-CSF filgrastim can help to prevent neutropenia (Wujcik, 2004). Studies in the 1990s showed significantly less treatment delays for neutropenia and fewer patients receiving dose reductions because of myelosuppression. Early studies in poor-risk patients with testicular cancer demonstrated increased dose intensity associated with the use of G-CSF and fewer deaths from neutropenic infections (Fossa et al., 1998). Despite these findings, a study by Fossa et al. concluded that although the use of filgrastim was associated with a significant reduction in the number of toxic deaths in the population studied, it did not support the routine use of G-CSF for standard chemotherapy with BEP (Collette et al., 1999; Fossa et al., 1998). NCCN (2009) recommends the use of G-CSF prophylaxis in all patients receiving chemotherapy who have a high (20% or greater) risk of developing febrile neutropenia. VIP, VeIP, BEP, and TIP are classified as high risk and EP as moderate risk (10%–20%). Other regimens are not addressed (NCCN). However, the American Society of Clinical Oncology recommends the use of G-CSF when the risk of neutropenia is approximately 20% (Khatcheressian et al., 2006).

Teaching is important in this group of active men, as treatment increases the risk of infection, anemia, and bleeding. CBC with differential should be monitored regularly. Men at risk for neutropenia and their families should be encouraged to be vaccinated for influenza. Despite the fact that 85% of neutropenic infections are caused by the patient's own normal flora (Wilkes, 2001), careful hand washing should be encouraged to help to prevent transmissible infections (Zitella et al., 2006). Nurses should instruct patients who are receiving chemotherapy to report fevers of greater than 38.3°C (100.5°F) and be evaluated for neutropenic fever.

Anemia occurs in almost all patients but rarely requires transfusion in chemotherapy-naïve patients (Bosl et al., 2005). The occurrence of clinically significant anemia can cause fatigue, hypotension, dyspnea, tachycardia, headaches, and irritability (Wilkes, 2001). Severe thrombocytopenia is not common in men receiving BEP or EP but is frequent in those receiving salvage therapies (Bosl et al., 2005). Men employed in jobs that put them at risk for injury, such as construction workers, police, and firefighters, and those involved in contact sports should be advised to adjust their activities accordingly. Patients should be taught to watch for signs of unusual bleeding or bruising. Frequent monitoring of blood counts should enable appropriate interventions before symptoms related to myelosuppression occur.

Gastrointestinal Toxicity

GI side effects are common during chemotherapy with testicular cancer treatments, in particular, nausea and vomiting. Other GI effects include constipation, mucositis, stomatitis, taste alterations, gastric reflux, and hiccups.

Cisplatin and etoposide are highly emetogenic, causing nausea and vomiting in 60%–90% of patients. Ifosfamide is moderately emetogenic; bleomycin, paclitaxel, and vinblastine are all mildly emetogenic (Camp-Sorrell, 2000). As most regimens include cisplatin and ifosfamide, chemotherapy-induced nausea and vomiting (CINV) occurs in many patients. The vomiting center in the brain is located near chemoreceptor trigger zone, which is sensitive to stimulation from emetogenic chemical substances in chemotherapy. The mechanism of CINV is not thoroughly understood, but damage to intestinal mucosa by chemotherapy releases serotonin ($5\text{-}HT_3$), which is implicated in stimulating the vomiting center. $5\text{-}HT_3$ antagonists like ondansetron and granisetron are considerably successful in helping to prevent and control acute CINV (Dougherty & Bailey, 2001). Antiemetics and dexamethasone should be given IV prior to chemotherapy, and patients should be given prescriptions for oral agents for delayed CINV. Lorazepam can be an effective addition to the antiemetic regimen, but patients should be cautioned about possible sedating effects (Tipton et al., 2006). Newer agents, such as the NK1 antagonist aprepitant, may offer additional clinical benefit (de Wit et al., 2004; Schwartzberg, 2007); however, studies were conducted in patients receiving emetogenic agents only one day per cycle. Little benefit has been found, though few studies were performed in patients who received highly emetogenic drugs daily over five days as given in testicular cancer regimens. Although these agents have potential for preventing CINV in patients receiving multiple-day chemotherapy, further research is needed to determine if NK-1 inhibitors will benefit this population (Navari, 2007).

Constipation during chemotherapy can have various causes. Chemotherapeutic drugs, $5\text{-}HT_3$ antagonists, decreased activity, diminished fluid and fiber intake, and electrolyte imbalances also can slow motility and increase fluid reabsorption (Massey, Haycock, & Curtiss, 2004). Men should be encouraged to increase fluid intake and maintain a high-fiber diet. Prophylactic stool softeners or stimulants can help to prevent constipation in patients who are at risk (Wilkes, 2001).

Chemotherapy for testicular cancer also can cause problems in the upper GI mucosa. *Mucositis*, inflammation and breakdown of the mucous membranes that line the GI tract, is referred to as *stomatitis* when it occurs in the oral cavity. It results from direct and indirect effects of chemotherapy—directly from the destruction of cells that are actively reproducing and indirectly from bone marrow suppression, particularly during the nadir. Objective signs are red, inflamed oral mucosa with or without ulcerations, blisters, cracks, or dryness, which can be accompanied by pain, hoarseness, and dysphagia (Beck, 2004; Wilkes, 2001). Mucositis should be distinguished from oral candidiasis and herpetic ulcers that also can occur in immunocompromised patients. Oral candidiasis, or thrush, and herpes simplex can occur when a patient's immunity is diminished by chemotherapy. Thrush, caused by *Candida albicans*, appears as small white cottage cheese-like patches on the tongue, buccal surfaces, and throat. Herpes simplex can occur on the mouth and lips and presents as vesicular lesions. Both can cause discomfort and pain. These lesions may not always be present in a classic manner, especially in immunosuppressed patients, and a culture may be the only way to obtain a precise diagnosis. Early intervention is important to prevent pain and dysphagia resulting in difficulty taking in foods and fluids and is particularly important with severe neutropenia, as a localized lesion can progress to a systemic and potentially life-threatening infection (Beck; Camp-Sorrell, 2000; Wilkes, 2001).

Altered taste sensations, ageusia, dysgeusia, and hypogeusia are common in patients receiving chemotherapy, especially in those receiving cisplatin. The onset and duration are variable and may begin as early as the first treatment. Symptoms may be intermittent or persistent and last from days to months following treatment (Sherry, 2002; Wickham et al., 1999). At least 50% of patients report taste changes, which include loss of taste, distorted or increased bitter and sweet taste, and metallic or cardboard taste. More than 70% of patients treated with cisplatin experience a metallic taste (Wickham et al.). The cause of these chemosensory distortions remains unclear. It is thought that the continuous cellular division that occurs in the mouth results in oral sensitivity during chemotherapy (Ackerman & Kasbekar, 1997). As taste alterations are not perceived as serious, the symptoms often are overlooked. However, these symptoms can cause or exacerbate anorexia, decrease caloric intake, and affect eating pleasure and quality of life (Ackerman & Kasbekar; Sherry).

Patients with dry mouth, disruptions of the oral mucosa, anorexia, nausea, and vomiting are at increased risk of developing taste alterations. Management should begin with treating underlying conditions. To increase saliva production, patients should be instructed to increase fluid intake with water or other nonirritating beverages, suck on sugar-free sour candies, and chew gum. Chewing mints and gum, switching from metal to plastic utensils, marinating foods in sweet sauces, using more herbs and spices, and eating chilled foods can decrease metallic taste. Frequent oral hygiene, smoking cessation, and avoiding noxious odors also should be encouraged (Sherry, 2002).

Hiccups and gastric reflux can be troublesome side effects, although these often are not discussed. A paucity of information is available in the literature concerning these symptoms in patients receiving chemotherapy. Intravenous dexamethasone is given to prevent CINV in patients receiving cisplatin-based regimens and can cause both of these conditions. Gastroesophageal reflux is common in men receiving prophylactic dexamethasone. Approximately 25% of patients

receiving steroid prophylaxis report moderate to severe symptoms (Vardy, Chiew, Galica, Pond, & Tannock, 2006). Symptoms can include burning, bloating, regurgitation, or a globus sensation (Katz, 2003).

Hiccups are involuntary contractions of the diaphragm that cause abrupt closure of the epiglottis. This can be uncomfortable and distressing and cause increased gastric discomfort and affect sleep, if persistent. It is thought that dexamethasone stimulates the hiccup reflex arc (Liaw et al., 2005; Ross, Eledrisi, & Casner, 1999; Vardy et al., 2006). Liaw et al. studied 277 patients receiving dexamethasone as part of their antiemetic therapy. Dexamethasone 20 mg IV was administered prior to chemotherapy and followed by dexamethasone 5 mg IV every 12 hours until completion of chemotherapy. Hiccups occurred in 41% of patients. When dexamethasone was discontinued, the incidence of hiccups decreased, and nausea and vomiting increased. Patients should be assured that hiccups are self-limiting, but if they cause distress or other GI symptoms, chlorpromazine and metoclopramide can be effective (Williams, 2003). To prevent heartburn and gastric reflux, lifestyle modifications such as avoiding reclining after eating or eating within three hours of bedtime, elevating the head of the bed, and avoiding tomato-based or acidic sauces, coffee, and spices can be beneficial. Histamine-2 antagonists can be helpful, but proton pump inhibitors have recently supplanted their use (Katz, 2003) and should be considered prophylactically at the initiation of therapy.

Neurologic and Otologic Effects

Cisplatin, paclitaxel, and vinblastine produce several types of neurotoxicities. Peripheral neuropathy, inflammation, injury, or degradation of the peripheral nerve fibers are common in patients treated with cisplatin-based chemotherapy. Symptoms can range from mild numbness and tingling to disabling sensory motor pain and weakness (Wilkes, 2004). The incidence of peripheral neuropathy has been reported to be as high as 76% (Chaudhary & Haldas, 2003). These are primarily sensory paresthesias and dysesthesias, which are believed to result from damage to the dorsal root ganglion (Chaudhary & Haldas). Symptoms may occur as early as the first cycle or may not present until months following the completion of treatment (Chaudhary & Haldas). Neuropathy is most common after cumulative doses of 300 mg/m^2, and at a cumulative dose of 500–600 mg/m^2 almost all patients have evidence of neurotoxicity (Oldenburg, Fossa, & Dahl, 2006). These effects can have a significant impact on activities of daily living, affecting the ability to walk, work, and perform fine motor skills. Therefore, nursing assessment is crucial for early recognition. Patients should be informed about the risk of peripheral neuropathy and advised to report any numbness, tingling, or unusual sensations in their extremities. Currently, no effective modality to prevent chemotherapy-induced neuropathy is available. Dose intensity is crucial, and dose reductions are not recommended. As neuropathy is more problematic after treatment, interventions will be discussed later in the section.

Ototoxicity, high-frequency hearing loss, and tinnitus occurs in 10%–30% of patients treated with cisplatin (Camp, Gilmore, Gullatte, & Hutcherson, 2007). This is thought to be related to cisplatin-induced death of hair cells in the organ of Corti (Bokemeyer, Berger, Kuczyk, & Schmoll, 1996). Most patients have only subclinical or mild symptoms. Interestingly, a significant discrepancy exists between the subjective complaints of hearing loss and audiometric results. Although data are inconclusive, patients with a history of preexisting hearing loss, exposure to noise, and cumulative cisplatin doses may be at increased risk (Chaudhary & Haldas, 2003; Strumberg et al., 2002; Vaughn et al., 2002). Additional exposure to noise and aminoglycosides can enhance ototoxicity (Fausti, Wilmington, Helt, Helt, & Konrad-Martin, 2005). Patients should be counseled to avoid excessive noise during chemotherapy by keeping music volumes low and wearing ear protection when exposed to significant occupational noise. Currently, no standards or recommendations for baseline or routine hearing assessments are available.

Nephrologic and Urologic Toxicities

Renal toxicity from cisplatin is caused by alterations of the renal vasculature, such as endothelial damage and narrowing, and a decrease in the glomerular filtration rate. This results in elevated creatinine, renal hypertension, altered renin levels, microalbuminuria, and chronic magnesium wasting (Bokemeyer et al., 1996; Meinardi, Gietema, van Veldhuisen, et al., 2000; Vaughn et al., 2002). The incidence of renal toxicity ranges 13%–30%. Acute damage may develop 3–21 hours following the infusion (Camp-Sorrell, 2000).

Patients treated with any cisplatin-based chemotherapy must receive hydration, often with at least two liters of a saline solution, and urine output must be monitored. Diuretic agents, such as mannitol, may be administered. Mannitol facilitates diuresis and may decrease the binding of cisplatin to renal tubules. Caution should be used with loop diuretics such as furosemide, as they are also nephrotoxic and ototoxic (Camp-Sorrell, 2000). Electrolyte wasting, in particular potassium and magnesium, can occur with cisplatin. Serum creatinine, potassium, and magnesium should be monitored closely and supplementation provided as needed. Concomitant use of nephrotoxic drugs should be avoided (King, 2001). Patients should be instructed to continue oral hydration during and following treatment. Failure of patients to report reduced urine output or nausea and vomiting that preclude good fluid consumption can result in acute renal failure that threatens future treatment with this agent, hence the necessity for intense patient education on renal function, hydration, and electrolyte replacement orally after discharge.

Ifosfamide, used in TIP and VIP regimens, can cause dysuria and hematuria ranging from microscopic hematuria to hemorrhagic cystitis. This is caused by a toxic metabolite,

acrolein. Acrolein has no antitumor activity but has irritant properties that affect the bladder epithelium. Regimens containing ifosfamide include the protective agent mesna, which binds acrolein and protects the bladder epithelium. Mesna may be administered before ifosfamide and 4 and 8 hours after for 24 hours (Camp-Sorrell, 2000; King, 2001; NCCN, 2009; Wilkes, 2001), although recommendations for mesna are not standardized (Schuchter, Hensley, Meropol, & Winer, 2002). Mesna also may be administered as a continuous infusion administered during ifosfamide therapy and continued for 12 hours after ifosfamide therapy is completed.

Pulmonary

Patients who are receiving BEP are at risk for pulmonary toxicity associated with bleomycin. This is the most serious and potentially fatal effect of bleomycin. It is fatal in approximately 2% of those affected (Keijzer & Kuenen, 2007). Fortunately, this is uncommon in patients without risk factors or preexisting lung disease who receive a total dosage of less than 300 units. The pathogenesis is not clear, but endothelial damage from leucocytes, in particular lymphocytes, neutrophils, and alveolar macrophages, infiltrating into the lung have been implicated in pulmonary fibrosis by secreting cytokines and growth factors (Hirata et al., 2008; Wilkes, 2001). The pulmonary dysfunction is restrictive and causes functionally decreased lung volumes and impaired gas exchange (Wilkes, 2001). As symptoms and radiographic findings are nonspecific, the diagnosis is often one of exclusion. Patients may present with dry hacking cough, dyspnea, decreased diffusion capacity, basilar rales, tachycardia, cyanoses, and sometimes fever. Chest x-ray findings vary and may show no abnormalities, bilateral basal infiltrates, or diffuse interstitial and alveolar infiltrates (Keijzer & Kuenen; Wilkes, 2001). Risk factors for developing bleomycin-induced pneumonitis include (Vaughn, 2007)
- Underlying pulmonary disease
- Age older than 70
- Impaired renal function
- History of smoking
- Cumulative dose.

Patients treated with three cycles of BEP will receive 30 units weekly for nine weeks for a total dose of 270 units, leaving them at low risk. Those requiring four cycles of BEP receive 30 units, weekly for a 12-week total dose of 360 units, which increases the risk (Vaughn, 2007).

Careful thought should be given when considering bleomycin for patients with risk factors. PFTs are performed at baseline and should include spirometry and diffusion capacity (DLCO). No generally accepted guidelines are available for monitoring PFTs during treatment. DLCO is the most sensitive indicator of injury. As lung damage can be progressive and irreversible, it is imperative to detect toxicity immediately. Health professionals should query patients about cough and dyspnea and observe for these symptoms. If symptomatic,

PFTs should be repeated, and if DLCO or FVC has fallen significantly, bleomycin should be discontinued. High-dose corticosteroids are the mainstay of treatment (Chaudhary & Haldas, 2003). For patients who will be undergoing subsequent RPLND, it must be ensured that the anesthesiologist, surgeon, and other healthcare providers are aware that they received treatment with bleomycin, as elevated concentrations of oxygen during surgery has been known to cause or increase bleomycin-related lung toxicity (Azambuja, Fleck, Batista, & Barreto, 2005; Ingrassia, Ryu, Trastek, & Rosenow, 1991). During surgery, it is recommended that adequate oxygenation be provided using the lowest oxygen concentration, average 40% fractional inspired oxygen (Donat & Levy, 1998). However, there is some controversy. Donat and Levy contend that FVC and operative time are significant predictive factors of procedure-related pulmonary morbidity, and perioperative oxygen restriction in patients treated with bleomycin is not necessary; rather, measures in management of IV fluids and transfusion are more significant in preventing postoperative pulmonary complications.

Dermatologic Effects

Chemotherapy can affect hair, nails, and skin. Some of these effects are the direct result of chemotherapy attacking rapidly proliferating cells or are an indirect effect caused by the skin's lack of an enzyme, bleomycin hydrolase, which leaves it vulnerable to dermatologic toxicity (Keijzer & Kuenen, 2007; Wilkes, 2001). Some skin effects occur because of the prophylactic steroids.

Alopecia will affect virtually all patients treated for testicular cancer. It is the most obvious effect of chemotherapy, though one of the least serious side effects, and is certainly one of the most distressing for patients. Hair loss is most complete on the scalp, as most scalp hair follicles are in anaphase, but also may involve facial, pubic, and body hair. Hair loss should be discussed before treatment begins, and patients should be reminded that alopecia is temporary and reversible. Hair loss can be preceded by some scalp discomfort and can begin as early two to three weeks after the first dose of chemotherapy and may begin to regrow about four to six weeks following the last dose, with much individual variability. It may take as long as a year for complete regrowth of hair. Scalp hair often grows back with slightly altered pigment and texture (Camp-Sorrell, 2000).

Skin and nail changes usually are related to bleomycin and the dexamethasone used to prevent CINV. Bleomycin can cause macular rashes, striae, pruritus, hyperpigmentation, and hyperkeratosis (Wilkes, 2001). Hyperpigmentation, which is more common in darker-skinned individuals, can occur over pressure points and in flagellate streaks from scratching. It can also occur on nail beds, oral mucosa, and along veins (Goodman, 2000). Hyperpigmentation is temporary. Dexamethasone is responsible for acne in 15% of patients (Vardy et al., 2006). Bothersome acne can be treated with topical antibiotics. In order to avoid exacerbating skin issues related to therapy, patients need to avoid sun exposure.

Quality of Life and Constitutional Symptoms

General quality of life is affected by all chemotherapy regimens used in treating testicular cancer. Physical and constitutional symptoms can impair individuals' ability to function as usual at home and at work and can interfere with their ability to maintain accustomed social and sexual relationships (Camp-Sorrell, 2000). A European Organisation for Research and Treatment of Cancer study of men with testicular cancer who received BEP found decreases in physical, emotional, and cognitive function, as well as role and social function (Fossa et al., 2003). This is particularly distressing in the population of active young men, some barely out of adolescence, and others with young families at the peak of their productive years. These men are accustomed to feeling in control and able to rely on their bodies, and now feel out of control. Every ache, unusual sensation, and body function can increase their sense of vulnerability and isolation (Dougherty & Bailey, 2001).

Fatigue is almost universal in patients receiving chemotherapy. NCCN describes chemotherapy-induced fatigue as "an unusual, persistent, subjective sense of tiredness related to cancer or cancer treatment that interferes with usual functioning" (Mock et al., 2000, p. 152). Fatigue occurs in 70%–100% of chemotherapy patients. Chemotherapy-induced fatigue is different from "normal" fatigue experienced after exercise, the flu, or excessive celebration. It is not relieved by rest and sleep and often involves weakness, lack of motivation, cognitive impairment, and reduced ability to continue usual social interactions (Morrow, 2007). Patients report that their fatigue is often more distressing than other symptoms such as pain, depression, and nausea. Fatigue undermines feelings of physical well-being and places formerly functional men in a position of dependence. They may have difficulty participating in their usual activities and frequently need to engage in unaccustomed behaviors, like lying down or napping during the day. This sedentary lifestyle can be demoralizing and discouraging (Morrow). Correcting comorbid conditions such as fluid and electrolyte imbalances, anemia, constipation, nausea, and depression is crucial, but behavioral interventions are important as well. Assisting patients in balancing activity and exercise with energy conservation modalities, napping with sleep interventions, and strategies for improving nutrition and hydration are some essential nursing interventions. Patients should be assured that fatigue is a common side effect of chemotherapy and their energy will gradually return when treatment is completed.

Many patients complain of difficulty with memory and concentration or just not feeling "sharp." Healthcare providers often overlook such complaints. These cognitive complaints are referred to as "chemo fog," "chemo brain," chemotherapy-induced cognitive impairment, and central neurotoxicity

(Coyne & Leslie, 2004). Patients can find the symptoms difficult to describe. Deficits can present as diminished information processing and reaction time and impaired organizational skills, language abilities, and attentiveness. Foresight and judgment also can be affected. High-functioning individuals appear to be more acutely aware of the deficits (Coyne & Leslie), making it especially problematic as these men are attending school, raising children, and starting careers. The mechanism for cognitive impairment is not understood. Subjective complaints do not always correlate with objective measures on cognitive testing. Supportive drugs given for testicular cancer treatments such as histamine-2 antagonists, opiates, and steroids can add to the effect, as can physiologic factors such as anemia, fatigue, and dehydration (Staat & Segatore, 2003). There is a paucity of information and research on this phenomenon in young men.

Flu-like symptoms can occur in patients receiving bleomycin. These symptoms include fatigue, headache, fever, chills, myalgias, arthralgias, and malaise. This is self-limiting and preventable with pretreatment using acetaminophen, antihistamines, and in some cases corticosteroids (Wilkes, 2001).

Sexuality and Fertility

Sexual dysfunction, which includes loss of libido, erectile dysfunction, and infertility, is a significant quality-of-life issue for men during chemotherapy (Wilkes, 2001). Loss of libido and erectile dysfunction can be the result of indirect effects of treatment. Changes in body image from weight loss, hair loss, nausea, fatigue, and altered role function, as well as depression, feelings of dependence, fear, and isolation, can rob men of their virility and interest in sex and intimacy (Wilkes, 2001). See Chapter 9 for more information regarding sexual rehabilitation.

Patients should be made aware that chemotherapy could be present in their seminal fluid. Semen entering the female reproductive tract during intercourse could have teratogenic effects and interfere with fetal development (Trasler & Doerksen, 1999). Men should be counseled to ensure that their female partners avoid pregnancy. Nurses should instruct patients to use condoms to prevent pregnancy and exposure of their partner to any toxic substances that may be present in the seminal fluid.

Follow-Up

Surveillance for disease recurrence following chemotherapy requires frequent visits with the oncologist for physical examinations, chest x-rays, CT scans, and blood draws for tumor markers (Vaughn et al., 2002). These visits are essential as early detection and treatment of recurrent disease can still result in cure rates of approximately 95% with second-line treatments (Kondagunta et al., 2003). Frequency and intensity of follow-up are determined by the pattern and probability of

recurrence based on patients' histology, stage of disease, and primary therapy. NCCN has outlined guideline recommendations; however, these are guidelines only. Currently, no consensus exists regarding a uniformly recommended follow-up schedule based on randomized data (Gospodarowicz, 2008; Kondagunta et al., 2003).

The current NCCN guidelines recommend frequent visits with imaging and tumor markers during the first two to three years following treatment. Visits and testing are recommended every one to every three months based on cell type, stage, and whether the patient has undergone orchiectomy alone or received chemotherapy or RPLND. Between the third and fifth year, the frequency of visits and testing decreases to approximately every three to six months, and then annually after five years. The specific current NCCN guidelines should be consulted and are available through NCCN and online (Kondagunta et al., 2003; NCCN, 2009; Oosterhof & Verlind, 2004; Vaughn et al., 2002).

Long-Term Effects

Since the 1980s, the body of literature that addresses the late effects of cancer treatment has been increasing. Results from long-term follow-up studies of childhood cancer survivors have increased the awareness of the potential for complications in the years following treatment. In adult oncology, much of this work has been conducted with testicular cancer because of the generally young age of the patients who are affected and the excellent chance for cure and long-term survival (Chaudhary & Haldas, 2003; Meinardi, Gietema, van Veldhuisen, et al., 2000; Vaughn et al., 2002). Potential late effects, which vary according to treatment, include increased risk factors for cardiovascular disease, nephrotoxicity, neurotoxicity, secondary cancers, and infertility (Efstathiou & Logothetis, 2006; Kondagunta et al., 2003; Vaughn et al.) (see Table 8-5). The most serious late effects are cardiovascular toxicities and secondary malignancies, with the risk being approximately 16% over 25 years (Efstathiou & Logothetis).

Cardiovascular Toxicity

Raynaud phenomenon (RP) is the most common postchemotherapy vascular toxicity in patients with germ cell cancer. RP is defined as transient episodes of vasoconstriction of the digital arteries precipitated by cold or stress, manifested by pain and color changes of the affected digits (Chaudhary & Haldas, 2003). The cause is believed to be bleomycin. The incidence of RP ranges 20%–60%. Symptoms can occur anytime during the treatment and up to 36 months after completion of chemotherapy. Some patients have gradual resolution of symptoms, but as many as 25% of patients with RP were found to have chronic symptoms lasting more than 10 years (Berger, Bokemeyer, Schneider, Kuczyk, & Schmoll, 1995; Gerl, 1994; Zoltick, Jacobs, & Vaughn, 2005). Although RP is not the most

Table 8-5. Long-Term Effects, Prevention, and Intervention

Toxicity	Effects	Prevention and Interventions
Cardiovascular toxicity	Raynaud phenomenon	Avoid exposing hands to cold.
	Endothelial damage	Diet
	Elevated cholesterol	Exercise
	Hypertension	Weight control
	Increased body mass index	Monitor blood pressure, lipids. Smoking cessation
Nephrotoxicity	Magnesium wasting	Hydration during treatment
	Elevated creatinine	Avoid nephrotoxic drugs.
	Decreased glomerular filtration rate	Monitor blood urea nitrogen, creatinine, magnesium.
Neurotoxicity	Peripheral neuropathy	Safety interventions Inspection of extremities Physical therapy Pain management Avoid neurotoxic drugs.
Ototoxicity	Hearing loss	Avoid noise.
	Tinnitus	Avoid ototoxic drugs.
Pulmonary effects	Pulmonary fibrosis	Avoid scuba diving. Appropriate fluid and oxygen management during anesthesia Avoid oxygen bars.
Secondary cancers	Leukemia	Routine medical follow-up
	Solid tumors	Age-appropriate cancer screening
Infertility	Impaired spermatogenesis	Sperm banking before treatment Referral to reproductive center Counseling

Note. Based on information from Bokemeyer et al., 1996; Camp-Sorrell, 2000; Chaudhary & Haldas, 2003; Donat & Levy, 1998; Efstathiou & Logothetis, 2006; Huls & ten Bokkel Huinink, 2003; Vaughn et al., 2002; Visovsky et al., 2007; Zoltick et al., 2005.

serious vascular effect, it does cause discomfort and can negatively affect quality of life. An association between RP and erectile dysfunction may exist, as they both involve angiopathy of the penile arteries (Hennessy, O'Connor, & Carney, 2002; Meinardi, Gietema, van Veldhuisen, et al., 2000; Zoltick et al.). Smoking cessation is important to reduce symptoms, as well as to help to prevent further vascular effects. Nurses should instruct men with symptoms of RP to stop smoking and to avoid exposure to cold. Calcium channel blockers also have been used to decrease symptoms of RP with some success (Chaudhary & Haldas).

Chemotherapy can have chronic damaging effects on the cardiovascular system that are more serious. Cardiovascular toxicity is likely a result of direct endothelial damage induced by cisplatin and indirect hormonal and metabolic changes (Efstathiou & Logothetis, 2006). Indirect side effects of chemotherapeutic agents used to treat testicular cancer have been found to contribute to developing increased cardiac risk factors and cardiovascular disease (Efstathiou & Logothetis; Meinardi, Gietema, van der Graaf, et al., 2000; Strumberg et al., 2002). Cardiac risk factors include elevated serum cholesterol, hypertension, and increased body mass index. The increased incidence of the metabolic syndrome identified in long-term survivors possibly is related to lower testosterone levels found in these men (Efstathiou & Logothetis). Smoking, obesity, diet, and family history of cardiac disease are predisposing factors that further increase the risks (Bosl et al., 1986; Boyer et al., 1990; Grundy, Pasternak, Greenland, Smith, & Fuster, 1999; Huddart et al., 2003; Strumberg et al.; Vaughn et al., 2002).

Survivors should be counseled regarding modifiable risk factors such as smoking cessation, diet, exercise, and weight control to help to prevent cardiac disease (Vaughn et al., 2002). Nurses should encourage men to have a primary healthcare provider who is aware of their cancer history to ensure they receive ongoing evaluation for risk factors such as hypertension and elevated cholesterol.

Nephrotoxicity

All patients who receive cisplatin-based chemotherapy will have some degree of chronic nephrotoxicity. Magnesium wasting related to subclinical renal damage following treatment with cisplatin has been implicated in the development of hypertension. Although altered renal function is not usually of clinical significance for the majority of patients, consequences can include hypomagnesemia, which can last for many years, and chronic renal failure. This can be significant for patients who might later require aminoglycosides or other potentially nephrotoxic agents, as well as patients who subsequently recur and require salvage therapy with ifosfamide (Chaudhary & Haldas, 2003). Possible risk factors for developing renal toxicity in patients with normal baseline creatinine have not been addressed in the literature. Survivors should have magnesium, creatinine, and BUN levels monitored routinely. Nephrotoxic drugs should be avoided whenever possible.

Neurotoxicity and Ototoxicity

Peripheral neuropathy that occurs during or immediately after treatment usually resolves over time but may persist in 20%–40% of patients. Severe neurotoxicity, particularly motor dysfunction, which is not common but does occur, has been linked to preexisting neuropathy and decreased levels of serum magnesium (Bokemeyer et al., 1996; Vaughn et al., 2002).

Numerous agents have been tested for the prevention of neuropathy without any established effectiveness. Supportive nursing recommendations for intervention are limited to education, support, safety (e.g., keeping rooms and hallways free of clutter and throw rugs, ensuring shower safety, avoiding excess temperatures), and careful inspection of hands and feet for signs of injury or infection as sensation may be diminished. The efficacy of acupuncture, physical exercise, and spinal stimulation are under investigation (Visovsky, Collins, Hart, Abbott, & Aschenbrenner, 2007). Referral to a physiatrist or a rehabilitation or pain specialist can help patients to learn compensatory measures and assist with pain control.

Past studies have cited that 20% of patients will experience chronic tinnitus and hearing loss in the high-frequency range (Bokemeyer et al., 1996; Vaughn et al., 2002). A recent study by Biro et al. (2006), which used a new, highly sensitive method for detecting hearing loss, found that not only high frequencies are affected. In patients who received at least 400 mg/m^2 of cisplatin, significant hearing impairment was detected at lower frequencies important for speech perception (Fausti et al., 2005). Patients should be counseled to avoid excessive noise and to have any new tinnitus or hearing deficits evaluated. They also should be advised to discuss prior cisplatin exposure with their healthcare providers to avoid the use of ototoxic drugs, if possible.

Pulmonary Effects

Pulmonary fibrosis caused by bleomycin is an acute rather than a late effect of chemotherapy (Carver et al., 2007; Vaughn et al., 2002) but does have implications for survivors. The period of time when oxygen administration is safe following treatment with bleomycin is not yet clear. Therefore, current safeguards for anesthesia in patients exposed to bleomycin should include the use of the lowest required concentration of inspired oxygen and fluid replacement to prevent pulmonary edema. Patients treated with bleomycin should be instructed to inform surgeons, anesthesiologists, and all future healthcare providers of their treatment history so safeguards can be taken. Men should be advised not to scuba dive, as there is a potential risk of pulmonary damage from exposure to the high concentrations of oxygen necessary for diving (Huls & ten Bokkel Huinink, 2003). Patients who have received bleomycin may be advised to wear medi-cal alert bracelets in case of events where emergency oxygen may be necessary. As always, smoking should be avoided.

Secondary Cancers

Men who have been treated with chemotherapy or radiation have an increased risk of treatment-related secondary cancers including leukemia, lymphomas, and solid tumors (Gospodarowicz, 2008; Kondagunta et al., 2003; Travis et al., 1997). Secondary leukemia is the most serious complication of cured GCTs, and treatment has been found to be largely ineffective. Etoposide appears to carry much of the risk and may have a synergistic effect with cisplatin (Chaudhary & Haldas, 2003; Gospodarowicz; Travis et al.). The risk also is increased slightly for non-Hodgkin lymphoma, bladder, stomach, thyroid, and kidney cancers (Kaufman & Chang, 2007; Vaughn & Meadows, 2002). Patients should be informed of these risks prior to therapy as part of chemotherapy patient teaching. Patients should be followed closely by their oncologists or primary care providers for routine laboratory work, symptom assessment, and age-appropriate cancer screening.

Infertility

Infertility, though not life threatening, is a very distressing issue (Vaughn & Meadows, 2002), as men are usually diagnosed in the prime of their reproductive lives (Chaudhary & Haldas, 2003). It is difficult to assess the impact of chemotherapy on fertility, as up to 59% of patients with GCTs have decreased sperm counts before they are treated. The reason for the gonadal dysfunction is not completely understood (Botchan et al., 1997; Lampe, Horwich, Norman, Nicholls, & Dearnaley, 1997). After orchiectomy, even before chemotherapy, approximately one-third of patients who had been fertile will have impaired spermatogenesis (Chaudhary & Haldas; Poirier & Rawl, 2000). Patients who have undergone RPLND may be infertile because of retrograde ejaculation (Lampe et al.). Chemotherapy can further impair spermatogenesis, although some studies suggest that treating testicular cancer may even improve fertility (Vaughn et al., 2002). For patients treated with chemotherapy, recovery of fertility is dependent on the patient's age, pretreatment fertility, and cumulative chemotherapy. The inability to father children can have a significant impact on a man's self-perception, relationships, and outlook on life. Counseling prior to treatment is imperative.

Recovery of fertility depends on many factors: pretreatment oligospermia, chemotherapy and number of cycles, RPLND, age, and hormonal status. Some individuals, though, do regain fertility and successfully father children naturally. Men need to be informed about the reproductive implications and options concerning reproductive issues and be encouraged to sperm bank before treatment. When that is not possible or successful, and fertility is an important issue, they should be referred to a center specializing in assisted reproductive technologies (Vaughn et al., 2002).

Summary

Patients with testicular cancer have an excellent chance for cure and long-term survival because of the introduction of cisplatin-based chemotherapy. Chemotherapy is an essential part of curative therapy for many patients, especially those with advanced disease, but it is not without cost—physically and emotionally, acutely, and over time. Despite side effects, dose intensity and intervals between treatments should not be altered in the absence of unusually severe effects because of the excellent chance for cure.

The time surrounding diagnosis is extremely stressful for patients and their families, whether their treatment will involve chemotherapy, surgery, radiation, close surveillance, or a combination of strategies. Patients who have treatment options and must choose between chemotherapy, radiation, RPLND, or surveillance may be even more anxious concerning which option to choose and whether it will ultimately be the best choice. Nurses involved in the care of these men must be familiar with treatment protocols and the potential risks and benefits of each treatment. Knowledge of the specific treatments, options, and acute and long-term effects of each treatment is important in developing an individualized profile based on the patient's stage, prognosis, and risk factors. This information is imperative in enabling the nurse to develop a plan of care with the patient and to provide support, teaching, treatment, symptom management, long-term follow-up care, assistance with lifestyle modifications, and referrals for additional psychosocial care as needed. Nurses should be acquainted with questions to ask and signs and symptoms to monitor. Patients need teaching prior to treatment to understand their options and the rationale and consequences for each treatment modality. Information about acute and long-term side effects is especially important. Survivors need ongoing education and support concerning surveillance for early detection of disease recurrence and potential treatment sequelae, as well as assistance with strategies to enhance appropriate lifestyle modifications and compliance for life.

References

Abdel-Aziz, K.F., Anderson, J.K., Svatek, R., Margulis, V., Sagalowsky, A.I., & Cadeddu, J.A. (2006). Laparoscopic and open retroperitoneal lymph node dissection for clinical stage I nonseminomatous germ cell testis tumor. *Journal of Endourology, 20*(9), 627–631.

Ablan, C.J., Littooy, F.N., & Freeark, R.J. (1990). Postoperative chylous ascites: Diagnosis and treatment. A series report and literature review. *Archives of Surgery, 125*(2), 270–273.

Ackerman, B., & Kasbekar, N. (1997). Disturbances of taste and smell induced by drugs. *Pharmacotherapy, 17*(3), 482–496.

American Joint Committee on Cancer. (2002). *AJCC cancer staging manual* (6th ed.). New York: Springer.

Azambuja, E., Fleck, J.F., Batista, R.G., & Barreto, S.S.M. (2005). Bleomycin lung toxicity: Who are the patients with increased risk? *Pulmonary Pharmacology and Therapeutics, 18*(5), 363–366.

Baniel, J., Foster, R.S., Rowland, R.G., Bihrle, R., & Donohue, J.P. (1995). Complications of post-chemotherapy retroperitoneal lymph node dissection. *Journal of Urology, 153*(3, Pt. 2), 976–980.

Becherer, A., De Santis, M., Karanikas, G., Szabo, M., Bokemyer, C., Dohmen, B.M., et al. (2005). FDG PET is superior to CT in the prediction of viable tumour in post-chemotherapy seminoma residuals. *European Journal of Radiology, 54*(2), 284–288.

Beck, S.L. (2004). Mucositis. In C.H. Yarbro, M.H. Frogge, & M. Goodman (Eds.), *Cancer symptom management* (3rd ed., pp. 276–292). Sudbury, MA: Jones and Bartlett.

Benedetto, P. (1999). Chemotherapy of testicular cancer. *Cancer Control, 6*(6), 549–559.

Berger, C.C., Bokemeyer, C., Schneider, M., Kuczyk, M.A., & Schmoll, H.J. (1995). Secondary Raynaud's phenomenon and other late vascular complications following chemotherapy for testicular cancer. *European Journal of Cancer, 31A*(13–14), 2229–2238.

Bhatia, S., Abonour, R., Porcu, P., Seshadri, R., Nichols, C.R., Cornetta, K., et al. (2000). High-dose chemotherapy as initial salvage chemotherapy in patients with relapsed testicular cancer. *Journal of Clinical Oncology, 18*(19), 3346–3351.

Bhayani, S.B., Allaf, M.E., & Kavoussi, L.R. (2004). Laparoscopic RPLND for clinical stage I nonseminomatous germ cell testicular cancer: Current status. *Urologic Oncology, 22*(2), 145–148.

Biro, K., Noszek, L., Prekopp, P., Nagyivanyi, K., Geczi, L., Gaudi, I., et al. (2006). Characteristics and risk factors of cisplatin-induced ototoxicity in testicular cancer patients detected by distorsion product otoacoustic emission. *Oncology, 70*(3), 177–184.

Bokemeyer, C., Berger, C.C., Kuczyk, M.A., & Schmoll, H.J. (1996). Evaluation of long-term toxicity after chemotherapy for testicular cancer. *Journal of Clinical Oncology, 14*(11), 2923–2932.

Bokemeyer, C., Nowak, P., Haupt, A., Metzner, B., Kohne, H., Hartmann, J.T., et al. (1997). Treatment of brain metastasis in patients with testicular cancer. *Journal of Clinical Oncology, 15*(4), 1449–1454.

Bosl, G.J., Bajorin, D.F., Sheinfeld, J., Motzer, R.J., & Chaganti, R.S.K. (2005). Cancer of the testis. In V.T. DeVita Jr., S. Hellman, & S.A. Rosenberg (Eds.), *Cancer: Principles and practice of oncology* (7th ed., pp. 1269–1293). Philadelphia: Lippincott Williams & Wilkins.

Bosl, G.J., Leitner, S.P., Atlas, S.A., Sealey, J.E., Preibisz, J.J., & Scheiner, E. (1986). Increased plasma renin and aldosterone in patients treated with cisplatin-based chemotherapy for metastatic germ-cell tumors. *Journal of Clinical Oncology, 4*(11), 1684–1689.

Bosl, G.J., & Motzer, R.J. (1997). Testicular germ-cell cancer. *New England Journal of Medicine, 337*(4), 242–253.

Botchan, A., Hauser, R., Yogev, L., Gamzu, R., Paz, G., Lessing, J.B., et al. (1997). Testicular cancer and spermatogenesis. *Human Reproduction, 12*(4), 755–758.

Boyer, M., Raghavan, D., Harris, P.J., Lietch, J., Bleasel, A., Walsh, J.C., et al. (1990). Lack of late toxicity in patients treated with cisplatin-containing combination chemotherapy for metastatic testicular cancer. *Journal of Clinical Oncology, 8*(1), 21–26.

Brown, C.G. (2004). Testicular cancer: An overview. *Urologic Nursing, 24*(2), 83–94.

Camp, M.J., Gilmore, J.W., Gullatte, M.M., & Hutcherson, D.A. (2007). Antineoplastic agents. In M.M. Gullatte (Ed.), *Clinical guide to antineoplastic therapy: A chemotherapy handbook* (2nd ed., pp. 77–362). Pittsburgh, PA: Oncology Nursing Society.

Camp-Sorrell, D. (2000). Chemotherapy: Toxicity management. In C.H. Yarbro, M.H. Frogge, M. Goodman, & S.L. Groenwald (Eds.), *Cancer nursing: Principles and practice* (5th ed., pp. 444–486). Sudbury, MA: Jones and Bartlett.

Carver, J.R., Shapiro, C.L., Ng, A., Jacobs, L., Schwartz, C., Virgo, K.S., et al. (2007). American Society of Clinical Oncology clinical evidence review on the ongoing care of adult cancer survivors: Cardiac and pulmonary late effects. *Journal of Clinical Oncology, 25*(25), 3991–4008.

Cepeda, M.S., Carr, D.B., Miranda, N., Diaz, A., Silva, C., & Morales, O. (2005). Comparison of morphine, ketorolac and their combination for postoperative pain: Results from a large, randomized double-blind trial. *Anesthesiology, 103*(6), 1225–1232.

Chang, S.S., Smith, J.A., Jr., Girasole, C., Baumgartner, R.G., Roth, B.J., & Cookson, M.S. (2002). Beneficial impact of a clinical care pathway in patients with testicular cancer undergoing retroperitoneal lymph node dissection. *Journal of Urology, 168*(1), 87–92.

Chapple, A., & McPherson, A. (2004). The decision to have a prosthesis: A qualitative study of men with testicular cancer. *Psycho-Oncology, 13*(9), 654–664.

Chaudhary, U.B., & Haldas, J.R. (2003). Long-term complications of chemotherapy for germ cell tumours. *Drugs, 63*(15), 1565–1577.

Choo, R., Thomas, G., Woo, T., Lee, D., Kong, B., Iscoe, N., et al. (2005). Long-term outcome of postorchiectomy surveillance for Stage I testicular seminoma. *International Journal of Radiation Oncology, Biology, Physics, 61*(3), 736–740.

Christoph, F., Weikert, S., Miller, K., & Schrader, M. (2005). New guidelines for clinical stage I testicular seminoma? *Oncology, 69*(6), 455–462.

Classen, J., Dieckmann, K.P., Loy, V., & Bamberg, M. (1998). Die testikuläre intraepitheliale Neoplasie (TIN). Indikation zur Strahlentherapie? [Testicular intraepithelial neoplasms (TIN). An indication for radiotherapy?] *Strahlentherapie und Onkologie, 174*(4), 173–177.

Classen, J., Dieckmann, K., Bamberg, M., Souchon, R., Kliesch, S., Kuehn, M., et al. (2003). Radiotherapy with 16 Gy may fail to eradicate testicular intraepithelial neoplasia: Preliminary communication of a dose reduction trial of the German Testicular Cancer Study Group. *British Journal of Cancer, 88*(6), 828–831.

Classen, J., Souchon, R., Hehr, T., & Bamberg, M. (2001). Treatment of early stage testicular seminoma. *Journal of Cancer Research and Clinical Oncology, 127*(8), 475–481.

Collette, L., Sylvester, R.J., Stenning, S.P., Fossa, S.D., Mead, G.M., de Wit, R., et al. (1999). Impact of the treating institution on survival of patients with "poor-prognosis" metastatic nonseminoma. European Organization for Research and Treatment of Cancer Genito-Urinary Tract Cancer Collaborative Group and the Medical Research Council Testicular Cancer Working Party. *Journal of the National Cancer Institute, 91*(10), 839–846.

Correa, J.J., Politis, C., Rodriguez, A.R., & Pow-Sang, J.M. (2007). Laparoscopic retroperitoneal lymph node dissection in the management of testicular cancer. *Cancer Control, 14*(3), 258–264.

Coyne, B.M., & Leslie, M.L. (2004). Chemo's toll on memory. *RN, 67*(4), 40–43.

Culine, S., Kerbrat, P., Bouzy, J., Theodore, C., Biron, P., Chevreau, C., et al. (2003). The optimal chemotherapy regimen for good-risk metastatic non seminomatous germ cell tumors (MNSGCT) is 3 cycles of bleomycin, etoposide and cisplatin: Mature results of a randomized trial [Abstract]. *Proceedings of the American Society of Clinical Oncology, 22,* 188.

Daugaard, G., Karas, V., & Sommer, P. (2006). Inguinal metastasis from testicular cancer. *BJU International, 97*(4), 724–726.

De Santis, M., Becherer, A., Bokemeyer, C., Stoiber, F., Oechsle, K., Sellner, F., et al. (2004). 2-18fluoro-deoxy-D-glucose posi-

tron emission tomography is a reliable predictor for viable tumor in postchemotherapy seminoma: An update of the prospective multicentric SEMPET trial. *Journal of Clinical Oncology, 22*(6), 1034–1039.

de Wit, R., & Fizazi, K. (2006). Controversies in the management of clinical stage I testicular cancer. *Journal of Clinical Oncology, 24*(35), 5482–5492.

de Wit, R., Herrstedt, J., Rapoport, B., Carides, A.D., Guoguang-Ma, J., Elmer, M., et al. (2004). The oral NK1 antagonist, aprepitant, given with standard antiemetics provides protection against nausea and vomiting over multiple cycles of cisplatin based chemotherapy: A combined analysis of two randomized, placebo controlled phase III clinical trials. *European Journal of Cancer, 40*(3), 403–410.

de Wit, R., Roberts, J.T., Wilkinson, P.M., de Mulder, P.H., Mead, G.M., Fossa, S.D., et al. (2001). Equivalence of three or four cycles of bleomycin, etoposide, and cisplatin chemotherapy and of a 3- or 5-day schedule in good-prognosis germ cell cancer: A randomized study of the European Organization for Research and Treatment of Cancer Genitourinary Tract Cancer Cooperative Group and the Medical Research Council. *Journal of Clinical Oncology, 19*(6), 1629–1640.

de Wit, R., Stoter, G., Kaye, S.B., Sleijfer, D.T., Jones, W.G., ten Bokkel Huinink, W.W., et al. (1997). Importance of bleomycin in combination chemotherapy for good-prognosis testicular nonseminoma: A randomized study of the European Organization for Research and Treatment of Cancer Genitourinary Tract Cancer Cooperative Group. *Journal of Clinical Oncology, 15*(5), 1837–1843.

Dieckmann, K.P., Classen, J., & Loy, V. (2003). Diagnosis and management of testicular intraepithelial neoplasia (carcinoma in situ)—surgical aspects. *APMIS: Acta Pathologica, Microbiologica, et Immunologica Scandinavica, 111*(1), 64–68.

Dodd, P.M.K., & Kelly, W.M. (2001). Testicular cancer. In R.E. Lenhard, R.T. Osteen, & T. Gansler (Eds.), *Clinical oncology* (pp. 419–426). Atlanta, GA: American Cancer Society.

Donat, S.M. (1999). Perioperative care in patients treated for testicular cancer. *Seminars in Surgical Oncology, 17*(4), 282–288.

Donat, S.M., & Levy, D.A. (1998). Bleomycin associated pulmonary toxicity: Is perioperative oxygen restriction necessary? *Journal of Urology, 160*(4), 1347–1352.

Donohue, J.P. (2003). Evolution of retroperitoneal lymphadenectomy (RPLND) in the management of non-seminomatous testicular cancer (NSGCT). *Urologic Oncology, 21*(2), 129–132.

Donohue, J.P., Leviovitch, L., Foster, R.S., Baniel, J., & Tognoni, P. (1998). Integration of surgery and systemic therapy: Results and principles of integration. *Seminars in Urologic Oncology, 16*(2), 65–71.

Donohue, J.P., Zachary, J.M., & Maynard, B.R. (1982). Distribution of nodal metastases in nonseminomatous testicular cancer. *Journal of Urology, 128*(2), 315–320.

Dougherty, L., & Bailey, C. (2001). Chemotherapy. In J.B. Corner & C. Bailey (Eds.), *Cancer nursing: Care in context*. London: Blackwell Science.

Eastham, J.A., Wilson, T.G., Russell, C., Ahlering, T.E., & Skinner, D.G. (1994). Surgical resection in patients with nonseminomatous germ cell tumor who fail to normalize serum tumor markers after chemotherapy. *Urology, 43*(1), 74–80.

Efstathiou, E., & Logothetis, C.J. (2006). Review of late complications of treatment and late relapse in testicular cancer. *Journal of the National Comprehensive Cancer Network, 4*(10), 1059–1070.

Einhorn, L.H. (1990). Treatment of testicular cancer: A new and improved model. *Journal of Clinical Oncology, 8*(11), 1777–1781.

Einhorn, L.H. (2002). Curing metastatic testicular cancer. *Proceedings of the National Academy of Sciences, 99*(7), 4592–4595.

Einhorn, L.H., & Donohue, J. (1977). Cis-diamminedichloroplatinum, vinblastine, and bleomycin combination chemotherapy in disseminated testicular cancer. *Annals of Internal Medicine, 87*(3), 293–298.

Einhorn, L.H., Williams, S.D., Chamness, A., Brames, M.J., Perkins, S.M., & Abonour, R. (2007). High-dose chemotherapy and stem-cell rescue for metastatic germ-cell tumors. *New England Journal of Medicine, 357*(4), 340–348.

Fausti, S.A., Wilmington, D.J., Helt, P.V., Helt, W.J., & Konrad-Martin, D. (2005). Hearing health and care: The need for improved hearing loss prevention and hearing conservation practices. *Journal of Rehabilitation Research and Development, 42*(4, Suppl. 2), 45–62.

Ferraz, A.A., Cowles, V.E., Condon, R.E., Carilli, S., Ezberci, F., Fraztzides, C.T., et al. (1995). Nonopioid analgesics shorten the duration of postoperative ileus. *American Surgeon, 61*(12), 1079–1083.

Finelli, A. (2008). Laparoscopic retroperitoneal lymph node dissection for nonseminomatous germ cell tumors: Long term oncologic outcomes. *Current Opinion in Urology, 18*(2), 180–184.

Fischbach, F., & Dunning, M.B. (2006). *Nurses' quick reference to common laboratory and diagnostic tests* (7th ed.). Philadelphia: Lippincott Williams & Wilkins.

Fossa, S.D., de Wit, R., Roberts, J.T., Wilkinson, P.M., de Mulder, P.H., Mead, G.M., et al. (2003). Quality of life in good prognosis patients with metastatic germ cell cancer: A prospective study of the European Organization for Research and Treatment of Cancer Genitourinary Group/Medical Research Council Testicular Cancer Study Group (30941/TE20). *Journal of Clinical Oncology, 21*(6), 1107–1118.

Fossa, S.D., Horwich, A., Russell, J.M., Roberts, J.T., Cullen, M.H., Hodson, N.J., et al. (1999). Optimal planning target volume for stage I testicular seminoma: A Medical Research Council randomized trial. Medical Research Council Testicular Tumor Working Group. *Journal of Clinical Oncology, 17*(4), 1146–1150.

Fossa, S.D., Kaye, S.B., Mead, G.M., Cullen, M., de Wit, R., Bodrogi, I., et al. (1998). Filgrastim during combination chemotherapy of patients with poor-prognosis metastatic germ cell malignancy. European Organization for Research and Treatment of Cancer, Genito-Urinary Group, and the Medical Research Council Testicular Cancer Working Party, Cambridge, United Kingdom. *Journal of Clinical Oncology, 16*(2), 716–724.

Foster, R., & Bihrle, R. (2002). Current status of retroperitoneal lymph node dissection and testicular cancer: When to operate. *Cancer Control, 9*(4), 277–283.

Friedman, H.M., Sheetz, S., Levine, H.L., Everett, J.R., & Hong, W.K. (1986). Combination chemotherapy and radiation therapy. The medical management of epidural spinal cord compression from testicular cancer. *Archives of Internal Medicine, 146*(3), 509–512.

Gerl, A. (1994). Vascular toxicity associated with chemotherapy for testicular cancer. *Anticancer Drugs, 5*(6), 607–614.

Goodman, M. (2000). Chemotherapy: Principles of administration. In C.H. Yarbro, M.H. Frogge, M. Goodman, & S.L. Groenwald (Eds.), *Cancer nursing: Principles and practice* (5th ed., pp. 385–443). Sudbury, MA: Jones and Bartlett.

Gospodarowicz, M. (2008). Testicular cancer patients: Considerations in long term care. *Hematology/Oncology Clinics of North America, 22*(2), 245–255.

Grande, N.R., Peao, M.N.D., de Sa, C.M., & Aguas, A.P. (1998). Lung fibrosis induced by bleomycin: Structural changes and overview of recent advances. *Scanning Microscopy, 12*(3), 487–494.

Gray, M. (2005). Management of men with reproductive disorders. In J.M. Black & J.H. Hawks (Eds.), *Medical-surgical nursing: Clinical management for positive patient outcomes* (7th ed., pp. 1013–1051). St. Louis, MO: Elsevier Saunders.

Grundy, S.M., Pasternak, R., Greenland, P., Smith, S., Jr., & Fuster, V. (1999). AHA/ACC scientific statement: Assessment of cardiovascular risk by use of multiple-risk-factor assessment equations: A statement for healthcare professionals from the American Heart Association and the American College of Cardiology. *Journal of the American College of Cardiology, 34*(4), 1348–1359.

Hawkins, C., & Miaskowski, C. (1996). Testicular cancer: A review. *Oncology Nursing Forum, 23*(8), 1203–1211.

Heidenreich, A. (2004). Organ preserving surgery in testicular tumors. In S.D. Graham, J.F. Glenn, & T.E. Keane (Eds.), *Glenn's urological surgery* (6th ed., pp. 501–504). Philadelphia: Lippincott Williams & Wilkins.

Heidenreich, A., Weissbach, L., Holtl, W., Albers, P., Kliesch, S., Kohrmann, K.U., et al. (2001). Organ sparing surgery for malignant germ cell tumor of the testis. *Journal of Urology, 166*(6), 2161–2165.

Hennessy, B., O'Connor, M., & Carney, D.N. (2002). Acute vascular events associated with cisplatin therapy in malignant disease. *Irish Medical Journal, 95*(5), 145–146, 148.

Herr, H.W., Sheinfeld, J., Puc, H.S., Heelan, R., Bajorin, D.F., Mecel, P., et al. (1997). Surgery for post-chemotherapy residual mass in seminoma. *Journal of Urology, 157*(3), 860–862.

Hickey, J. (2003). Overview of neuroanatomy and neurophysiology. In J. Hickey (Ed.), *The clinical practice of neurological and neurosurgical nursing* (pp. 45–87). Philadelphia: Lippincott Williams & Wilkins.

Hirata, H., Arima, M., Fukushima, Y., Ishii, Y., Tokushisa, T., & Fukuda, T. (2008). Effects of Th2 pulmonary inflammation in mice with bleomycin-induced pulmonary fibrosis. *Respirology, 13*(6), 788–798.

Horwich, A., Shipley, J., & Huddart, R. (2006). Testicular germ-cell cancer. *Lancet, 367*(9512), 754–765.

Huddart, R.A., Norman, A., Shahidi, M., Horwich, A., Coward, D., Nicholls, J., et al. (2003). Cardiovascular disease as a long-term complication of treatment for testicular cancer. *Journal of Clinical Oncology, 21*(8), 1513–1523.

Huls, G., & ten Bokkel Huinink, D. (2003). Bleomycin and scuba diving: To dive or not to dive. *Netherlands Journal of Medicine, 61*(2), 50–53.

Ingrassia, T.S., III, Ryu, J.H., Trastek, V.F., & Rosenow, E.C., III. (1991). Oxygen-exacerbated bleomycin pulmonary toxicity. *Mayo Clinic Proceedings, 66*(2), 173–178.

International Germ Cell Cancer Collaborative Group. (1997). International germ cell consensus classification: A prognostic factor-based staging system for metastatic germ cell cancers. *Journal of Clinical Oncology, 15*(2), 594–603.

Janetschek, G., Hobisch, A., Peschel, R., & Bartsch, G. (2000). Laparoscopic retroperitoneal lymph node dissection. *Urology, 55*(1), 136–140.

Jankilevich, G. (2004). BEP versus EP for treatment of metastatic germ-cell tumours. *Lancet Oncology, 5*(3), 146–147.

Jones, R.H., & Vasey, P.A. (2003). Part II: Testicular cancer—management of advanced disease. *Lancet Oncology, 4*(12), 738–747.

Jones, W.G., Fossa, S.D., Mead, G.M., Roberts, J.T., Sokal, M., Horwich, A., et al. (2005). Randomized trial of 30 versus 20 Gy in the adjuvant treatment of stage I testicular seminoma: A report on Medical Research Council Trial TE18, European Organisation for the Research and Treatment of Cancer Trial 30942 (ISRCTN 18525328). *Journal of Clinical Oncology, 23*(6), 1200–1208.

Katz, P.O. (2003). Disorders of the esophagus, dysphagia, noncardiac chest pain, and gastric reflux. In L. Barker, J.R. Burton, & P.D. Zieve (Eds.), *Principles of ambulatory medicine* (6th ed., pp. 571–583). Philadelphia: Lippincott Williams & Wilkins.

Kaufman, M.R., & Chang, S.S. (2007). Short- and long-term complications of therapy for testicular cancer. *Urologic Clinics of North America, 34*(2), 259–268.

Keijzer, A., & Kuenen, B. (2007). Fatal pulmonary toxicity in testicular cancer with bleomycin containing chemotherapy. *Journal of Clinical Oncology, 25*(23), 3543–3549.

Khatcheressian, J.L., Wolff, A.C., Smith, T.J., Grunfeld, E., Muss, H.B., Vogel, V.G., et al. (2006). American Society of Clinical Oncology 2006 update of the breast cancer follow-up and management guidelines in the adjuvant setting. *Journal of Clinical Oncology, 24*(31), 5091–5097.

King, R.S. (2001). Drug interactions in the cancer chemotherapy patient. In M. Barton-Burke, G.M. Wilkes, & K.C. Ingwersen (Eds.), *Cancer chemotherapy: A nursing process approach* (3rd ed., pp. 534–558). Sudbury, MA: Jones and Bartlett.

Kollmannsberger, C., Nichols, C., & Bokemeyer, C. (2006). Recent advances in management of patients with platinum-refractory testicular germ cell tumors. *Cancer, 106*(6), 1217–1226.

Kondagunta, G.V., Bacik, J., Donadio, A., Bajorin, D., Marion, S., Sheinfeld, J., et al. (2005). Combination of paclitaxel, ifosfamide, and cisplatin is an effective second-line therapy for patients with relapsed testicular germ cell tumors. *Journal of Clinical Oncology, 23*(27), 6549–6555.

Kondagunta, G.V., & Motzer, R.J. (2006). Chemotherapy for advanced germ cell tumors. *Journal of Clinical Oncology, 24*(35), 5493–5502.

Kondagunta, G.V., & Motzer, R.J. (2007). Adjuvant chemotherapy for stage II nonseminomatous germ cell tumors. *Urologic Clinics of North America, 34*(2), 179–185.

Kondagunta, G.V., Sheinfeld, J., & Motzer, R.J. (2003). Recommendations of follow-up after treatment of germ cell tumors. *Seminars in Oncology, 30*(3), 382–389.

Kopp, H.G., Kuczyk, M., Classen, J., Stenzl, A., Kanz, L., Mayer, F., et al. (2006). Advances in the treatment of testicular cancer. *Drugs, 66*(5), 641–659.

Lampe, H., Horwich, A., Norman, A., Nicholls, J., & Dearnaley, D.P. (1997). Fertility after chemotherapy for testicular germ cell cancers. *Journal of Clinical Oncology, 15*(1), 239–245.

Lasky, J., & Ortiz, L. (2005). *Bleomycin induced lung toxicity* [UpToDate]. Retrieved June 24, 2008, from http://www.uptodate.com/online/content/topic.do?topicKey=cc_medi/20009&selectedTitle=3~150&source=search_result#11

Lee, J.T., & Calcaterra, T.C. (1998). Testicular carcinoma metastatic to the neck. *American Journal of Otolaryngology, 19*(5), 325–329.

Leibovitch, I., Mor, Y., Golomb, J., & Ramon, J. (2002). The diagnosis and management of postoperative chylous ascites. *Journal of Urology, 167*(2, Pt. 1), 449–457.

Liaw, C.C., Wang, C.H., Chang, H.K., Wang, H.M., Huang, J.S., Lin, Y.C., et al. (2005). Cisplatin-related hiccups: Male predominance, induction by dexamethasone, and protection against nausea and vomiting. *Journal of Pain and Symptom Management, 30*(4), 359–366.

Link, R.E., Amin, N., & Kavoussi, L.R. (2006). Chylous ascites following retroperitoneal lymphadenectomy for testes cancer. *Nature Clinical Practice: Urology, 3*(4), 226–232.

Loehrer, P.J., Sr., Johnson, D., Elson, P., Einhorn, L.H., & Trump, D. (1995). Importance of bleomycin in favorable-prognosis disseminated germ cell tumors: An Eastern Cooperative Oncology Group trial. *Journal of Clinical Oncology, 13*(2), 470–476.

Malhotra, A., Schwartz, D., & Schwartzstein, R. (2007). *Oxygen toxicity* [UpToDate]. Retrieved June 24, 2008, from http://www.uptodate.com/online/content/topic.do?topicKey=cc_medi/20009&selectedTitle=3~150&source=search_result#11

Massey, R.L., Haycock, P.J., & Curtiss, C. (2004). Constipation. In C.H. Yarbro, M.H. Frogge, & M. Goodman (Eds.), *Cancer symptom management* (3rd ed., pp. 512–524). Sudbury, MA: Jones and Bartlett.

Masters, J.R., & Koberle, B. (2003). Curing metastatic cancer: Lessons from testicular germ-cell tumours. *Nature Reviews Cancer, 3*(7), 517–525.

McCullagh, J., & Lewis, G. (2005). Testicular cancer: Epidemiology, assessment and management. *Nursing Standard, 19*(25), 45–53.

McKiernan, J.M., Motzer, R.J., Bajorin, D.F., Bacik, J., Bosl, G.J., & Sheinfeld, J. (2003). Reoperative retroperitoneal surgery for nonseminomatous germ cell tumors: Clinical presentation, patterns of recurrence and outcomes. *Urology, 62*(4), 732–736.

Meinardi, M.T., Gietema, J.A., van der Graaf, W.T., van Veldhuisen, D.J., Runne, M.A., Sluiter, W.J., et al. (2000). Cardiovascular morbidity in long-term survivors of metastatic testicular cancer. *Journal of Clinical Oncology, 18*(8), 1725–1732.

Meinardi, M.T., Gietema, J.A., van Veldhuisen, D.J., van der Graaf, W.T., de Vries, E.G., & Sleijfer, D.T. (2000). Long-term chemotherapy-related cardiovascular morbidity. *Cancer Treatment Reviews, 26*(6), 429–447.

Mock, V., Atkinson, A., Barsevick, A., Cella, D., Cimprich, B., Cleeland, C., et al. (2000). NCCN practice guidelines for cancer-related fatigue. *Oncology, 14*(11A), 151–161.

Morrow, G.R. (2007). Cancer-related fatigue: Causes, consequences, and management. *Oncologist, 12*(Suppl. 1), 1–3.

Morton, G.C., & Thomas, G.M. (2004). Testis. In C. Perez, L. Brady, E. Halperin, & R. Schmidt-Ullrich (Eds.), *Principles and practice of radiation oncology* (4th ed., pp. 1763–1784). Philadelphia: Lippincott Williams & Wilkins.

Murphy, B.R., Breeden, E.S., Donohue, J.P., Messemer, J., Walsh, W., Roth, B.J., et al. (1993). Surgical salvage of chemorefractory germ cell tumors. *Journal of Clinical Oncology, 11*(2), 324–329.

Nail, L.M. (2004). Fatigue. In C.H. Yarbro, M.H. Frogge, & M. Goodman (Eds.), *Cancer symptom management* (3rd ed., pp. 47–60). Sudbury, MA: Jones and Bartlett.

National Cancer Institute. (2009, January 15). *Testicular cancer treatment.* Retrieved February 2, 2008, from http://www.cancer.gov/cancertopics/pdq/treatment/testicular/healthprofessional

National Comprehensive Cancer Network. (2009). *NCCN Clinical Practice Guidelines in Oncology™: Testicular cancer* [v.2.2009]. Retrieved January 30, 2009, from http://www.nccn.org/professionals/physician_gls/PDF/testicular.pdf

Navari, R.M. (2007). Prevention of emesis from multiple-day and high dose chemotherapy regimens. *Journal of the National Comprehensive Cancer Network, 5*(1), 51–59.

Neill, M., Warde, P., & Fleshner, N. (2007). Management of low-stage testicular seminoma. *Urologic Clinics of North America, 34*(2), 127–136.

Neyer, M., Peschel, R., Akkad, T., Springer-Stohr, B., Berger, A., Bartsch, G., et al. (2007). Long-term results of laparoscopic retroperitoneal lymph node dissection for clinical stage nonseminomatous germ cell testicular cancer. *Journal of Endourology, 21*(2), 180–183.

Ohl, D.A., & Sonksen, J. (1996). What are the chances of infertility and should sperm be banked? *Seminars in Urologic Oncology, 14*(1), 36–44.

Oliver, R.T., Mason, M.D., Mead, G.M., von der Maase, H., Rustin, G.J., Joffe, J.K., et al. (2005). Radiotherapy versus single-dose carboplatin in adjuvant treatment of stage I seminoma: A randomised trial. *Lancet, 366*(9482), 293–300.

Oliver, R.T., Mead, G.M., Fogarty, P.J., Stenning, S.P., & MRC TE19 and EORTC 30982 Trial Collaborators. (2008). Radiotherapy versus carboplatin for stage I seminoma: Updated analysis of the MRC/EORTC randomized trial (ISRCTN27163214) [Abstract]. *Journal of Clinical Oncology, 26*(15S), Abstract 1.

Oldenburg, J., Fossa, S.D., & Dahl, A.A. (2006). Scale for chemotherapy-induced long-term neurotoxicity (SCIN): Psychometrics, validation, and findings in a large sample of testicular cancer survivors. *Quality of Life Research, 15*(5), 791–800.

Oosterhof, G.O., & Verlind, J. (2004). Testicular tumours (nonseminomatous). *BJU International, 94*(8), 1196–1201.

Polovich, M., White, J., & Kelleher, L.O. (Eds.). (2005). *Chemotherapy and biotherapy guidelines and recommendations for practice* (2nd ed.). Pittsburgh, PA: Oncology Nursing Society.

Poirier, S.M., & Rawl, S.M. (2000). Testicular germ cell cancer. In C.H. Yarbro, M.H. Frogge, M. Goodman, & S.L. Groenwald (Eds.), *Cancer nursing: Principles and practice* (5th ed., pp. 1494–1510). Sudbury, MA: Jones and Bartlett.

Putra, L., Lawrentschuk, N., Ballok, Z., Hannah, A., Poon, A., Tauro, A., et al. (2004). 18F-fluorodeoxyglucose positron emission tomography in evaluation of germ cell tumor after chemotherapy. *Urology, 64*(6), 1202–1207.

Raghavan, D. (2006, June). *Bladder, renal, and testicular cancer: Germ cell tumors of the testis.* Retrieved August 25, 2007, from http://www.medscape.com/viewarticle/534555

Ross, J., Eledrisi, M., & Casner, P. (1999). Persistent hiccups induced by dexamethasone. *Western Journal of Medicine, 170*(1), 51–52.

Schmoll, H.J., Souchon, R., Krege, S., Albers, P., Beyer, J., Kollmannsberger, C., et al. (2004). European consensus on diagnosis and treatment of germ cell cancer: A report of the European Germ Cell Cancer Consensus Group (EGCCCG). *Annals of Oncology, 15*(9), 1377–1399.

Schwartzberg, L.S. (2007). Chemotherapy induced nausea and vomiting: Which antiemetic for which therapy? *Oncology, 21*(8), 946–953.

Schuchter, L.M., Hensley, M.L., Meropol, N.J., & Winer, E.P. (2002). Update of recommendations for the use of chemotherapy and radiotherapy protectants: Clinical practice guidelines of the American Society of Clinical Oncology. *Journal of Clinical Oncology, 20*(12), 2895–2903.

Sherry, V.W. (2002). Taste alterations among patients with cancer. *Clinical Journal of Oncology Nursing, 6*(2), 73–77.

Sheinfeld, J., Bartsch, G., & Bosl, G.J. (2007). Surgery of testicular tumors. In A.J. Wein, L.R. Kavoussi, A.C. Novick, A.W. Partin, & C.A. Peters (Eds.), *Campbell-Walsh urology* (9th ed., pp. 936–958). Philadelphia: Saunders.

Smalley, S.R., Earle, J.D., Evans, R.G., & Richardson, R.L. (1990). Modern radiotherapy results with bulky stages II and III seminoma. *Journal of Urology, 144*(3), 685–689.

Sobin, L.H., & Whittekind, C. (Eds.). (1997). *International Union Against Cancer TNM classification of malignant tumours* (5th ed.). New York: John Wiley and Sons.

Staat, K., & Segatore, M. (2003). The phenomenon of chemo brain. *Clinical Journal of Oncology Nursing, 9*(6), 713–721.

Steele, G.S., & Richie, J. (2007, May 29). *Retroperitoneal lymph node dissection* [UpToDate]. Retrieved June 24, 2008, from http://utdonline.com

Stein, M.E., Leviov, M., Drumea, K., Moshkovitz, B., Nativ, O., Milstein, D., et al. (1998). Radiation induced tumors in irradiated stage I testicular seminoma: Results of a 25-year follow-up (1968-1993). *Journal of Surgical Oncology, 67*(1), 38–40.

Stephenson, A.J., & Sheinfeld, J. (2004). The role of retroperitoneal lymph node dissection in the management of testicular cancer. *Urologic Oncology, 22*(3), 225–235.

Stephenson, A.J., Tal, R., & Sheinfeld, J. (2006). Adjunctive nephrectomy at post-chemotherapy retroperitoneal lymph node dissection for nonseminomatous germ cell testicular cancer. *Journal of Urology, 176*(5), 1996–1999.

Stevenson, T.D., & McNeill, J.A. (2004). Surgical management of testicular cancer. *Clinical Journal of Oncology Nursing, 8*(4), 355–359.

Strumberg, D., Brugge, S., Korn, M.W., Koeppen, S., Ranft, J., Scheiber, G., et al. (2002). Evaluation of long-term toxicity in patients after cisplatin-based chemotherapy for non-seminomatous testicular cancer. *Annals of Oncology, 13*(2), 229–236.

Tipton, J., McDaniel, R., Barbour, L., Johnston, M.P., LeRoy, P., Kayne, M., et al. (2006). *Putting evidence into practice: Nausea and vomiting.* Pittsburgh, PA: Oncology Nursing Society.

Trasler, J.M., & Doerksen, T. (1999). Teratogen update: Paternal exposures-reproductive risks. *Teratology, 60*(3), 161–172.

Travis, L.B., Curtis, R.E., Storm, H., Hall, P., Holowaty, E., Van Leeuwen, F.E., et al. (1997). Risk of second malignant neoplasms among long-term survivors of testicular cancer. *Journal of the National Cancer Institute, 89*(19), 1429–1439.

Turkoski, B.B., Lance, B.R., & Bonfiglio, M.F. (2007). *Drug information handbook for advance practice nursing* (8th ed., pp. 950–953). Philadelphia: Lippincott Williams & Wilkins.

van Leeuwen, F.E., Stiggelbout, A.M., van den Belt-Dusebout, A.W., Noyon, R., Eliel, M.R., van Kerkhoff, E.H., et al. (1993). Second cancer risk following testicular cancer: A follow-up study of 1,909 patients. *Journal of Clinical Oncology, 11*(3), 415–424.

Vardy, J., Chiew, K.S., Galica, J., Pond, G.R., & Tannock, I.F. (2006). Side effects associated with the use of dexamethasone for prophylaxis of delayed emesis after moderately emetogenic chemotherapy. *British Journal of Cancer, 94*(7), 1011–1015.

Vaughn, D.J. (2007). Chemotherapy for good-risk germ cell tumors: Current concepts and controversies. *Urologic Clinics of North America, 34*(2), 171–177.

Vaughn, D.J., Gignac, G.A., & Meadows, A.T. (2002). Long-term medical care of testicular cancer survivors. *Annals of Internal Medicine, 136*(6), 463–470.

Vaughn, D.J., & Meadows, A.T. (2002). Cancer survivorship research: The best is yet to come. *Journal of Clinical Oncology, 20*(4), 888–890.

Visovsky, C., Collins, M.L., Hart, C., Abbott, L.I., & Aschenbrenner, J.A. (2007). *Putting evidence into practice: Peripheral neuropathy.* Pittsburgh, PA: Oncology Nursing Society.

Wickham, R.S., Rehwaldt, M., Kefer, C., Shott, S., Abbas, K., & Glynn-Tucker, E. (1999). Taste changes experienced by patients receiving chemotherapy. *Oncology Nursing Forum, 26*(4), 697–706.

Wilkes, G.M. (2001). Potential toxicities and nursing management. In M. Barton-Burke, G.M. Wilkes, & K.C. Ingwersen (Eds.), *Cancer chemotherapy: A nursing process approach* (3rd ed., pp. 89–186). Sudbury, MA: Jones and Bartlett.

Wilkes, G.M. (2004). Peripheral neuropathy. In C.H. Yarbro, M.H. Frogge, & M. Goodman (Eds.), *Cancer symptom management* (3rd ed., pp. 333–358). Sudbury, MA: Jones and Bartlett.

Willan, B.D., & McGowan, D.G. (1985). Seminoma of the testis: A 22-year experience with radiation therapy. *International Journal of Radiation Oncology, Biology, Physics, 11*(10), 1769–1775.

Williams, M.F. (2003). Selected disorders of the nose and throat: Epistaxis, snoring, anosmia, hoarseness, and hiccups. In L. Barker, J.R. Burton, & P.D. Zieve (Eds.), *Principles of ambulatory medicine* (6th ed., pp.1698–1711). Philadelphia: Lippincott Williams & Wilkins.

Williams, S.D., Birch, R., Einhorn, L.H., Irwin, L., Greco, F.A., & Loehrer, P.J. (1987). Treatment of disseminated germ-cell tumors with cisplatin, bleomycin, and either vinblastine or etoposide. *New England Journal of Medicine, 316*(23), 1435–1440.

Williams, S.D., Einhorn, L.H., Greco, F.A., Oldham, R., & Fletcher, R. (1980). VP-16-213 salvage therapy for refractory germinal neoplasms. *Cancer, 46*(10), 2154–2158.

Williams, S.D., Stablein, D.M., Einhorn, L.H., Muggia, F.M., Weiss, R.B., Donohue, J.P., et al. (1987). Immediate adjuvant chemotherapy versus observation with treatment at relapse in pathologic stage II testicular cancer. *New England Journal of Medicine, 317*(23), 1433–1438.

Wood, D.P., Herr, H.W., Motzer, R.J., Reuter, V., Sogani, P.C., Morse, M.J., et al. (1992). Surgical resection of solitary metastases after chemotherapy in patients with nonseminomatous germ cell tumors and elevated serum tumor markers. *Cancer, 70*(9), 2354–2357.

Wujcik, D. (2004). Infection. In C.H. Yarbro, M.H. Frogge, & M. Goodman (Eds.), *Cancer symptom management* (3rd ed., pp. 252–275). Sudbury, MA: Jones and Bartlett.

Yossepowitch, O., & Baniel, J. (2004). Role of organ-sparing surgery in germ cell tumors of the testis. *Urology, 63*(3), 421–427.

Zack, E. (2005). Testicular Cancer. In C.H. Yarbro, M.H. Frogge, & M. Goodman (Eds.), *Cancer nursing: Principles and practice* (6th ed., pp. 1630–1646). Sudbury, MA: Jones and Bartlett.

Zagars, G.K., Ballo, M.T., Lee, A.K., & Strom, S.S. (2004). Mortality after cure of testicular seminoma. *Journal of Clinical Oncology, 22*(4), 640–647.

Zitella, L., Friese, C., Gobel, B.H., Woolery-Antill, M., O'Leary, C., Hauser, J., et al. (2006). *Putting evidence into practice: Prevention of infection.* Pittsburgh, PA: Oncology Nursing Society.

Zoltick, B.H., Jacobs, L.A., & Vaughn, D.J. (2005). Cardiovascular risk in testicular cancer survivors treated with chemotherapy: Incidence, significance, and practice implications. *Oncology Nursing Forum, 32*(5), 1005–1009.

Sexual Function and Sexual Rehabilitation With Genitourinary Cancer

Jeffrey Albaugh, PhD, APRN, CUCNS, Susan Kellogg-Spadt, PhD, CRNP,
Linda U. Krebs, PhD, RN, AOCN®, FAAN, Jean H. Lewis, BSN, APRN-C, ANP, and
Denise Kramer-Levien, BA, CURN

Introduction

Sexuality and intimacy are an integral part of the human experience, which is shaped by biologic, psychological, spiritual, and social factors. Human beings crave intimate relationships with others, and most Americans prefer a long-term commitment with a sexual partner (Laumann, Gagnon, Michael, & Michaels, 2000). Intimacy is a process by which people move toward deeper communication and understanding on multiple levels (Hatfield, 1982). Although sexual function and intimacy are important aspects of life, it is probably one of the least addressed aspects of patient care. Among men already seeking medical care in an office setting, less than 50% sought treatment for sexual dysfunction because they thought it might get better or was a normal part of the aging process, or they were embarrassed (Shabsigh, Perelman, Laumann, & Lockhart, 2004). Even in urology care settings, many patients are unlikely to bring up the subject of sexual dysfunction (Baldwin, Ginsberg, & Harkaway, 2003). Healthcare providers are no better at addressing sexual issues with patients. Haboubi and Lincoln (2003) found that even though more than 90% of healthcare professionals thought it was essential to address sexual issues with patients, 94% did not readily discuss these issues. Nurses are unlikely to ask patients about sexual issues for multiple reasons, including lack of time, expecting the patient to bring it up, and not knowing what to do with the information or how to help the patient with these concerns (Magnan & Reynolds, 2006). If patients are afraid to ask and healthcare professionals are not addressing sexual issues, how will patients ever resolve their sexual issues? Sexual dysfunction seems to be a neglected problem that healthcare providers are not discussing, leaving patients without options for sexual problems. Patients continue to suffer in silence, waiting for someone to address these most private issues. Nurses are the best healthcare providers to address the issues, as nurses spend a significant amount of time with patients and are identified by the public as the most trusted professional in *USA Today/Gallup* polls year after year (United Press International, 2007).

Many individuals with urologic cancers may struggle with sexual problems, and it is essential that the nurse address these sexual issues with patients.

Sexual Dysfunction

Sexual dysfunction can be any problem related to sex that prevents the individual and/or couple from enjoying intimacy or sexual relations. Male sexual dysfunction can be further categorized into desire disorders, arousal disorders, erectile dysfunction (ED), orgasmic disorders, delayed ejaculation, rapid or premature ejaculation, and pain disorders. Several categories have been defined and are used universally for female sexual dysfunction, including desire disorders, arousal disorders, orgasmic disorders, and sexual pain disorders (Basson et al., 2000). A desire disorder in men or women can be further differentiated into a hypoactive sexual desire disorder or a sexual aversion disorder. A *hypoactive sexual desire disorder* manifests as a persistent or recurrent decreased desire for sex and decreased fantasizing thoughts about sex. *Sexual aversion disorder* is more of a phobic avoidance of sexual activity. *Arousal disorders* relate to an inability to attain or maintain excitement during sexual relations, which may result in distress. This may mean a lack of clitoral or penile engorgement. In men, ED is the inability to attain or maintain an erection sufficient for sexual performance (National Institutes of Health Consensus Development Panel on Impotence, 1993). *Orgasmic disorders* relate to the ability to experience orgasm and may be problems with delayed orgasm or an inability to orgasm. In men, premature or rapid ejaculation occurs when the orgasm occurs sooner than desired and may be as rapid as 30–60 seconds of intravaginal penetration time. *Sexual pain disorders* are associated with painful sexual relations. In women, these may be further delineated into the following (Basson et al.).

- Dyspareunia, which is the recurrent or persistent presence of genital pain during sex

- Vaginismus, which is the recurrent or persistent presence of involuntary pelvic floor spasms while trying to have penetrative sex
- Noncoital sexual pain disorder, which involves recurrent or persistent pain from nonpenetrative sexual stimulation

Peyronie disease in men is associated with a curvature of the penis related to a postinflammatory plaque formation that may or may not be associated with pain. These disorders may be lifelong or acquired, and in the case of patients with urogenital cancer, they are most often acquired.

Sexual dysfunction can occur in greater than 80% of patients with cancer after treatment (Andersen, 1990; Jensen et al., 2003). Changes may be related to the cancerous growth that presses on nerves and blood vessels; pelvic or genital surgery; or radiation to the pelvic area, which may cause desire disorder, ED, sensory changes, or decreased vaginal lubrication and expansion. Hormonal changes associated with some medications may cause decreased desire, decreased vaginal lubrication, increased pain, and decreased pleasure, as well as ED. Any or all of these factors may affect sexual function, and it is essential to address these issues with patients.

Approach to Patients

The idea of talking with patients about their sexuality often is fraught with multiple concerns by both patients and healthcare providers. Lally (2006) identified that "patients want and need to know how cancer and its treatment may affect their sexual feelings and function" (p. 1). However, patients rarely bring up the topic of sexual problems, often considering it to be a taboo or unimportant topic (Baldwin et al., 2003; Krebs, 2005). Providers often are reluctant to broach sexuality concerns with patients because of (Katz, 2005; Magnan & Reynolds, 2006; Magnan, Reynolds, & Galvin, 2005)

- Fears of embarrassment
- Inadequate training or education
- Fears of overstepping patient or provider boundaries
- Lack of time
- Other issues and side effects seeming much more important during the brief time for the patient consultation.

Gott, Galena, Hinchliff, and Elfor (2004) noted that some nurses fear "opening a can of worms" (p. 528) if they begin to discuss sexuality; thus, they do not even broach the topic. Strategies that benefit both patients and providers need to be incorporated into daily clinical practice if the important topic of sexuality is to be addressed. Providers must become comfortable bringing up the subject and must help their patients to overcome any sense of embarrassment or discomfort, so that adequate assessment and appropriate interventions can be included in the plan of care.

For oncology nurses, Wilmoth (2006) suggested the following four key processes for addressing sexual issues with patients.

- Become comfortable talking about sex.

- Increase one's personal knowledge about sexual issues.
- Learn to use effective communication skills.
- Identify and facilitate the patient's use of appropriate resources to manage any identified sexual dysfunction.

Katz (2005) stated that providers need to understand their own sexual attitudes and beliefs to recognize what may be preventing them from discussing sexual issues with their patients. Others (Krebs, 2005; Nusbaum, Lanahan, & Sadovsky, 2005) have suggested that knowing one's own beliefs and attitudes will help providers to assess and manage any personal discomforts that they may have with some sexual topics or activities, such as same-sex partners, and oral or anal sex, so that they can more comfortably address sexuality with each patient. Oncology nurses may find the use of role models, such as other nurses who are able to talk with patients about sexuality with relative ease, and role playing to be very helpful in learning how to communicate about sexual issues related to cancer and cancer therapy. Journal clubs, grand rounds, seminars, and multidisciplinary presentations may facilitate both an understanding of potential sexual problems that can occur in those with cancer and can provide tools and strategies to enable nurses to talk with the patient and family without discomfort (Katz, 2005; Krebs, 2005, 2006; Wilmoth, 2006). Additionally, it may be difficult for nurses to talk with patients of the opposite gender about sexual issues. Practice and time may make this easier, or nurses may wish to enlist a colleague of the appropriate gender to handle the discussion (Krebs, 2005, 2006; Magnan & Reynolds, 2006).

Nurses who actively discuss sexuality issues with patients recognize the need for a sensitive but matter-of-fact approach, making questions about sexuality a part of routine assessment and follow-up. Krebs (2005, 2006, 2008) and Nusbaum et al. (2005) suggested that the most important aspects of approaching the topic of sexuality with patients and families are ones that

- Use both sensitivity and timing
- Take cues from the patient
- Include appropriate family members or significant others
- Provide factual information
- Move from less sensitive to more sensitive topics
- Avoid medical jargon
- Are sensitive and nonjudgmental
- Give patients permission to be sexually active and engage in sexual activities that fit their and their sexual partners' personalities and lifestyles.

Lally (2006) noted that it is important to ask "the right questions at the right time" (p. 4), including questions about current sexual activity, if the current level is desired, and what, if anything, would be more desirable or could be different or improved. Answers to these questions will both guide the next questions and provide information for identifying appropriate resources to meet the patient's identified needs. Goals to be integrated into a plan of care include (Krebs, 2005, 2006)

- Helping the patient to find acceptance of himself or herself as a sexual being
- Facilitating the patient's ability to give and receive affection
- Providing the confidence and resources for the patient to maintain his/her usual level of sexual confidence despite the cancer diagnosis.

According to Krebs (2008), it is important to recognize the cultural differences that each person brings to a discussion of sexuality and sexual intimacy. Not only race and ethnicity, but age, sexual orientation, cultural beliefs, and background, as well as myriad other aspects will affect how sexuality is approached and discussed with each patient and his or her partner (if applicable). Specific consideration should be given to young adults who will require appropriate, age-specific assessments, education, and interventions. Older adults also may have life challenges and comorbidities that affect their abilities or desire to be sexually intimate regardless of their cancer status. Additionally, because of the potential for bias and discrimination based on sexual orientation or gender identity, particular consideration needs to be given to lesbian, gay, and transgender patients. Finally, special consideration needs to be provided to those in their final stages of the illness, as these individuals may need—or choose to focus—their sexual functioning solely on intimacy and physical closeness (Krebs, 2008).

Assessment Tools

A comprehensive sexual assessment may incorporate a variety of methods or models along with specific discussion questions and evaluation instruments. The assessment may be brief or intensive. Topics that may be discussed include current sexual activity, intimacy, communication styles, current relationships, disease and treatment issues, satisfaction with current activities, and coping skills (Krebs, 2008). Several tools are available for both assessment of sexual function and for intervention once sexuality has been assessed. Assessment models include the ALARM model developed by Andersen and Lamb (1995), the Schover Method developed by Schover (1998), and the BETTER model developed by Mick, Hughes, and Cohen (2004). The most commonly used intervention model, the PLISSIT model, was developed by Annon (1974). The ALARM model and the Schover Method focus on patients' objective and subjective evaluation of their sexuality, as well as their current medical condition. The BETTER model focuses on general discussion, education, and resource referral. The PLISSIT model generally is used to focus interventions to manage sexual dysfunction by giving patients permission to be sexually active and by providing appropriate, individualized information, and explicit suggestions for managing problems. Referral for intensive therapy is included for those whose dysfunction cannot be resolved by the first three steps (Annon). The BETTER and PLISSIT models have been used for both assessment and intervention and easily can be employed by oncology nurses to begin to address the topic of sexuality with their patients. An extension of the PLISSIT model, called EX-PLISSIT, was recently proposed by Davis and Taylor (2006). This model incorporates permission-giving at each step, as well as including sexuality discussion review with the patient and partner and reflecting on the discussion and outcomes by the provider (see Figure 9-1).

Figure 9-1. Methods of Assessment and Intervention

Assessment
ALARM Model (Anderson & Lamb, 1995)
Activity (sexual)
Libido/desire
Arousal/orgasm
Resolution/release/relaxation
Medical information (cancer and past and concomitant health status)

Schover Method (Schover, 1998)
Evaluate past and present:
- Sexual practices
- Sexual function
- Sexual relationships.
Evaluate current:
- Status of cancer
- Status of cancer treatment
- Concomitant medical condition
- Psychological condition.
Identify sexual knowledge, desires, and goals.

BETTER (Mick et al., 2004)
Bring up issues of sexuality.
Explain that sexuality is part of quality of life for many; is important to discuss.
Tell patients that resources are available; you will assist them to obtain those needed.
Timing is important; facilitate discussions/provide information when the patient/family desires it.
Educate the patient/family about potential changes in sexual response/side effects that may affect response/reproduction.
Record discussions, assessments, interventions, and outcomes in the patient's healthcare record.

Intervention
PLISSIT (Annon, 1974)
Permission (to have sexual feelings and relationships)
LImited Information (about treatment/cancer on sexuality)
Specific **S**uggestions (to manage sexual side effects)
Intensive **T**herapy
(First three can usually be accomplished by the healthcare provider; the last may require referral to sex therapist or counselor.)

Note. From "What Should I Say?" by L.U. Krebs, 2006, *Clinical Journal of Oncolcogy Nursing, 10*(3), p. 315. Copyright 2006 by Oncology Nursing Society. Adapted with permission.

Specific Urologic Cancers and Their Effect on Sexuality

Penile Cancer

Penile cancer is fairly uncommon, comprising less than 0.2% of all cancers in men in the United States (Jemal et al., 2008). Diagnosis and treatment for penile cancer can have a profound impact on sexuality and sexual function. Men older than 18 years, especially those at risk for infection, need to be taught to check regularly for lesions, indurations, papules, or growths on the penis (Blanco-Yarosh, 2007). Risk factors include human papillomavirus infection, genital warts, lack of circumcision, and tobacco use. These factors are discussed in greater detail in Chapter 4.

Treatment for penile cancer includes surgical excision of the lesion, laser surgery, subtotal penectomy, or total penectomy. The goal of treatment is to remove the cancer so there are tumor-free margins. Obviously, the less invasive or extensive the surgery performed, the less chance of sexual dysfunction. Depending on how much of the glans or shaft is removed, men may have decreased sensation and pleasure, leading to ED, orgasmic disorders, and decreased overall sexual satisfaction. In addition, the psychological influences of body image changes related to any portion of the penis being removed can lead to sexual dysfunction.

When penile cancer is diagnosed and treated early, the impact on sexual function is less dramatic. In a study of 40 men who underwent laser treatment for penile cancer, 72% reported no change in erectile function after treatment, with 6% of the men reporting improved function (Windahl, Skeppner, Andersson, & Fugl-Meyer, 2004). Unfortunately, men often delay treatment of penile lesions because of a lack of knowledge about this disease. Disease progression requires more aggressive treatment and thus causes a greater impact on sexuality and sexual function. Sexual function is affected most by a total penectomy and also may be greatly affected by a partial penectomy. Romero et al. (2005) found that after penectomy, only 33.3% of men were able to maintain their preoperative frequency of intercourse and were satisfied with their sexual relationship with their partners. However, 55.6% of patients reported erectile function sufficient for penetrative sexual relations.

The change in sexual function is related to physiologic factors as well as psychological factors related to a change in body image. Some patients may accept the new body image because they view the treatment as life saving, whereas other patients may be devastated by the partial or entire loss of their penis. Each patient will respond differently to sexuality and sexual dysfunction issues with penile cancer and after treatment. It is essential that patients are appropriately counseled from diagnosis through treatment and that they play an active role in each decision, as well as have a full understanding of the possible consequences of each decision. Nurses play a

vital role in helping patients to explore feelings about their diagnosis and treatment and in moving forward in the future with sexual goals and intimacy. Counseling to discuss body image changes and feelings of loss is essential. If a patient has ED, he can try any of the treatment options, depending on his particular circumstance, to determine what is most effective. The treatment options for ED are outlined later in this chapter.

Testicular Cancer

Testicular cancer is the most common malignancy in young men ages 20–34. In the United States, there are about 8,090 new cases yearly, with approximately 380 deaths per year (Jemal et al., 2008). Although it accounts for only about 1% of all cancers in men, testicular cancer is the number-one cancer killer among men in their 20s and 30s. Most testicular cancers are self-discovered by patients as a painless or uncomfortable lump in the testicle. When found early, testicular cancer is almost always curable. Early-stage testicular cancer generally is treated with surgery and radiation therapy. Late-stage testicular cancer can be treated with a combination of surgery, radiation therapy, or chemotherapy. The prognosis for men with testicular cancer is very good, even for patients with advanced disease. The chances of recovery are excellent with surgery and radiotherapy for early-stage disease. If the cancer has not spread outside the testicle, the five-year relative survival rate is 99% (American Cancer Society, 2007a).

Psychologically, patients with testicular cancer may experience altered sexuality, altered body image, altered role function, fertility issues, grief, and concerns related to mortality (Brown, 2004). Many men who have recurrent disease can be cured with chemotherapy or radiation; however, some may opt for an orchiectomy and then will have to deal with the adverse effects associated with the removal of the testes. After the removal of one or both testes and the spermatic cord(s), the scrotum will look and feel empty. To offset these side effects, a testicular prosthesis can be implanted during the orchiectomy procedure. Commercially available testicular prostheses come in many sizes, so matching the remaining testicle is possible (see Figure 9-2). The prosthesis is filled with liquid (usually normal saline) and feels normal. In addition, because the incision of the surgery typically is at the inguinal area, the scar usually is covered by pubic hair, and, without close observation, one cannot tell that a patient has undergone such surgery. Patients undergoing unilateral orchiectomy who have one remaining healthy testicle can still have normal erections and can still produce sperm. Sperm cell concentrations often are reduced, however, when compared to presurgery concentrations (Petersen, Skakkebaek, Vistisen, Rorth, & Giwercman, 1999). When a retroperitoneal lymph node dissection (RPLND) is necessary, it will not alter a man's ability to have an erection or an orgasm but can cause infer-

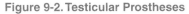

Figure 9-2. Testicular Prostheses

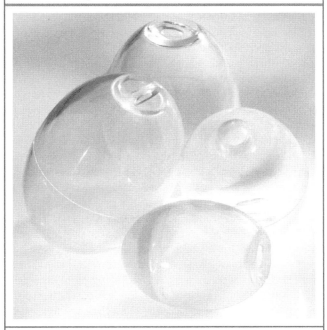

Note. Photo courtesy of Coloplast Corp. Used with permission.

tility because it interferes with ejaculation. Currently, most surgeons attempt to perform a nerve-sparing RPLND.

Radiation therapy can interfere with sperm production. Usually, the effect will be temporary, and most patients will regain their fertility within a matter of months.

Chemotherapy frequently causes *azoospermia*, which is a complete absence of sperm in the ejaculate, resulting in infertility (Dearnaley, Huddart, & Horwich, 2001). This infertility is frequently temporary, but infertility can be a permanent problem for some men following chemotherapy, especially when cisplatin and alkylating agents are used together (Lampe, Horwich, Norman, Nicholls, & Dearnaley, 1997).

Contemporary reproductive technology allows men receiving sterilizing cancer treatments to remain optimistic about future fertility issues. In emergent cases, such as the need to initiate chemotherapy treatment immediately, adequate samples of sperm can be obtained with only 24–48 hours between collection times, to allow for the storage of samples prior to treatment (Schover, Brey, Lichtin, Lipshultz, & Jeha, 2002). Cryopreservation (sperm banking) of sperm must be discussed with patients before treatment, and this will be discussed in detail later in the chapter. In men considering future paternity, treatments that are less gonadotoxic can be considered, and semen cryopreservation should be undertaken. Patients with preexisting fertility problems, such as azoospermia or anejaculation, should be offered sperm retrieval techniques so that recovered sperm cells can be cryopreserved for future use. In patients with

suspected testicular cancer, fertility-preserving measures should be initiated before testicular surgery.

Bladder Cancer

Bladder cancer is the fourth most common cancer in men and the ninth most common cancer in women (Dalbagni & Herr, n.d.; Jemal et al., 2008). Bladder cancer can be superficial, invasive, or metastatic. The stage of the cancer dictates the treatment, including transurethral surgery, chemotherapy, radiation, and partial or full cystectomy (American Cancer Society, 2007b). Each treatment has a unique effect, both physically and psychologically, on the patients' sexuality. When discussing possible treatments, it is important to discuss the potential impact on the patients' sexual function. Patients may be too embarrassed to mention their concerns or may not understand that the disease process and treatment can affect sexual functioning. They need to be reassured of the treatment options available for sexual dysfunction.

Transurethral resection of bladder tumors (TURBT) is used for superficial bladder cancers. Side effects include bleeding and pain for a short time after the surgery. The initial burning, bleeding, and discomfort pass within a short time. During that time, patients usually are not sexually active. In some instances, even after the discomfort passes, patients are fearful of having sexual activity. They may fear discomfort with intercourse or worry about inadvertently damaging the bladder or urethra with thrusting. Patients need to be educated that sexual activity is safe once their postoperative healing is complete. Men may notice some discomfort the first few times they ejaculate. They should be reassured that this will resolve (American Cancer Society, 2007b).

Intravesical immunotherapy involves giving medication through a catheter into the bladder instead of intravenously. Intravesical therapy is used with patients who are at high risk for disease recurrence and progression to more invasive disease. It often is recommended for patients after resection of tumors to prevent recurrence (UpToDate, 2008). Bacillus Calmette-Guérin, often used to vaccinate against tuberculosis, is considered to be the most effective intravesical immunotherapy medication for bladder cancer. After treatment, patients may have flu-like symptoms as well as a burning sensation in the bladder. Even after patients expel the medication, residual drug still may be excreted through the urine for up to seven days (Durek et al., 2001). Patients and their partners are instructed to abstain from intercourse or use a condom during this period for partner protection. Reassurance should be given that after seven days it is safe to have intercourse. Some patients find abstaining initially after treatment to be preferable, especially if they have residual burning in the bladder and urethra.

Systemic chemotherapy also can be used as a treatment for bladder cancer. This may be employed instead of intravesical therapy for low-risk superficial bladder cancers and also can be used to shrink a large tumor before surgery. Because the medication is systemic, there are more potential side effects. Temporary side effects include nausea and vomiting, loss of appetite, hair loss, and mouth sores (American Cancer Society, 2007b). During this period, many patients will have decreased sexual interest. Some of this is because of the physical trauma the body undergoes during chemotherapy. Patients generally are tired and lack energy, and many may have body image concerns as well. The loss of hair and potential weight loss may make the patient feel unattractive or "not themselves." Counseling patients and their partners through this time is important. Reassurance that the side effects of chemotherapy are temporary and usually disappear within months after chemotherapy is completed will give patients and their partners hope. It is helpful to encourage them to keep their intimate connection through hugging, cuddling, and touching even if the idea of intercourse seems overwhelming. The intimate connection with each other will make them feel less alone during this difficult period. Patients may experience permanent complications such as infertility and premature menopause secondary to the anticancer medications (American Cancer Society, 2007b). Patients need to be counseled of this possibility before starting treatment. If patients are still of childbearing age and are planning to have children, steps can be discussed to store sperm or eggs. If the female patient does become menopausal, it is important to discuss potential vaginal changes such as dryness and tissue atrophy. Patients should be counseled regarding use of a water-soluble lubricant or vaginal moisturizers during intercourse and foreplay.

External beam radiation therapy has been used after TURBT as an alternative to intravesical therapy for select patients (Weiss et al., 2006). It may be used in conjunction with chemotherapy or alone. Similar to patients receiving chemotherapy, patients receiving radiation therapy may not feel they have the energy for or interest in sexual activity. It is important to counsel patients and partners in a similar manner as previously described (Schover, 2006).

Because the nerves for erections in men surround the prostate directly below the bladder, damage can occur during radiation therapy. This can result in ED. If this occurs, patients need to be counseled regarding treatment options for ED.

Women may experience dryness and shortening or narrowing of the vagina from radiation therapy. This can result in painful intercourse and subsequent difficulty reaching orgasm. During radiation therapy, the tissue in the vagina may become inflamed and tender. Penetration during this time may be uncomfortable. Patients need to be counseled to use water-soluble lubricants for vaginal dryness. Local introital application of an estrogen hormonal cream often can keep the vaginal tissue supple and less dry. If shortening or narrowing of the vagina occurs, patients and their partners need to be counseled regarding techniques to improve function. A frank discussion regarding positioning and educational tools such as sexual education books can be helpful. Most women find that if they use the female superior position during intercourse, they can more easily control the depth of the thrusting to prevent pain. If narrowness is severe, patients may need to learn dilation techniques to slowly stretch the vaginal vault (American Cancer Society, 2007b; Mayo Clinic, 2007). Frequent intercourse and/or dilation will help keep the vaginal walls stretched and pliable.

For infiltrating and high-grade, organ-confined, multifocal bladder cancer, radical cystectomy is the gold-standard treatment (Martis, D'Elia, Massimo, Ombres, & Mastrangeli, 2005). This surgery removes the entire bladder and nearby local lymph nodes. In men, the prostate is also removed. In women, the uterus, ovaries, a small portion of the vagina, and the fallopian tubes are removed. Sexual dysfunction complications of these surgeries are more serious. Men often suffer ED after surgery because of the removal of the prostate and loss of associated nerve bundles. Because of the lack of prostate, the man will no longer produce seminal fluid, which will result in a "dry" orgasm. As a result of the removal of ovaries, female patients will become hypoestrogenic. This can result in vaginal dryness and atrophy. The partial removal of the vagina may cause difficulty with intercourse, including pain, especially with deep thrusting. Women may notice a narrowing of the vagina if it was necessary to also remove the urethra, which can lead to painful intercourse. Referral to a trained physical therapist or healthcare provider for vaginal stretching exercises will benefit these patients.

Newer nerve-sparing procedures have shown improvement in maintaining erectile function (Martis et al., 2005). Not all patients are candidates for this type of surgery, and even with nerve-sparing techniques, not all will regain erectile function. It is important to prepare patients for this possibility.

Reconstructive surgery after cystectomy can provide some normalcy to life. Several options are available for reconstructive surgery. One possibility is a urostomy. In this situation, the urine drains into a pouch attached to the skin of the abdomen. A small piece of colon is relocated as a conduit for the urine to pass from the kidney to the urostomy. Urine drains continuously into the urostomy pouch, which is worn under clothing. A continent diversion, also known as a Kock pouch, is another type of urostomy, in which the pouch is created from the colon and has a valve that allows urine to be stored for a time. The patient catheterizes the stoma several times a day to empty. Many patients prefer this, as a bag is not needed. The most natural surgery option is the formation of a neobladder constructed of intestine. The neobladder is then attached to the ureters and to the urethra. This procedure allows patients to urinate normally (American Cancer Society, 2007b).

Sexual issues around the presence of a stoma are both emotional and physical. Patients who wear a pouch may be self-conscious and struggle with body image. Patients with a stoma, but no bag or pouch, will still have these issues. It is important for patients and partners to have counseling on adjusting their sexual activity. Patients need an outlet to voice their concerns. They need reassurance that, with planning, sex can again be pleasurable. See Figure 9-3 for tips to share with

---

Figure 9-3. Tips for Patients With a Stoma Regarding Sexual Activity

- Make sure the pouch fits correctly around the stoma to reduce the chance of leakage.
- Empty the pouch immediately before sexual activity to decrease leakage.
- Wear a pouch cover or a wide sash to stabilize it and to make it appear less like a medical appliance.
- Wear a comfortable shirt or nightgown during sexual activity.
- Choose positions that minimize the partner's weight on the appliance.
- Catheterize continent diversion immediately before sexual activity. Cover the stoma to minimize leakage.

---

patients with a stoma regarding sexual activity. All treatments for bladder cancer have the potential to change patients' sexual life. It is important for nurses to take the time to initiate the discussion, answer questions, and offer solutions.

Kidney Cancer

Kidney cancer is the third leading genitourinary cancer and the twelfth leading cause of cancer in the United States; an estimated 54,390 new cases and 13,010 deaths occurred from kidney cancer in 2008 (Jemal et al., 2008). During the past two decades, there has been a 2% per year increase in the number of new cases (Ries et al., 2006). According to Pow-Sang (2007), the majority of new kidney cancer diagnoses are made incidentally when investigating another medical complaint. Because tumors tend to be small at diagnosis, those with tumors smaller than 4 cm generally are treated with nephron-sparing surgery (NSS), usually some type of partial nephrectomy. Other possible NSS procedures include renal cryoablation, radiofrequency ablation (hyperthermic ablation), or high-intensity focused ultrasound ablation. Radical nephrectomy still is used for select patients (Al-Qudah, Rodriguez, & Sexton, 2007; Hafron & Kaouk, 2007a, 2007b; Park & Cadeddu, 2007; Rini & Campbell, 2007; Tobisu, 2006). For those with advanced or metastatic disease, current treatment consists of debulking the tumor through a surgical approach followed by administration of one of the vascular endothelial growth factor (VEGF) inhibitors (Garcia & Rini, 2007; Rini & Campbell).

Little has been written about the sexual side effects of treatment for kidney cancer. A review of the literature for the past 10 years located only one article specifically addressing sexual dysfunction in those with kidney cancer (Anastasiadis et al., 2003) and an additional two articles (Clark et al., 2001; Shinohara et al., 2001) investigated the effect of NSS on quality of life without a specific focus on sexuality. Anastasiadis et al. specifically investigated sexual functioning in 301 randomly selected patients with kidney cancer through an anonymous, cross-sectional, mailed survey. The questionnaire explored the topics of depression, sexuality, general

health, and adjustment to illness. Analysis of the returned questionnaires (N = 84) showed that although respondents maintained sexual activity, women who responded (N = 42) had lower scores on the Watts Sexual Function Questionnaire than healthy participants and age-comparable patients with breast cancer, indicating worse sexual functioning. Additionally, both male and female responders had scores on the Center for Epidemiologic Studies Depression Scale that indicated mild depression. The number of participants was insufficient to further analyze these data or make any conclusions about the combination of decreased sexual function and depression (Anastasiadis et al.). Of note, all three studies found that quality of life was improved in those with NSS versus those who underwent total nephrectomy (Anastasiadis et al.; Clark et al.; Shinohara et al.).

Patients with minimal disease that requires surgery might be expected to have body image changes based on surgical scars and the sense of loss experienced when losing a body part (regardless of whether that loss is apparent to others). If depression is significant, sexual function, including decreasing interest and frequency, as well as communication patterns could be affected (although this was not confirmed by the Anastasiadis et al. data from 2003). Patients with advanced disease who require more extensive surgery, as well as those requiring the administration of immunotherapy or biotherapy, might experience sexual side effects, including fatigue, body image changes, and decreased libido in both men and women; ED, impotence, and gynecomastia in men; and pelvic pain, mucous membrane dryness, and amenorrhea in women. Additionally, pregnant women receiving biologics are at risk for spontaneous abortion and fetal malformation, as the VEGF-inhibitor drugs are considered teratogenic and embryotoxic (Krebs, 2005, 2006; Wilkes & Barton-Burke, 2007).

Evaluation of Sexual Dysfunction in Men and Women With Urologic Cancer

A comprehensive history and physical examination are paramount in determining the presence of sexual dysfunction in men and women with specific urologic cancers. It also is essential to understand sexuality from both the patients' and partners' (if the patient is partnered) perspectives. Insight into the sexual relationship can help to identify areas of greatest concern and to determine how treatment options might be integrated into the sexual relationship. Whenever possible, it is important to include patients' partners.

Evaluation of Women for Sexual Dysfunction After Urologic Cancer

Today more than ever in the specialties of urology and oncology, comprehensive sexual health care is available for women. Women typically are seen by a team of specialty physicians, advanced practice nurses, sexologists, psychologists, and physical therapists who can assist them in maintaining or regaining sexual function after cancer. Of the 43% of American women with sexual dysfunction, lack of desire for physical intimacy is the most common sexual complaint and can be the most difficult to assess and treat (Nappi, Ferdeghini, & Polatti, 2006). This can be especially true for women who have a urologic cancer and who suffer from chronic pain as a result of their cancer.

Desire Disorders

Desire disorders are divided into two major categories: hypoactive sexual desire disorder and sexual aversion disorder. *Hypoactive sexual desire disorder* (HSDD) is a persistent or recurring deficiency or absence of sexual fantasies, thoughts, and/or receptivity to sexual activity that causes personal distress. *Sexual aversion disorder* (SAD) is a persistent or recurring phobic aversion to and avoidance of sexual contact with a partner that causes personal distress. Several situational phenomena can contribute to desire disorders, including physiologic, psychosexual, and cultural factors. The more dramatic aversion responses often are emotionally based and may result from trauma. A final desire issue that many women describe is "desire discrepancy." In this circumstance, women verify that they experience fantasy thoughts and are interested in sexual activity, but at a far less frequent interval than their partners. When this creates personal and interpersonal distress, intervention may be warranted (Levy, 2002; Maurice, 1999; Nappi et al., 2006).

To understand the desire disorder, the clinician must perform an assessment. An initial step in assessing complaints of lack of interest is to identify a woman's baseline or normal pattern of initiation and receptivity to sex play; contrast it with her current patterns of initiation and receptivity to sex play; and identify if, how, and when patterns changed. Non-partner–oriented sexual expressions, such as desire for and enactment of self-stimulation, incidence of erotic nighttime dreams, and spontaneous sexual thoughts during the day, also are factors that identify the extent of the disorder. Asking about partner response to the cancer diagnosis, support for seeking treatment, and relationship conflict issues is key (Levy, 2002).

It is important to check medication profiles for drugs that are known to adversely affect desire, including selective serotonin reuptake inhibitors, tricyclic antidepressants, anticonvulsants, antihypertensives, and tranquilizers. Altering medications or adding prosexual drugs, such as bupropion, to current regimens may reawaken desire (Hensley & Nurnberg, 2006).

Pelvic Floor Dysfunction

Normal function of the pelvic floor musculature is essential in maintaining appropriate function of the bladder, trigone, and urethra, as well as appropriate sexual functioning. Alteration in the function of this musculature often is seen in women who have had excisional or reconstructive surgery or radiation during the treatment for urologic cancer (Ali-El-Dein, Gomha, & Ghoneim, 2002). *Pelvic floor dysfunction* (PFD) refers to conditions in which the pelvic floor muscular support system is functioning suboptimally (see Table 9-1). PFD can be caused by muscular support that is lax and suboptimal, termed *low-tone pelvic floor dysfunction* (LT-PFD), or disorders that cause spasticity and too much tightness of the pelvic floor, termed *high-tone pelvic floor dysfunction* (HT-PFD). Either can be closely associated with sexual dysfunction (Barral, 1993; Lukban & Whitmore, 2000; Srinivasan, Kaye, & Moldwin, 2007; Travell & Simons, 1992).

Table 9-1. Pelvic Floor Dysfunction		
Type	**Causes**	**Pelvic Floor Dysfunction (PFD) Symptoms**
Low-tone PFD	• Childbirth • Injury • Senescence • Surgical trauma	• Incontinence (during or outside intercourse) • Pelvic organ prolapse • Thrusting dyspareunia • Vaginal laxity
High-tone PFD	• Adhesions • Childbirth • Infection • Microtrauma • Postural stressors • Surgical trauma • Visceral inflammation	• Dysuria • Fecal retention • Frequency • Muscular tightness that prohibits penetration • Penetrative dyspareunia that prohibits penetration • Urgency • Urinary retention

Note. Based on information from Fitzgerald & Kotarinos, 2003; Lukban & Whitmore, 2000; Whitmore et al., 1998.

Assessment of tone in the pelvic floor muscles is performed to determine a woman's ability to isolate, contract, and relax the pelvic floor muscles. While conducting a digital examination by exerting light pressure on the inferior lateral walls of the vagina, the woman is asked to squeeze the examining finger and to "lift" the pelvic floor, without simultaneously tightening the abdominal, gluteal, or adductor muscle groups. If the patient is unable to produce sufficient muscle strength to "squeeze" the finger or to sustain that squeeze for a period of five seconds, she may be exhibiting an LT-PFD pattern. If, conversely, the woman experiences muscle tenderness or pain when pressure is applied to the lateral vaginal wall or during an attempted squeeze against resistance, she may be exhibiting a spastic or HT-PFD pattern (Fitzgerald & Kotarinos, 2003; Lukban & Whitmore, 2000; Whitmore, Kellogg-Spadt, & Fletcher, 1998).

Pain and Hypersensitivity Disorders Associated With Urologic Cancers

Hypersensitivity or sensory disorders of the lower urinary tract represent a spectrum of symptoms and conditions that include urgency and frequency syndrome, sensory urgency, urethral syndrome, and interstitial cystitis. Frequent and painful voiding, as well as anticipation of genital pain during sex play, can result in pelvic floor muscle guarding, which, over time, can result in a spastic or high-tone pelvic floor (Curhan, Speizer, Hunter, Curhan, & Stampfer, 1999; Williams & Lloyd, 1998).

Estrogen Deficiency

Women with urologic cancers may experience atrophic urogenital symptoms as a result of being peri- or postmenopausal, or as a result of chemotherapy or radiation therapy. Trauma or increased fragility of the urogenital tissues can alter a woman's ability to lubricate during sexual arousal and may contribute to pain during penetration or coital thrusting. Estrogen deficiency symptoms include dryness, itching, burning, penetrative pain, irritative leukorrhea, urethral pressure, urinary urgency, and fissures associated with loss of tissue elasticity. In addition, poor estrogen binding in genitourinary tissues can lead to ischemia with a decreased urethral mucosal cushion and increased susceptibility of the bladder to bacterial adherence and development of recurrent urinary tract infections. Treatment of atrophic genital and urethral mucosal changes is of paramount importance. Topical or intravaginal estrogen cream application and locally acting estrogen pills and rings are options to address estrogen deficiency and preserve sexual arousal and comfort (McKay, 1991; Sarrell, 1990; Stewart & Spencer, 2002). The amount of systemic absorption from estrogen-containing vaginal creams, rings, and tablets depends on the type of hormone used and the dosage. Patients should be reassured that low doses of estradiol given vaginally (via topical introital cream or intravaginal tablet) achieve local vaginal effects without detectable systemic absorption. One study using an ultrasensitive estradiol bioassay detected small increases in plasma estrogen values after administration of 10 mcg of vaginal creams, but levels remained well within the postmenopausal range of 3–10 pg/ml (Santen et al., 2002). Similarly, Rioux, Devlin, Gelfand, Steinberg, and Hepburn (2000) found no detectable increments in estradiol levels with the 25 mcg vaginal estradiol tablet.

Evaluation of Men for Sexual Dysfunction After Urologic Cancer

Loss of sexual function is embarrassing, frightening, and devastating to male patients. Many cancer treatments can result in loss of sexual function. It is important that male patients are diagnosed and offered treatment as soon as possible. Making a diagnosis may be as simple as completing a sexual and medical history, physical examination, and basic testing, or it may be complex and involve more extensive specialized testing. A basic understanding of the diagnostic evaluation patients undergo will enable the healthcare provider to better prepare and discuss treatment options. After the basic assessment is completed, a decision can be made whether further, more specialized testing is necessary.

One of the most important first steps in the diagnostic process is a complete medical and sexual history. The medical history should include presence of chronic disease (e.g., diabetes, renal failure, hepatic failure, hypertension, cardiac/pulmonary disease), surgical history, radiation treatment history, current and past medications (including any chemotherapy or biotherapy), and trauma. Social habits such as smoking, alcohol use, and recreational drug use are also important. Family history, particularly vascular, endocrine, or cancer diagnoses, should be sought (Kandeel, Koussa, & Swerdloff, 2001). Sexual history should include precise questions about the quality of sexual functioning both before and after cancer treatment. Specific questions about erections should include rigidity, sustainability, presence of nighttime or early morning erections, or any physical abnormality (e.g., bend or curvature), changes in orgasm, amount or absence of ejaculate, discomfort during orgasm, and ability to reach orgasm (Kandeel et al.). This assessment should be performed once cancer treatment has been completed.

If possible, partner involvement during these discussions can provide a better and clearer picture of the problem. Partners often notice changes in function before patients do, but remain silent to protect patients' feelings. It is important to confirm the presence or absence of any change in functioning before cancer treatment to determine the amount of change linked to the treatment itself. Many patients are within the age group where changes in function caused by other health issues are common. In addition, patients may remember and focus on the warning of sexual dysfunction as a possible side effect and be suffering from psychological dysfunction. This is why the physical examination and diagnostic testing are important.

The physical examination should include a thorough vascular assessment with palpation of ankle, femoral, and dorsal penile arteries. Physical signs of muscular atrophy, pallor, and loss of hair growth in the lower extremities also can be indicative of a vascular pathology (Kandeel et al., 2001). An evaluation of the patient's neurologic system should include presence of motor deficits, changes in deep tendon reflexes, loss of sphincter tone, or decrease in light touch or pinprick sensations (particularly in the genital area). The bulbocavernosus reflex should be confirmed by squeezing the glans penis and assessing the evoked contractions of the external anal sphincter or bulbocavernosus muscles. This reflex response is detectable in 70% of healthy males (Goldstein, 1985). A careful examination of the genitalia that focuses on any decrease in testicular size or abnormality of the penile shaft or glans is necessary. Any decrease in secondary sexual characteristics may indicate hypogonadism or androgen resistance (Kandeel et al.).

Some common blood tests may include a hormonal panel that includes measurement of testosterone (both serum and bioavailable or free), luteinizing hormone (LH), prolactin, and sex hormone-binding globulin (SHBG) to assess hypogonadism. Treatment of hypogonadism will be dependent on the type of cancer and length of time the patient has been cancer-free. A blood chemistry panel, including lipids, can help to rule out diabetes, renal disease, and vascular changes secondary to hypercholesterolemia (Archer, Gragasin, Webster, Bochinski, & Michelakis, 2005).

More specific testing may be needed on a case-by-case basis to further assess the sexual dysfunction. See Table 9-2 for an overview of male sexual dysfunction assessments.

It is important to take the time to carefully assess and diagnose the male patients with cancer who experience sexual dysfunction. Although the etiology of the sexual dysfunction may seem obviously caused by the cancer treatment the patient has undergone, it is still important to have a thorough diagnostic evaluation to rule out other factors. The diagnostic findings also may assist in steering the patient to a more effective treatment. Generally speaking, the more accurate the diagnosis, the faster the treatment can be initiated. Proper diagnosis will give the patient the emotional security he needs to have reliable sexual functioning and an improved quality of life.

Consensus Panel Overview for Approach to Men With Erectile Dysfunction

A consensus panel met in 2001 to develop provider guidelines for the management of ED (Albaugh et al., 2002). The panel evaluated recent literature on the causes and treatments of ED and developed evidence-based guidelines for office management of ED by qualified clinicians. Nurses and advanced practice nurses play a major role in the identification, assessment, and management of ED, working in close collaboration with physicians and other healthcare providers. Although the broad principles involved might be applied to other sexual problems in men or women, these guidelines focused on ED.

The panel included registered nurses, advanced practice nurses, physician assistants, diabetes educators, and physicians. A broad range of specialties was represented, including urology, cardiology, endocrinology, diabetology, psychiatry, family medicine, and rehabilitation medicine. Each participant had significant clinical and professional experience in sexual healthcare and ED management, and most had published in peer-reviewed journals on this topic. Common themes included a patient-centered, multidisciplinary approach (Hatzichristou et al., 2004) and a thorough assessment that includes review of current medications; medical, sexual, and psychosocial histories; a focused physical examination; and select laboratory tests as appropriate. The need for discussion of the patient and his partner's relationship, the partner's health as an important contribution to successful assessment and treatment, and the need to educate both the patient and the partner about ED and the treatments available were mentioned often. Modifying reversible causes

Table 9-2. Tests to Assess Male Sexual Dysfunction		
Test	**Purpose**	**Comments**
Duplex (color) ultrasonography or penile Doppler examination	To assess the arterial and venous function of the penis	Can be performed either in a clinic or an outpatient setting
Dynamic infusion cavernosography and cavernosometry	To diagnose veno-occlusive dysfunction (traumatic versus congenital)	Performed in conjunction with radiology utilizing injection of vasoactive agents, infusing the corpora with heparinized saline to check pressures, and finally infusing radiocontrast material into the corpora to obtain radiographic images of the penis and perineum
Penile angiography	Usually reserved for younger patients who are being considered for reconstructive vascular surgery such as those who have sustained blunt trauma leading to a blockage of the origin of the cavernosal artery.	Rarely done on a patient after cancer treatment
Nocturnal penile tumescence monitoring	May help to assess the absence or presence and quality of nocturnal erectile activity in order to determine an organic versus psychological etiology	Monitoring performed over several nights in a sleep lab with direct observation or by a take-home unit that records the patient's nocturnal erectile activity, which is then downloaded to a computer

Note. Based on information from Archer et al., 2005; Kandeel et al., 2001.

of ED and managing underlying risk factors and comorbidities are equally important. A systematic stepwise approach, starting with the least invasive treatment that has proven to be effective, is imperative (Lue et al., 2004), as is stressing the importance of follow-up to assess treatment effectiveness and modify the treatment plan as necessary (Process of Care Consensus Panel, 1999). Therefore, the panel proposed the following key steps in the management of ED.

Problem Identification and Recognition

Problem identification should be a routine component of medical care for all men. Sexual inquiry may be especially indicated following surgery or hospitalization, diagnosis of a new disease or illness, medication initiation or adjustment, or major life changes (e.g., divorce, death of a spouse). Sexual function is assessed most often by direct interview with the patient, although partner interviews, paper-and-pencil questionnaires, or computer-based methods may be of value. Perhaps most important is the style or manner in which sexual inquiry is conducted. This should always reflect sensitivity to each individual's ethnic, cultural, and personal background. Simple questions such as "Are you currently sexually active? Do you have any difficulty getting or keeping an erection?" generally are recommended but should be adapted to the age, health, literacy, culture, ethnicity, and demographic background of the patient. Some patients may prefer to talk with someone of the same gender, and this option should be offered when available.

Assessment and Diagnosis

Assessment includes a sexual, psychosocial, medical, and medication history, selected laboratory tests, and a focused physical examination. The guidelines recommend that the sexual and psychosocial history include such key topics as erectile function, ejaculation, orgasm, libido, sexual interest, partner sexual function and relationship, and the patient's self-esteem and mood. Medical history should include any chronic medical or psychiatric illnesses, pelvic or perineal trauma or surgery, spinal cord or head trauma or surgery, radiotherapy, prescription drugs, smoking history, alcohol use, recreational drug use, and lifestyle. A focused physical examination should include secondary sexual characteristics and cardiovascular, endocrine, and neurologic systems, as well as a genitourinary examination. Highly recommended blood tests include serum chemistries, complete blood count, lipids and total and free testosterone. Optional tests may include prolactin, LH, thyroid-stimulating hormone, prostate-specific antigen, liver enzymes, or urinalysis as deemed necessary (Albaugh et al., 2002).

Intervention, Counseling, and Education

The guidelines strongly recommend education and counseling for all patients (and partners) prior to initiation of specific therapies for ED. Patients frequently have misconceptions about their genital anatomy and physiology, causes of ED, and risks and benefits of various treatments. Education can be provided through various modalities, including printed or electronic materials and personal presentation in individual or group formats.

Follow-Up and Reassessment

An active program of follow-up and reassessment should occur at regular intervals. Initial follow-up visits should be scheduled within one month after the initial visit. The partner should be involved whenever possible. During the follow-up visit, a healthcare provider can discuss patient and partner satisfaction with the treatment, compliance with and correct use of the treatment, adverse events, dosage adjustment as necessary, and the couple's overall health and relationship status.

This model is problem oriented and cost-effective. The importance of communication and involvement of the sexual partner in all phases of treatment is emphasized. Healthcare providers need to be sensitive to patients' cultural backgrounds and lifestyle choices. Alternatives to medical or surgical treatment should be considered, including referral for couples or individual counseling when indicated. Potential advantages of identification and management of ED include benefits in improved quality of life and interpersonal relationships, increased compliance with medical treatment for other conditions, and improved patient/clinician relationships.

Treatment Options for Men and Women

Relationship Issues and Counseling

The more that is known about what sexual changes to expect, the better an individual can cope with what happens. Everyone has the right to know about his or her own sexual health. The following are possible questions men and women may want to ask depending on their specific cancer. This information could be easily produced as a handout for patient education.
- Will this treatment (surgery, chemotherapy, radiation) affect my desire for sex?
- Will this treatment affect my ability to feel pleasure when my genital areas are touched?
- Will this treatment affect my ability to reach an orgasm?
- Will I have pain during sex as a result of this treatment?
- Will this treatment affect my ability to have an erection and ejaculation?
- Will this treatment affect my ability to have children in the future?
- Will these effects be temporary or permanent?
- What will I look like? Can you show me pictures?

- Are there any other alternative treatments or options available to me?
- Will I be able to have sex while undergoing treatment?

Counseling

An open, frank discussion about sex and sexual dysfunction treatment options with the patient and partner helps to bring everything into the open, thus encouraging questions and discussion and ultimately reducing stress. The more relaxed and comfortable the couple, generally the better the outcome. Partners often wonder about how their sex lives will be affected but are afraid to open the topic for fear of hurting their partner's feelings. This gives partners a forum to discuss the issue without causing emotional strife for either of them. When the diagnosis includes the word *cancer*, much of the information presented by the healthcare provider is lost. Written materials that the patient can refer to later will provide information and reassurance. Patients also may benefit from individual counseling regarding the role of stress and lifestyle factors, partner issues or problems, and medication effects. Patients who are not counseled may very well avoid sexual activity. This can lead to tragic end results with relationships and emotional health. With time and education, this can be avoided.

The emotional stress of cancer treatment and dealing with chronic pain can sometimes result in patients becoming unable to work or unable to contribute meaningfully to the day-to-day maintenance of the home and family. This may result in lowered self-esteem and feeling unattractive and "unlovable" and can create an emotional and physical distance in the relationship.

The first step in reclaiming intimacy may be for a woman or man to reestablish patterns of communication with their partner (Maliski, Heilemann, & McCorkle, 2001). The work for individuals and couples struggling with ED issues is further described in Figure 9-4. Couples who are working on ED-related issues should choose a neutral setting without sexual overtones. They should be encouraged to talk about feelings, fears, and desires. Often, patients interpret a partner's fear of hurting them as lack of interest. Discussing these issues can lead to better understanding and negotiation of expectations, and can begin to rekindle a gentle, loving spark between cancer survivors and their partners (Mayo Clinic, 2007).

Whether it is the cancer itself, the treatment, or general anxiety, many people experience decreased libido during cancer treatment. Loving yourself is particularly hard when the "cancer is contagious" myth creates a "caste of untouchables." This unfortunate misunderstanding makes many people feel unlovable and rejected. Sexual intercourse is certainly an important part of loving for many people. But loving means much more than intercourse. It encompasses all the social interaction that takes place in an intimate relationship, including touching, holding, hugging, and sharing intimacies. Many people with cancer report that one of the hardest aspects of

---

Figure 9-4. Individuals' and Couples' Work in the Management of Erectile Dysfunction

His Work: Regaining Mastery
- Confronting erectile dysfunction and putting it in perspective
- Prioritizing
- Gaining control over associated physical problems
- Purposeful networking (e.g., speaking with peers with similar problems and with medical professionals)

Our Work: Going Through It Together
- Establishing a routine
- Strengthening intimacy (e.g., sharing thoughts and feelings, expressing comfortable physical affection)

Her Work: Supportive Presence
- Managing anxiety—his and hers
- Facilitating his control
- Gaining perspective and reassuring him

Note. From "Mastery of Postprostatectomy Incontinence and Impotence: His Work, Her Work, Our Work," by S.L. Maliski, M.V. Heilemann, and R. McCorkle, 2001, *Oncology Nursing Forum, 28*(6), p. 988. Copyright 2001 by Oncology Nursing Society. Adapted with permission.

---

adjusting to the illness is learning how to receive love and support without feeling guilty.

Sexuality, broadly defined, encompasses all aspects of feeling close to the important people in our lives. It is a part of who we are and what we do. How we view ourselves as sexual beings influences our overall concept of self-worth, as well as our ability to make and keep meaningful intimate relationships. Some important areas to discuss when working with patients with urologic cancers are that survival overshadows sexuality, total worth is not based on physical attributes, the most potent sex organ is the brain, patience with themselves and others, they do not have to do it alone, and communicate, communicate, communicate (Johnson & Klein, 1994). Establishing a healthy sexual relationship may require professional help for some. A referral to a qualified intimacy or marital therapist helps to address psychosexual and interpersonal concerns that underlie sexual problems and can assist in the assessment of the patients and partners. Counseling sessions with a therapist can be particularly helpful with couples who have desire discrepancies, where negotiation of acceptable "middle ground" is the key for resolution. This can be a valuable adjunct to medical management (Maurice, 1999). Couples or individuals who participate in sexual counseling can learn effective ways to communicate feelings. Counseling can ease some of the stress associated with sexual dysfunction and infertility and can dispel myths.

Any discussion should include sexual changes that occur either from the cancer and its treatment or from medications. Many chemotherapy drugs cause changes in the reproductive system. If fertility will be affected by treatment, men and women may want to consider banking eggs or sperm before treatment if they think they may be interested in starting a family later.

Referral to a Specialist in Sexual Health

Sex therapy is a brief type of psychotherapy or counseling focused on solving a sexual problem. Sex therapists believe that lovemaking skills are learned and that bad habits can be corrected by learning different sexual techniques. They may practice in a clinic or independently. It is not always easy to find a well-trained sex therapist, but a professional society, such as the American Association of Sexuality Educators, Counselors, and Therapists, can provide information about members who have specific training in sex therapy.

Encourage patients to ask their cancer specialists for help with sexual problems. If they are not able to help, a family physician or member of the healthcare team may be able to offer a referral to a specialist in sexual problems. Cancer centers often offer sexual rehabilitation programs with experts who can assess and treat sexual problems. In recent years, university medical schools and even some private practice groups have begun to treat sexual problems. They may provide psychological and medical examinations through many different types of healthcare providers. When a patient is in a committed relationship, some clinics require both sexual partners to participate in the evaluation.

Fertility and Sperm Cryopreservation

Male patients with cancer who are at risk for permanent or long-lasting post-treatment infertility and who have not ruled out post-treatment paternity should be offered cryopreservation of sperm cells. This also should be offered to men with high-grade oligospermia and those with azoospermia. In some men with azoospermia, sperm cells can be retrieved by testicular sperm extraction (Schrader et al., 2003). Ideally, semen cryopreservation should be performed before treatment is initiated, and if possible, multiple samples should be preserved. Semen cryopreservation also can be considered after chemotherapy for patients in whom intensive cytotoxic treatment is planned because of tumor recurrence. Clinicians should recommend that cryopreservation be performed before orchiectomy (Peterson et al., 1999).

Although offering pretreatment semen cryopreservation is routine in many cancer centers, only a minority of patients ever use their frozen semen because they do not attempt post-treatment paternity, or they become fathers through natural conception or by using their oligospermic, post-treatment ejaculates for assisted reproductive techniques (Magelssen et al., 2005). In a retrospective study of 821 newly diagnosed male patients with cancer ages 14–30 who cryopreserved samples of semen from 1995–2005, only 146 (17.8%) used the cryopreserved sperm. Of these 146 patients, the success rate for intrauterine insemination was 36.4% with a clinical pregnancy rate of 50% in those using in vitro fertilization and intracytoplasmic sperm injection (Neal et al., 2007). The current average cost of sperm banking is more than $1,000, which includes three sperm donations and several years of storage.

Costs vary from center to center, so it is important for patients to compare costs at different centers. Many sperm banks offer financing and payment plans for patients with cancer to help with the yearly costs (American Cancer Society, 2008).

Nurses caring for patients with testicular cancer should focus on any issues surrounding the patients' altered sexuality, altered body image, altered role function, and fertility, as well as grief and concerns related to mortality. Men may view the removal of their testicle as castration, potentially affecting their masculinity, self-worth, and ability to father children. These patients should understand that neither their sexual function nor their fertility is usually decreased as a result of an orchiectomy (Poirier & Rawl, 2000). These men also might be embarrassed to discuss issues regarding their sexuality and their genitalia. Nurses should approach patients openly with the ultimate goal of creating an atmosphere where they will feel comfortable discussing sexuality.

Nurses and other healthcare professionals must be knowledgeable about the fertility hazard of oncologic treatments. Additionally, they must be informed about cryopreservation of sperm or eggs to include the actual procedure of cryopreservation, coupled with the monetary cost of storage. In some instances, because of the aggressiveness of the cancer, patients opt to forego cryopreservation. It is imperative that patients have the proper information so they can make an educated and informed decision. The process of preserving fertility in patients with urologic cancer starts with a pretreatment discussion of issues related to fertility. Depending on a patient's age and circumstances, a partner or parents also might be involved in this discussion. Patients must recognize both the possibility of a cure for their cancer and the risk of infertility, and they need to be included in the final choice of therapy. No particular fertility-preserving measures are necessary in patients who do not wish to become a parent in the future.

Sensate Focus

Sensate focus involves planned love-play exercise sessions for couples and consists of touching, caressing, and sensual massage. Sensate focus exercises consist of home exercises aimed at body exploration through sensual touching, stroking, embracing, caressing, and kissing in ways that are mutually gratifying for a couple. The sessions last approximately 30–60 minutes. Sensate focus involves various levels or phases that begin with nongenital sensual touch in the first phase, which may last for a week or longer. The next phase involves some genital touch, but no intercourse or penetrative sex, and the final phase involves anything the couple desires, including penetrative sex. Each phase or level lasts a week or longer depending on the couple's individual situation; the healthcare provider and the couple determine the length of each phase. *Sensate focus* also may be used as a phrase to describe intimate touch that may be sensual or sexual. An important concept in sensate focus is that individuals are responsible for teaching their own pleasure and orgasms to their partner. Pleasure is the goal, rather than orgasm, and this may alleviate stress related to performance anxiety. This technique was first described by Masters and Johnson (1970, 1986) and has been used in sex therapy since its introduction. Levine (1976) described sensate focus as being an essential element in sex therapy, and it has been shown to be an effective treatment for couples with sexual dysfunction (Renshaw, 1996; Sarwer & Durlak, 1997). The goal of sensate focus is to promote intimacy through positive touch and body exploration without performance anxiety for participants. This treatment option may be used in conjunction with other therapies.

Lifestyle Changes

Instructing patients about lifestyle changes can be an important part of the education process. Patients need to understand that a regular physical examination with blood work is crucial to understanding factors that may affect sexual function. Aside from the urogenital cancer, many other factors affect sexual function, including cardiovascular disease, hypertension, neurologic disorders, endocrine disorders, obesity, psychiatric illness, and high cholesterol. In addition, many medications such as antihypertensives, antidepressants, antihistamines, antiandrogens, medications used to treat benign prostate hyperplasia, and histamine-2 blockers affect sexual function. Many recreational drugs can cause ED such as alcohol, tobacco, opiates, methadone, and ecstasy. A sedentary lifestyle also can be a risk factor for sexual dysfunction in men and women (Rosen, Friedman, & Kostis, 2005; Rosen et al., 2009). A complete evaluation of the patient's history is important to understand all factors influencing sexual function.

In general, a healthy heart equals sexual health. The genitals are dependent on good blood flow for engorgement during arousal, and the blood vessels of the penis and clitoris are very small and, therefore, sensitive to any vascular changes or damage (Thompson et al., 2005). In fact, emerging scientific evidence indicates that ED may be an early indicator of cardiovascular disease (Billups, Bank, Padma-Nathan, Katz, & Williams, 2005). Patients need to be informed about the triad of sexual health-promoting lifestyle, which includes a heart-healthy diet, regular exercise, and smoking cessation. Proper weight management also is essential (Riedner, Rhoden, Ribeiro, & Fuchs, 2006). Lifestyle changes such as decreasing caloric intake, increasing physical activity, and decreasing body mass index have been shown to improve sexual function in obese men (Travison et al., 2007). Nurses play a crucial role in educating patients about eating a diet low in fat and cholesterol and high in fiber, with an appropriate caloric count. Nurses also can educate patients about the importance of regular cardiovascular exercise and smoking cessation. A healthy lifestyle can be an essential component to improving erectile function. Nurses can play a pivotal role in educating patients about healthy lifestyle choices to promote sexual health.

Treatment Options for Women

Hormonal and Nonhormonal Management

Hypoactive desire for any woman during perimenopause often is related to declining serum estradiol and testosterone levels but can be exacerbated by a diagnosis of genitourinary cancer. Adjuvant chemotherapy can cause precipitous drops in endogenous serum hormone production, and a woman's sense of self as a sexual being can be radically challenged as she faces a cancer diagnosis and potential discomfort associated with sexual activity. Healthcare providers, and women themselves, may see a prescription for hormones as a "quick fix" for sexual complaints, but in reality, hormone supplementation may or may not increase sexual desire. Cancer survivors with sexual complaints may benefit more from engaging in behavioral strategies to augment sexual desire. These may include activities such as reading erotic literature, active use of fantasy, regular exercise that increases blood flow to the pelvis, and self-stimulation of the genitals (Levy, 2002; Maurice, 1999). Women can be reminded that feeling "sexual" usually requires more than a cream or pill, and that thinking sexual thoughts and feeling the effects of arousal and exercise in their body are part of increasing libido.

Some women benefit from supplementation with estrogen, testosterone, or progesterone creams or pills. After baseline levels are assessed, the goal is to raise levels into the upper quartile of the normal range but never to supraphysiologic levels. Hormone regimens with the greatest efficacy and lowest risk often are chosen in conjunction with a compounding pharmacist and/or a reproductive endocrinologist (Davis, 1998; Goldstein, Meston, Davis, & Traish, 2006; Guay et al., 2001).

Although hormone replacement may be of great benefit to some women, it should not be considered a panacea. Research suggests that equal or greater libidinal enhancement can be achieved by combining behavior modification techniques with over-the-counter (OTC) products containing the amino acid L-arginine (e.g., ArginMax®, Daily Wellness Co.) or topical nutraceutical compounds (e.g., Zestra® arousal oil for women, Zestra Laboratories, Inc.) (Boone & Shields, 2005; Trant & Polan, 2000).

Pelvic Floor Dysfunction

Conservative therapy for either type of PFD is aimed at muscle reeducation. For HT-PFD, directed massage of the pelvic floor can be performed to elongate shortened muscles and decrease spasm of the pelvic floor muscles. Pelvic floor massage can precede and facilitate the gradual introduction of vaginal dilators and movement toward sexual penetration for patients who are having difficulty accommodating penile penetration. For LT-PFD, which can manifest as incontinence with sex, decreased sensation, or poor orgasm amplitude, a program focusing on progressive pelvic floor muscle strengthening using Kegel exercises, biofeedback, and/or electrical stimulation is often sufficient for return of function (Costello, 1998; Fitzgerald & Kotarinos, 2003; Lukban & Whitmore, 2000; Thiele, 1963; Travell & Simons, 1992).

For some women, participating in coitus or other forms of sexual play may result in a flare of urinary or pain symptoms for hours or days, which can become a negative reinforcer of future sexual activity. Prolonged lack of physical intimacy also can result in generalized loss of interest in sex, decreased ability to respond sexually, and feelings of depression. Nurses should encourage women and their partners to develop a unique definition of adequate pleasuring, which may or may not involve genital contact, and to make a commitment to pleasure each other with agreed-upon regularity. Encourage couples to follow their own sexual script, not one that society has written for them (Kellogg-Spadt, 2002; Leiblum, 1993).

For some couples, oral and manual pleasuring of the clitoris and/or penis (without penetration) are viable options, whereas others find the option of "outercourse" appealing and pain free. In this technique, a man mounts a woman in a traditional intercourse fashion, but instead of thrusting his penis inside of her vagina, he thrusts on the outside. By rubbing against the woman's lubricated lower abdomen and pubic bone area or between her inner thighs, friction is often sufficient enough to result in both male and female orgasm (Herman, 2000; Kellogg-Spadt & Whitmore, 2006; Leiblum, 1993; Webster & Brennan, 1995).

For other women, sexual intercourse can be accomplished on a limited basis. Comfort measures that facilitate intimate expression may include (Kellogg-Spadt & Albaugh, 2002; Kellogg-Spadt & Whitmore, 2006)

- Applying 2%–5% lidocaine jelly to the vaginal introitus 20 minutes before stimulation to decrease hypersensitivity of the urethra and vestibular gland areas
- Applying liberal amounts of a water-soluble lubricant or a small amount of estrogen-based vaginal cream to aid with penetration
- Premedicating with a sublingual smooth muscle relaxant or an anticholinergic agent to decrease sensory urinary or fecal urgency
- Premedicating with a skeletal muscle relaxant (either oral tablets or compounded vaginal or rectal suppositories) approximately one hour before sex play to decrease muscle spasm and calm both the bladder and pelvic floor.

In addition, many women find that precoital pelvic floor massage, pre- and postcoital voiding, and postcoital application of an icepack to the genital/suprapubic area enhance comfort (Fitzgerald & Kotarinos, 2003; Webster & Brennan, 1995; Whitmore et al., 1998).

Coital positions that are least likely to affect the pelvic floor include side-lying and female inferior with raised hips. Circular movement thrusting and limiting thrusting time to 5–10 minutes helps to minimize discomfort (Kellogg-Spadt & Albaugh, 2002; Kellogg-Spadt & Whitmore, 2006; Leiblum, 1993).

Incontinence

Women may experience involuntary loss of urine and/or feces after urologic cancer. Factors that predispose a woman to incontinence include age, birth trauma, pelvic/vaginal surgery, radiation therapy, menopausal status, strenuous lifting, obesity, and constipation. Assessment strategies for incontinence include evaluation of voiding diaries, urinalysis, cytology, and urodynamic testing (Parker, Rosenman, & Parker, 2002). Incontinence can be improved in 8 of 10 women by multimodal treatment approaches, including behavioral bladder retraining, pelvic floor muscle retraining, pessary placement, use of smooth muscle relaxants, anticholinergics, antimuscarinics, and reconstructive surgical procedures (Berglund & Fugl-Meyer, 1996; Hampel, Weinhold, Benken, Eggersmann, & Thuroff, 1997; Parker et al.).

Managing Sexuality With Incontinence

Estimates of incontinence during intercourse range from 20%–56% (Bo, Talseth, & Vinsnes, 2000; Clark & Romm, 1993; Gordon et al., 1999). Studies suggest that the effect of incontinence upon sexual activity varies widely. For example, Barber et al. (2002) and Gordon et al. noted that the frequency of sexual activity is reduced in incontinent patients, and because of the attendant embarrassment that accompanies urine loss, these patients avoid intercourse. Data from other sources suggest that women with mild to moderate incontinence report a commensurate frequency of sexual activity, comfort, and enjoyment with sex, as do women without incontinence (Berglund & Fugl-Meyer, 1996; Roe & May, 1999). Parker et al. (2002) noted that stress urinary incontinence associated with pelvic organ prolapse may be less problematic in terms of sexuality (because herniated tissues often are pushed into the vagina with penile penetration), whereas urine loss associated with sensory urgency may be more distressing because of the physical discomfort caused by pressure and the unpredictability of urine loss.

Women who experience urinary incontinence during intercourse express concerns about feeling unclean, undesirable, and "unsexy." They fear embarrassment, rejection, and possible subsequent vaginal or urinary tract infection (Coyne et al., 2007). Encouraging a woman to be open and communicative with her partner about incontinence will often decrease anxiety by bringing the issue into the forefront. Educating the woman with urinary leakage that urine is sterile and poses little true health threat often will decrease fear associated with unavoidable leakage. Other strategies for women who experience any type of incontinence during sexual activity include (Kellogg-Spadt & Albaugh, 2002; Kellogg-Spadt & Whitmore, 2006; LeCroy, 2006; Parker et al., 2002)

- Daily performance of Kegel exercises
- Use of biofeedback or electrical stimulation before intimacy
- Emptying the bladder or colon before sexual activity
- Avoiding ingestion of fluids for one hour before lovemaking
- Coital positioning to decrease leakage (e.g., female in superior or side-lying position with minimal-depth thrusting)
- Using a water-soluble lubricant or vaginal estrogen before penetration to decrease urethral trauma and facilitate comfortable entry.

An individual's sense of well-being after urologic cancer may be closely tied to the quality of her intimate physical relationships. By taking the time to assess and address patients' sexual concerns, healthcare providers can help people with genitourinary cancers to reclaim a sense of self as a woman capable of intimacy, enabling active participation in a loving relationship (Kellogg-Spadt & Albaugh, 2002; LeCroy, 2006; Parker et al., 2002).

Treatment Options for Men

Erectile Dysfunction Treatment Options

Several options are available to men with cancer who are experiencing ED. See Table 9-3 for a comprehensive description of treatment modalities.

Vacuum Constriction Devices

Vacuum constriction devices (VCDs) are the least invasive and least expensive of all ED treatment options and can be used regardless of etiology. The VCD consists of an acrylic cylinder with a pump that may be applied directly to the penis, and several tension/constriction bands or rings of various sizes and tensions (see Figure 9-5). These devices operate manually or are battery powered. Water-soluble lubricant also is needed. The cylinder's open base is large enough to fit over the penis. All devices have pressure release valves on either the pump or the cylinder. To use the device, the cylinder, with a tension band stretched over the open end, is placed over the flaccid penis. A vacuum suction is created from negative pressure drawing blood into the shaft of the penis and causing it to become erect. Once the penis is erect, the constriction band is slid off the base of the cylinder and onto the penis. The pump then is removed from the penis, lubricant is applied, and intercourse can be attempted with the constriction band in place to maintain the erection. The band can remain safely in place for up to 30 minutes. Studies suggest that about 80%–90% of men are satisfied with the results of VCD (DeWolf & Heney, 1997; Sidi & Lewis, 1992). In one study (Cookson and Nadig, 1993), patient and partner satisfaction rates were 84% and 89%, respectively, in a group of 115 men followed

at 11–63 months (mean follow-up 29 months). As with any other method of treatment for ED, satisfaction rates may decrease with time. In a study comparing self-injection therapy using papaverine and phentolamine and VCDs, the group using self-injection therapy had a 59% dropout rate, whereas the VCD group had only a 16% dropout rate (Turner et al., 1992).

VCDs are safe and can be used by patients with ED caused by various etiologies. Men who may have a significant congenital bleeding disorder or a disorder that predisposes them to a condition called priapism (a prolonged, sometimes painful erection lasting several hours) should not use VCDs. Examples include sickle cell anemia, some forms of leukemia, blood conditions, and clotting disorders. An erection obtained by the VCD is not the same as an erection achieved naturally. The penis tends to be purplish or bluish in color, can be cold to the touch, and may have less sensation. Other side effects can include hematoma, ecchymosis, petechiae, blocked or retrograde ejaculation, pulling on scrotal tissue, and pivoting of the base of the penis. VCDs vary in cost and are approximately $300–$500, depending on the brand and type. The battery-powered versions tend to be more expensive. It is more difficult to control the amount of vacuum pressure, but they tend to work a little faster. Battery-powered devices are especially helpful for men who do not have good hand strength or coordination or who have arthritis. Several devices are available that work effectively, and some can be obtained without a prescription. Most insurance policies, including Medicare, cover at least part of the costs of a VCD, especially if a medical cause for ED has been documented. Medicaid, however, does not cover these devices.

The use of VCDs for treating ED appears straightforward, yet patients need thorough initial instruction if the therapy is to be successful. They also need ongoing medical and emotional support to understand and manage associated problems, such as difficulty achieving or maintaining an erection and pain or discomfort during use of a vacuum device. Success with the VCD requires a period of "reconditioning" that consists of 5–10 minutes of daily practice for approximately 14 days before proceeding to sexual intercourse (Albaugh & Lewis, 2005). The use of easily understood analogies (e.g., explaining how the process is similar to training any other muscle in the body to become accustomed to a new kind of exercise with conditioning for a few minutes a day to build tolerance) can help the patient to understand the reason for the "reconditioning" period and the need to become familiar with the device.

The value of individualized education, and technical and emotional support for both the patient and partner, often is critical in determining the success of this treatment. Couples who receive proper initial instruction on the use of the VCD and assistance with problems that arise during its use are more likely to see this therapy succeed.

Table 9-3. Erectile Dysfunction Treatments

Treatment	Dosage	Contraindications	Precautions	Side Effects	Teaching/Instruction
Sildenafil (Viagra®, Pfizer Inc.) Onset: 30–60 minutes Duration: 4 hours; may be in system for up to 12–14 hours	25–100 mg Adjust to 25 mg for hepatic or severe renal impairment	Not with nitrates	Start at 25 mg in patients > 65 years old. Use caution with CHF or MI within 6 months, resting hypotension, and if on alpha-blockers, or with retinitis pigmentosa. See PI for information on use with alpha-blockers. Have patient report changes in vision that might indicate NAION.	Headache, dyspepsia, visual disturbances, flushing, nasal congestion, dizziness	No fat in diet for 2 hours before. Must have stimulation. Not approved for females. Does not protect against STDs. Use no more than once a day. Take 30–60 minutes prior to sexual activity. May need multiple attempts. No effect on libido, ejaculation, or orgasm.
Vardenafil (Levitra®, Bayer Healthcare Pharmaceuticals Inc.) Onset: 25–30 minutes Duration: 4–5 hours; may last in system for up to 12–14 hours	10–20 mg	Not with nitrates	A starting range of 5 mg is recommended for patients 65 or older. Adjust dose to 5 mg and advance to no greater than 10 mg with moderate renal impairment. Levitra has not been evaluated in men with severe renal impairment. Use caution with QT prolongation. Caution with alpha-blockers (see PI for how to dose with alpha-blockers). Have patient report changes in vision that might indicate NAION.	Headache, flushing, dyspepsia, rhinitis, indigestion, dizziness, visual changes	Very high fat intake may affect absorption. Not approved for females. Does not protect against STDs. Use no more than once a day. Take 30–60 minutes prior to sexual activity. May need multiple attempts. No effect on libido, ejaculation, or orgasm. Must have stimulation.
Tadalafil (Cialis®, Eli Lilly and Co.) Onset: 30 minutes Duration: 12–24 hours; may last in system up to 36 hours	5–20 mg	Not with nitrates	Not if MI in last 90 days, unstable angina, class 2 or greater heart failure, uncontrolled arrythmias, hypotension or uncontrolled HTN, stroke within last 6 months. Caution with QT prolongation. Caution with alpha-blockers (see PI for how to titrate with alpha-blockers). Have patient report changes in vision that might indicate NAION.	Headache, dyspepsia, dizziness, flushing, nasal congestion, back pain, myalgia	No food restrictions. Not approved for females. Does not protect against STDs. Use no more than once a day. Take 30–60 minutes prior to sexual activity. May need multiple attempts. No effect on libido, ejaculation, or orgasm. Must have stimulation.
ACTIS® (Vivus, Inc.) Duration: 30 minutes duration max.	N/A	Latex or rubber hypersensitivty Abnormally formed penis Sickle cell, leukemia, tumor of bone marrow, or conditions that increase or decrease blood clotting	–	Pain in or redness of penis Bruising Prolonged erection	Do not keep on more than 30 minutes at a time. Do not fall asleep using product. Allow 60 minutes between uses.

(Continued on next page)

Table 9-3. Erectile Dysfunction Treatments (Continued)

Treatment	Dosage	Contraindications	Precautions	Side Effects	Teaching/Instruction
Vacuum therapy	N/A	History of priapism, sickle cell, bleeding disorders	–	Hematoma, ecchymosis, petechiae, numbness of penis, pain, pulling of scrotal tissue, blocked or painful ejaculation	Requires thorough initial instruction, good dexterity, lots of water-soluble jelly, and reconditioning for up to 2 weeks. Do not use the tension ring for more than 30 minutes at a time.
MUSE® (Vivus, Inc.) Onset: 5–10 minutes Duration: 30–60 minutes	250–1,000 mcg	Hypersensitivity to drug Abnormally formed penis Conditions causing prolonged erections like sickle cell, leukemia, tumor of bone marrow Not for intercourse with pregnant women without a barrier	–	Aching in penis, testicles, or perineum Warmth or burning in urethra Redness of penis Hypotension Bleeding Prolonged erection Swelling of leg veins Lightheadedness/ dizziness Fainting Rapid pulse	Monitor the patient. He may be uncomfortable or hypotensive. If lightheadedness occurs, have the patient lie down until it passes. Patient must move around to get blood circulating immediately after instilled. Refrigerate unopened pacakage. Can be kept at room temperature for up to 14 days at < 86°.
Intracavernosal injection (PGE1) Onset: 5–20 minutes Duration: 30 minutes–4 hours	5–40 mcg or as prescribed with compounds	Hypersensitivity Conditions that may lead to priapism like sickle cell, multiple myeloma, leukemia, deformed penis Penile implants	–	Priapism (prolonged erection) Pain Peyronies (curvature) Ecchymosis Injection site hematoma Upper respiratory infection	Comprehensive one-on-one teaching and in-office titration Regular follow-up Store at or below 77°. Single-use item Rotate sites; avoid visible veins. Once in 24 hours, 3 times/week max What to do when erection lasts > 3–4 hours
Penile implant	N/A	Poor surgical risk	–	Postoperative pain Possibility of infection Erosion Mechanical failure Risks of any surgery like blood clot or bleeding Unrealistic expectations	Always a final irreversible choice

CHF—congestive heart failure; HTN—hypertension; mcg—microgram; mg—milligram; MI—myocardial infarction; N/A—not applicable; NAION—nonarteritic anterior ischemic optic neuropathy; PI—package insert; STD—sexually transmitted disease

Note. From *Understanding Erectile Dysfunction: Patient Evaluation and Treatment Options* (pp. 11–14), by J.A. Albaugh and J.H. Lewis, 2007, Pitman, NJ: Society of Urologic Nurses and Associates. Copyright 2007 by Society of Urologic Nurses and Associates. Adapted with permission.

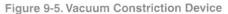

Figure 9-5. Vacuum Constriction Device

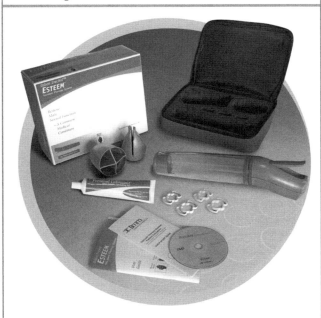

Note. Photo courtesy of Timm Medical Technologies, Inc. Used with permission.

Venous Flow Constriction Therapy

These devices are helpful for men with difficulty maintaining their erection. They are bands of various designs and materials that are placed around the base of the penis, allowing the penis to stay fully erect. They are placed on the penis after achieving an erection to assist in the maintenance of the erection. They are easy to use, comfortable, and fully adjustable. Vivus, Inc. (2003) offers a constriction band, ACTIS® (see Figure 9-6), that can be applied at the base of the penis to decrease venous flow return back into the body. This

Figure 9-6. Venous Flow Constriction Band

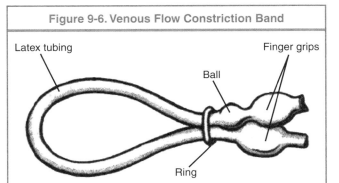

Latex tubing   Finger grips

Ball

Ring

Note. Figure courtesy of Vivus, Inc., manufacturer and marketer of ACTIS® venous flow constriction band. Used with permission.

device can be used in conjunction with alprostadil (MUSE® suppositories, Vivus, Inc.) to improve erectile function.

Oral Agents

Sildenafil, tadalafil, and vardenafil are potent, reversible, competitive inhibitors of phosphodiesterase type 5 (PDE5). At this time, evidence is insufficient to support the superiority of one agent over the others (Montague et al., 2006). Many patients prefer oral therapy because its convenience decreases the embarrassment of discussing ED (Hatzichristou et al., 2000).

Sildenafil (Viagra®, Pfizer Inc.): Sildenafil citrate is the first oral medication that was approved by the U.S. Food and Drug Administration for the treatment of ED. Sildenafil is a PDE5 inhibitor that increases cyclic guanosine monophosphate levels, a chemical present in the penis to relax the erectile tissue and dilate the arteries, thus increasing blood flow during the erectile process (Boolell, Gepi-Attee, Gingell, & Allen, 1996).

Sildenafil is available in three doses: 25 mg, 50 mg, and 100 mg (Pfizer Inc., 2007). The usual starting dose is 50 mg one hour prior to sex as needed, no more than one time in 24 hours. If needed, patients can receive a dose as low as 25 mg or be escalated to a dose of 100 mg. In a dose escalation study, sildenafil was found to be successful in 69% of men with mixed etiology ED (Goldstein et al., 1998). The success rate falls to 50% after nerve-sparing radical prostatectomy (Zippe, Kedia, Kedia, Nelson, & Agarwal, 1998).

Individualized patient instruction is the key to the success of the oral medications. Patients need to be instructed to take the medication one hour prior to initiating sexual activity. Although some patients may notice results in as little as 30 minutes to as long as four hours, one hour is the usual reaction time after medication ingestion. It should preferably be taken on an empty stomach or after a low-fat meal. High-fat food and a full stomach interrupt absorption of sildenafil. It is essential when starting sexual activity that the patient has direct physical stimulation to the penis; without stimulation, sildenafil will not be effective.

Sildenafil is a vasodilator that lowers blood pressure by about 8 mm Hg (Kloner, 2000). Because of the vasodilation effect of sildenafil, it is recommended that patients not take an alpha-blocker within four hours of sildenafil. The combination of sildenafil and nitrates can result in severe hypotension and syncope (Webb et al., 2000). As a result, sildenafil is contraindicated for any patient carrying an active nitrate prescription. These patients should be referred for consideration of alternate therapies.

Patients need to be cautioned regarding potential side effects of sildenafil. Side effects include cutaneous flushing, headache, dyspepsia, dizziness, and visual disturbances (Pfizer Inc., 2007). The most common side effects are flushing and headache. The visual change often called "blue haze" is rare, only seen in approximately 3% of patients (Archer et al., 2005). Patients with this side effect may complain of their vision taking on a blue hue or a blue hue around bright lights. They should be reassured that it is a temporary effect and will resolve when the medication leaves the system. If patients notice a headache, they may take an OTC medication for it. Although no studies support the use of OTC headache medications (e.g., acetaminophen, aspirin, ibuprofen) for PDE5 inhibitor–induced headaches, many patients anecdotically have reported that premedicating with an OTC headache medication before taking sildenafil may help to prevent the headache as well as decrease headache pain.

Vardenafil (Levitra®, Bayer Healthcare Pharmaceuticals Inc.): Vardenafil was the second oral medication made available for ED. As a selective PDE5 inhibitor, vardenafil was found to be more biochemically potent than sildenafil in both in vitro and in vivo studies when tested under the same conditions (Saenz de Tejada et al., 2001). Vardenafil is available in 5 mg, 10 mg, and 20 mg doses. Most patients are started on 10 mg and may dose down to 5 mg or up to 20 mg as needed. Vardenafil may be active from 30 minutes to four hours. As with other PDE5 medications, it should be taken one hour prior to sexual activity. Vardenafil can be taken with food in the stomach, but taking it after eating a large meal will slow down absorption and may affect efficacy. It is recommended not to mix alcohol and vardenafil. Patients should be counseled to have direct physical stimulation at the start of sexual activity to activate the vardenafil. Patients who have an active prescription for nitrates are contraindicated for vardenafil. The combination of vardenafil and nitrates can cause severe syncope that could be life threatening. Patients on large amounts of alpha-blockers will need to be managed carefully, beginning with the lowest dose of vardenafil and slowly titrating as needed. Patients should not take vardenafil and alpha-blockers within a four-hour time period (Bayer Healthcare Pharmaceuticals Inc., 2008).

The most common side effects seen with vardenafil include headache, rhinitis, cutaneous flushing, and dyspepsia. No "blue haze" effect has been shown with vardenafil (Hellstrom et al., 2002). If patients notice a headache, anecdotal reports from patients support that taking an OTC medication for headache usually helps to relieve the discomfort. In the rare cases in which the side effects are severe, the patient should be referred for other treatment options.

Vardenafil is another choice for patients with ED after cancer treatment. It is commonly used as a daily medication after nerve-sparing surgery to maintain tissue integrity during the healing process. The medication can be discontinued if spontaneous erections return. As with other ED treatments, counseling on the use of vardenafil is recommended for both the patient and partner when possible (Bayer Healthcare Pharmaceuticals Inc., 2008).

Tadalafil (Cialis®, Eli Lilly and Co.): Tadalafil is a potent, selective, reversible PDE5 inhibitor with proven efficacy in men with mild to severe ED of psychogenic, organic, or mixed origins. It is rapidly absorbed but longer lived than sildenafil and vardenafil. Food consumption has no effect on the adsorption of tadalafil (Eli Lilly and Co., 2005). These factors may translate into a more convenient, comfortable sexual experience by virtually eliminating the need for planning intercourse. It is important to involve the spouse or partner in processes that help the patient to achieve success. This also may strengthen their relationship.

The recommended starting dosage is 10 mg once a day and can be increased to 20 mg or decreased to 5 mg based on efficacy and tolerability. Dosing change is not necessary based on patient age. As with all PDE5 inhibitors, sexual stimulation, both visual and physical, is needed. Success does not always happen on the first try or even the first couple of attempts. Some patients require seven or eight attempts before intercourse is successfully completed. In men receiving tadalafil 20 mg, more than 70% of intercourse attempts were successfully completed from more than 30 minutes to 36 hours after dosing (Brock et al., 2002). Tadalafil has a longer half-life (16–18 hours) than the other PDE5 inhibitors. It is contraindicated in patients who take nitrates in any form or frequency, as PDE5 inhibitors potentiate the profound and rapid vasodilation caused by nitrates. Caution should be used with alpha-blockers, and patients should notify their healthcare providers of any loss of vision and stop taking tadalafil immediately. The most common adverse events include headache, flushing, dyspepsia, and back pain. Back pain is infrequently problematic, leading to discontinuation in less than 1% of men. Other adverse events generally are mild and transient. Rare reports of prolonged erections greater than four hours and priapism have been documented (Eli Lilly and Co., 2005). The relatively low incidence of side effects is consistent with the approximately 100-fold greater PDE5:PDE6 selectivity of tadalafil.

As with all PDE5 inhibitors, sexual stimulation is needed, multiple sexual attempts may be required, and follow-up visits are essential. Adjust the dose or timing if necessary, advise patients regarding food interactions, and remember that risk factor modification may improve treatment outcomes.

Efficacy rates vary from patient to patient with the use of each of the three oral agents. After a patient and healthcare provider select a medication, it is important to try the medication several times under medical supervision for dosing titration. If patients are unsatisfied with the results of one oral medication, they may want to try a different agent. The goal with the oral agents is to find the most effective agent that is best tolerated in the particular patient.

Hormone Therapy for Men

Alterations in hormone levels in response to cancer treatment are common. Hormone replacement seems an obvious approach, but it is not without concern or controversy. Hormone therapy in men with genitourinary cancer may be given to either actively treat disease or to manage the side effects of disease and treatment.

Androgen replacement therapy with testosterone has been used by both men and women to increase libido, elevate mood, and reestablish sexual functioning (Shah & Montoya, 2007). In men, it is recommended that testosterone therapy be tried when clinical complaints are accompanied by decreased testosterone levels (Ohl & Quallich, 2006). It is well recognized that as men age, their testosterone levels will fall, regardless of whether they have a cancer diagnosis. The name attributed to this and its accompanying decrease in libido and sexual functioning is *andropause* (Katz, 2004; Thompson, Shanafelt, & Loprinzi, 2003). A variety of testosterone preparations can be used, including buccal testosterone (Striant®, Columbia Laboratories) given twice daily; intramuscular injections of testosterone cypionate (Depo®-Testosterone, Pfizer Inc.) given every two, three, or four weeks; and two topical forms as a transdermal testosterone patch (Androderm®, Watson Urology) or transdermal hypoalcoholic gel (Testim®, Auxillium Pharmaceuticals) administered daily. The topical preparations generally are without side effects but tend to be relatively expensive. Most believe that the oral agents are of no to limited value. The injectable form is most commonly used, but the patient may experience cyclical highs and lows right after and just prior to injections. This cycling effect is modified by altering administration schedules (Margo & Winn, 2006; Ohl & Quallich).

Alprostadil (MUSE, Vivus, Inc.)

MUSE (Medicated Urethral Suppository for Erection) was introduced in 1997. At the time it was the first FDA-approved medication for ED that did not require an injection into the penis. MUSE consists of a very small pellet containing alprostadil (prostaglandin E1). MUSE is supplied in an applicator (see Figure 9-7) for ease of use. MUSE is supplied in 125, 250, 500, and 1,000 mcg doses. It must be refrigerated. Alprostadil is a potent vascular dilator. When applied transurethrally, the medication is absorbed into the corpus spongiosum and then passed on to the corpus cavernosum. The alprostadil suppository aids in dilating vascular arteries and relaxing the smooth muscle tissue of the

penis. This results in erectile activity. MUSE should be used approximately 10–15 minutes prior to the beginning of sexual foreplay. Direct stimulation to the penis during foreplay will enhance the effects of the medication.

Careful instruction is essential for successful results with MUSE. Patients should be instructed to urinate immediately before applying the MUSE. The residual urine left in the urethra will help with insertion and dispersion. Patients are then advised to apply a constriction band, ACTIS, to the base of the penis. It has been shown that using the constriction band during application ensures better absorption in the penis, less loss of medication through venous outflow, and a more effective result (Padma-Nathan, Tam, & Place, 1997). The band should be very snug; assure the patient it will only be on during the MUSE application process. After pulling the penis out on a stretch, the patient should then carefully slide the applicator into the collar. If the patient is finding the insertion difficult, a small amount of water-soluble lubricant may be placed on the applicator. It is important to stress the need to keep the penis on a full stretch to elongate the urethra, thus preventing inadvertent scraping with the applicator. Once inserted, the patient should press the button on the end of the applicator to dislodge the pellet into the urethra. He can then slowly withdraw the applicator and discard. While keeping the penis in an upright position, the patient should slowly massage, downward only, along the urethra for approximately 15 seconds. The penis can then be left down. After five minutes, it is recommended that the penis be physically stimulated. After 10 minutes the ACTIS band can be removed.

Side effects of MUSE are mild penile pain, hypotension, and rare syncope (Padma-Nathan, Hellstrom, et al., 1997). Because of the risk of hypotension and the need for careful instruction, it is recommended that the first dose be given in the clinic setting under supervision. The usual first dose is 250 or 500 mcg. If patients notice a mild aching from the alprostadil, they should be encouraged to continue the therapy, because patients often report that the aching diminishes and disappears with time and use. Risks of penile scarring and priapism are rare with this treatment. Patients and partners may be concerned that the MUSE will pass to the partner during orgasm. Patients need to be reassured that the risk is rare. MUSE is absorbed quickly and is no longer present in any substance by the time the patient reaches orgasm. However, if this is a serious concern, patients can use a condom to alleviate the fear.

Use of the combination of a PDE5 inhibitor such as sildenafil and MUSE has shown very favorable results. In a study of 28 patients with ED, 17 of which had undergone radical prostatectomy, all patients had failed therapy with MUSE or sildenafil alone. However, with the combination therapy of sildenafil one hour before and MUSE immediately before sexual activity, all 28 patients were able to have successful intercourse at 30 months (Nehra, Blute, Barrett, & Moreland, 2002). Use of this combination of medications is a good alternative, particularly for motivated patients who are uncomfortable with the idea of injection therapy.

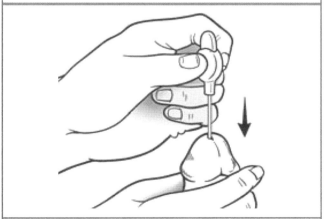

Figure 9-7. MUSE (Medicated Urethral Suppository for Erection) Hormone Therapy

Note. Figure courtesy of Vivus, Inc., manufacturer and marketer of MUSE®. Used with permission.

Intracavernosal Penile Injection Therapy

Penile injections have been utilized as a local penile treatment for ED since they were introduced in the early 1980s, and can be effective in patients with all types of ED (Brindley, 1986). Injections have an efficacy rate of 85%–95% in patients with ED caused by psychological, hormonal, neurologic, vascular, or iatrogenic dysfunction (Linet & Ogring, 1996; Shabsigh et al., 2000). They cause a direct vasodilatory response and, therefore, they may be effective in patients with urologic cancer who have undergone radiation or surgery affecting the neurovascular response to erections, patients who are on medications that affect erectile function, or patients who have impaired hormonal influences. The pharmacologically produced erection may occur with or without stimulation and may improve with stimulation. Injectable agents include monotherapy with alprostadil (prostaglandin) in the form of Caverject Impulse® (Pfizer Inc.) (see Figure 9-8), Edex® (Schwarz Pharma), or a compounded generic off-label use of prostaglandin E1. Off-label compounded injectable formulas have been used the longest, but must be produced in a special compounding pharmacy. These injectable agents include bi-mixtures, tri-mixtures, and quad-mixtures of prostaglandin E1, papaverine, phentolamine, and atropine. Penile injections utilize vasoactive agents to cause direct vasodilation of the blood vessels within the penis, causing penile engorgement and leading to an erection. Injections are contraindicated in the following individuals (Pharmacia, 2002; Schwarz Pharma, 2004).

- Anyone with a hypersensitivity to alprostadil or prostaglandins (if using tri-mixture or quad-mixture, also hypersensitivity to papaverine, phentolamine, and atropine)
- Men with a condition that would predispose them to priapism (sickle cell anemia or trait, multiple myeloma, leukemia, polycythemia, thrombocytopenia, hyperviscosity, prone to venous thrombosis)
- Men with an anatomic deformity of the penis (e.g., curvature, angulation, Peyronie disease, or fibrosis of the penis)
- Men with penile implants
- Men with conditions in which sexual activity is prohibited
- Women or children

The key to success with penile injections is one-on-one teaching with men and their partner, when appropriate. The partner can be involved in the injection process at whatever level the couple agrees will work best for them. Patient education includes instruction on how to prepare and mix the medication, how to safely inject it, and what to do if problems occur, including prolonged erection, pain, and curvature of the penis. Teaching modalities should be multidimensional including written, verbal, video, and demonstration techniques. After teaching is complete, the patient should demonstrate appropriate technique for injecting himself. A healthcare provider that is proficient in penile injection techniques should teach injections.

The most common side effects (in order of incidence) include penile pain/ache, prolonged erection, facial flushing or dizziness, bleeding, hematoma, ecchymosis, penile angulation, penile fibrosis, scarring or deformity of the penis, and difficulty attaining ejaculation (Pharmacia, 2002; Schwarz Pharma, 2004). With proper instruction from a healthcare provider, most side effects can be minimized. It is important to teach clients to seek immediate medical help if they have an erection lasting longer than three to four hours in duration.

Penile Prosthesis

Surgical implantation of a penile prosthesis, which was at one time the mainstay of treatment for ED, currently is performed when conservative treatments are not effective or desired by the patient. For patients who fail pharmacologic therapy or who prefer a permanent solution for the problem, surgical implantation of a semirigid or inflatable penile prosthesis is available. It should be emphasized that this is the only irreversible form of treatment for ED. Various types of surgical prostheses have been described in the literature. The inflatable penile prosthesis provides a more aesthetic erection and better concealment than semirigid prostheses. The penis may be slightly smaller and lack increased girth or tumescence with the malleable or positionable prostheses.

Erection with the inflatable prosthesis will be more normal in size and girth. The inflatable penile prosthesis consists of two cylinders—a reservoir and a pump—which are placed surgically in the body (see Figure 9-9). The two cylinders are inserted in the penis and connected by tubing to a separate reservoir of fluid. The reservoir is implanted under the groin muscles. A pump also is connected to the system and sits under the loose skin of the scrotal sac, between the testicles.

To inflate the prosthesis, the pump is pressed. The pump transfers fluid from the reservoir to the cylinders in the penis, inflating them and causing an erection. Pressing on a deflation valve at the base of the pump returns the fluid to the reservoir, deflating the penis and returning it to the normal flaccid state.

Figure 9-8. Caverject Impulse Syringe

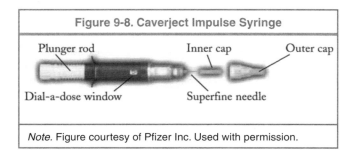

Plunger rod   Inner cap   Outer cap

Dial-a-dose window   Superfine needle

Note. Figure courtesy of Pfizer Inc. Used with permission.

Figure 9-9. Inflatable Penile Prosthesis	Figure 9-10. Positionable Penile Prosthesis
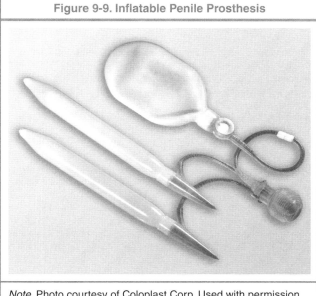	
Note. Photo courtesy of Coloplast Corp. Used with permission.	*Note.* Photo courtesy of Coloplast Corp. Used with permission.

When the penis is inflated, the prosthesis makes the penis stiff and thick, similar to a natural erection. Most men rate the erection as shorter than their normal erection; however, newer models have cylinders that may increase the length, thickness, and stiffness of the penis.

The positionable penile prosthesis has an innovative design providing three features: ease of positioning, cosmetic concealment, and rigidity for sexual intercourse (see Figure 9-10). The erection produced by an implant is not exactly "natural" and is particularly different in length. The patient can expect a post-implant length that is approximately the same as when the flaccid penis is stretched. Montague and Angermeier (2006) studied the utility of preoperative stretched penile length (SPL) as a predictor of post-implant functional length and concluded that preoperative SPL was useful for counseling patients on expected penile lengths with the implant.

A penile prosthesis does not change sensation on the skin of the penis or the ability to reach orgasm. Ejaculation is not affected. Once a penile prosthesis is implanted, men usually cannot get an erection without inflating the prosthesis. Implantation is irreversible, thus preventing men from returning to the less-invasive treatment options (Albaugh & Lewis, 2005).

About 90%–95% of inflatable prosthesis implants produce erections suitable for intercourse. Patient-partner satisfaction rates with the prosthesis are very high, and typically 80%–90% of men are satisfied with the results and say they would choose the surgery again (Govier, 1998; McLaren & Barrett, 1992). The failure rate for inflatable penile prostheses is approximately 2.5% (Goldstein, Newman, & Baum, 1997).

No surgery is totally free of complications. Complications associated with implanting a penile prosthesis include infection, scar tissue formation, prolonged pain, perforation, urethral or corporal perforation, device malfunction, and the need for further surgery. Men with diabetes have slightly higher complication rates. No attempt at sexual intercourse should be made for four to six weeks after surgery. Informed consent is essential to ensure that the patient makes a wholly personal, intelligent, unencumbered, and free choice. Insurance coverage for these operations is possible, as long as a medical cause of ED is established. Currently, Medicare covers the surgery, but Medicaid does not. Despite the cost, invasiveness, and potential medical complications involved, penile implant surgery has been associated with high rates of patient satisfaction in previous studies (Brinkman et al., 2005; Govier, 1998; McLaren & Barrett, 1992).

Treatment of Ejaculatory Problems in Men

Patients treated for urogenital cancer may exhibit problems with delayed or rapid ejaculation. Delayed ejaculation may occur in these patients from diminished sensation to the penis related to nerve damage or blood flow changes after pelvic surgery or radiation, or from side effects related to various medications such as selective serotonin reuptake inhibitor (SSRI) antidepressants or pain medications (Rosen, Lane, & Menza, 1999). It is important to determine the underlying cause of delayed ejaculation, and if it is a medication, the prescribing healthcare provider may want to consider other medication options. Patients should never be taken off or take themselves off antidepressants without qualified supervision. Sensate focus, utilizing planned love-play, and learning new ways of pleasure can be helpful in treating delayed orgasm/ejaculation. Unfortunately, no approved medications are available to treat this condition. Rapid or premature ejaculation can occur related to sensory nerve changes. This condition can be treated many ways including teaching the patient distraction techniques to use during sexual relations, along with other treatments such as using squeeze techniques just before ejaculation, wearing layered condoms to decrease sensation, using numbing gels or creams inside a condom to decrease sensation, and off-label use of SSRI antidepressants that may delay orgasm/ejaculation (Schuster, 2006). Treatment of ejaculatory and orgasmic problems can be successful under the supervision of a trained healthcare provider.

Summary

Sexuality and intimacy are integral to the human experience, yet healthcare providers often do not address these crucial functions. Nurses spend the greatest amount of time with patients and are a trusted source for patient education, which positions them perfectly to discuss sexual issues with patients. Nurses need not worry about offending patients, if they approach each patient with a sensitive, nonjudgmental attitude, provide appropriate privacy, and use excellent communication skills to determine a patient's comfort level with discussing sexual issues. The first steps are asking patients if they have any sexual or intimacy issues and giving the patient permission to talk about sexual issues. These steps are essential because so many patients with urogenital cancers have sexual dysfunction and are suffering in silence. Provide privacy and ease your way into these sensitive questions. It might be helpful to utilize a bridge statement such as "some women have experienced problems with sexual dysfunction after radiation." Patients typically are extremely pleased to have someone to talk to about private issues. If a nurse is uncomfortable helping a patient to resolve sexual issues, the patient can be referred to a more appropriate healthcare provider, such as a psychologist, psychiatrist, gynecologist, urologist, advanced practice nurse, physical therapist, or endocrine specialist. Patients struggling with urogenital cancer deserve the very best possible care, including addressing their sexual issues with their partners by their side. Nurses can make all the difference in patients' lives if they are willing to just ask one simple question about sexual function. The patients are waiting. It is up to every nurse to facilitate a patient's journey toward healing by asking about sexual issues. Providing this crucial, life-changing care to patients with urogenital cancer can radically improve their quality of life.

References

Albaugh, J., Amargo, I., Capelson, R., Flaherty, E., Forest, C., Goldstein, I., et al. (2002). Health care clinicians in sexual health medicine: Focus on erectile dysfunction. *Urologic Nursing, 22*(4), 217–231.

Albaugh, J.A., & Lewis, J.H. (2005). *Understanding erectile dysfunction: Patient evaluation and treatment options.* Pitman, NJ: Society of Urologic Nurses and Associates.

Ali-El-Dein, B., Gomha, M., & Ghoneim, M.A. (2002). Critical evaluation of the problem of chronic urinary retention after orthotopic bladder substitution. *Journal of Urology, 168*(2), 587–592.

Al-Qudah, H.S., Rodriguez, A.R., & Sexton, W.J. (2007). Laparoscopic management of kidney cancer: Updated review. *Cancer Control, 14*(3), 218–230.

American Cancer Society. (2007a). *Overview testicular cancer: Survival rates.* Retrieved February 14, 2009, from http://www.cancer.org/docroot/CRI/content/CRI_2_4_1X_What_are_the_key_statistics_for_testicular_cancer_41.asp

American Cancer Society. (2007b). *Detailed guide: Bladder cancer.* Retrieved February 14, 2009, from http://www.cancer.org/docroot/CRI/CRI_2_3x.asp?dt=44

American Cancer Society. (2008). *Coping with physical and emotional changes: Preserving fertility in men.* Retrieved June 22, 2008, from http://www.cancer.org/docroot/MBC/content/MBC_2_3X_preserving_fertility_in_men.asp?sitearea=MBC

Anastasiadis, A.G., Davis, A.R., Sawczuk, I.S., Fleming, M., Perelman, M.A., Burchardt, M., et al. (2003). Quality of life aspects in kidney cancer: Data from a national registry. *Supportive Care in Cancer, 11*(11), 700–706.

Andersen, B.L. (1990). How cancer affects sexual functioning. *Oncology, 4*(6), 81–88.

Andersen, B.L., & Lamb, M. (1995). Sexuality and cancer. In G.P. Murphy, W. Lawrence, & R.E. Lenhard (Eds.), *American Cancer Society textbook of clinical oncology* (2nd ed., pp. 699–713). Atlanta, GA: American Cancer Society.

Annon, J.S. (1974). *The behavioral treatment of sexual problems* (pp. 43–47). Honolulu, HI: Mercantile Printing.

Archer, S., Gragasin, F., Webster, L., Bochinski, D., & Michelakis, E. (2005). Aetiology and management of male erectile dysfunction and female sexual dysfunction in patients with cardiovascular disease. *Drugs and Aging, 22*(10), 823–844.

Baldwin, K., Ginsberg, P., & Harkaway, R.C. (2003). Under-reporting of erectile dysfunction among men with unrelated urologic conditions. *International Journal of Impotence Research, 15*(2), 87–89.

Barber, M., Visco, A., Wyman, J., Fantl, J., Bump, R., & the Continence Program for Women Group. (2002). Sexual function in women with urinary incontinence and pelvic organ prolapse. *Obstetrics and Gynecology, 99*(2), 281–289.

Barral, J.P. (1993). *Urogenital manipulation.* Seattle, WA: Eastland Press.

Basson, R., Berman, J., Burnett, A., Derogatis, L., Ferguson, D., Fourcroy, J., et al. (2000). Report of the international consensus development conference on female sexual dysfunction: Definitions and classifications. *Journal of Urology, 163*(3), 888–893.

Bayer Healthcare Pharmaceuticals Inc. (2008). Levitra [Package insert]. Wayne, NJ: Author. Retrieved February 13, 2009, from http://www.univgraph.com/bayer/inserts/levitra.pdf

Berglund, A., & Fugl-Meyer, K. (1996). Some sexological characteristics of stress incontinent women. *Scandinavian Journal of Urology and Nephrology, 30*(3), 207–301.

Billups, K.L., Bank, A.J., Padma-Nathan, H., Katz, S., & Williams, R. (2005). Erectile dysfunction is a marker for cardiovascular disease: Results of the minority health institute expert advisory panel. *Journal of Sexual Medicine, 2*(1), 40–50.

Blanco-Yarosh, M. (2007). Penile cancer: An overview. *Urologic Nursing, 27*(4), 286–291.

Bo, K., Talseth, T., & Vinsnes, A. (2000). Randomized controlled trial on the effect of pelvic floor muscle training on quality of life and sexual problems in genuine stress incontinent women. *Acta Obstetrica et Gynegologica Scandinnavica, 79*(7), 598–603.

Boolell, M., Gepi-Attee, S., Gingell, J.C., & Allen, J.M. (1996). Sildenafil, a novel effective oral therapy for male erectile dysfunction. *British Journal of Urology, 78*(2), 257–261.

Boone, S.A., & Shields, K.M. (2005). Dietary supplements for female sexual dysfunction. *American Journal of Health-System Pharmacy, 62*(6), 574–580.

Brindley, G.S. (1986). Pilot experiments on the actions of drugs injected into the human corpus cavernosum penis. *British Journal of Pharmacology, 87*(3), 495–500.

Brinkman, J.J., Henry, G.D., Wilson, S.K., Delk, J.R., II, Denny, G.A., Young, M., et al. (2005). A survey of patients with inflatable penile prostheses for satisfaction. *Journal of Urology, 174*(1), 253–257.

Brock, G.B., McMahon, C.G., Chen, K.K., Costigan, T., Shen, W., Watkins, V., et al. (2002). Efficacy and safety of tadalafil in the treatment of erectile dysfunction: Results of integrated analyses. *Journal of Urology, 168*(4, Pt.1), 1332–1336.

Brown, G.B. (2004). Testicular cancer: An overview. *Urologic Nursing, 23*(2), 83–94.

Clark, A., & Romm, J. (1993). Effect of urinary incontinence on sexual activity in women. *Journal of Reproductive Medicine, 38*(9), 679–683.

Clark, P.E., Schover, L.R., Uzzo, R.G., Hafez, K.S., Rybicki, L.A., & Novick, A.C. (2001). Quality of life and psychological adaptation after surgical treatment for localized renal cell carcinoma: Impact of the amount of remaining renal tissue. *Urology, 57*(2), 252–256.

Cookson, M.S., & Nadig, P.W. (1993). Long-term results with vacuum constriction devices. *Journal of Urology, 149*(2), 290–294.

Costello, K. (1998). Myofascial syndromes. In J.F. Steege, D.A. Metzger, B.A. Levy, R.E. Blackwell, & D.L. Olive (Eds.), *Chronic pelvic pain: An integrated approach* (pp. 251–265). Philadelphia: Saunders.

Coyne, K.S., Margolis, M.K., Jumadilova, Z., Bavendam, T., Mueller, E., & Rogers, R. (2007). Overactive bladder and women's sexual health: What is the impact? *Journal of Sexual Medicine, 4*(3), 656–666.

Curhan, G., Speizer, F., Hunter, D., Curhan, S., & Stampfer, M. (1999). Epidemiology of interstitial cystitis: A population based study. *Journal of Urology, 161*(2), 549–554.

Dalbagni, G., & Herr, H. (n.d.). *Treatment of superficial bladder cancer* [UpToDate]. Retrieved June 12, 2007, from http://www.UpToDate.com/physicans/index.asp

Davis, S. (1998). The clinical use of androgens in female sexual disorders. *Journal of Sex and Marital Therapy, 24*(3), 153–163.

Davis, S., & Taylor, B. (2006). From PLISSIT to Ex-PLISSIT. In S. Davis (Ed.), *Rehabilitation: The use of theories and models in practice* (pp. 101–129). Edinburgh: Elsevier.

Dearnaley, D., Huddart, R., & Horwich, A. (2001). Regular review: Managing testicular cancer. *BMJ, 322*(7302), 1583–1588.

DeWolf, W., & Heney, N. (1997). Impotence. *Harvard Men's Health Watch, 2*(2), 1–6.

Durek, C., Richter, E., Basteck, A., Rusch-Gerdes, S., Gerdes, J., Jocham, D., et al. (2001). The fate of bacillus Calmette-Guerin after intravesical instillation. *Journal of Urology, 165*(5), 1765–1768.

Eli Lilly and Co. (2005). Cialis [Package insert]. Indianapolis, IN: Author.

Fitzgerald, M.P., & Kotarinos, R. (2003). Rehabilitation of the short pelvic floor II: Treatment of the patient with the short pelvic floor. *International Urogynecology Journal of Pelvic Floor Dysfunction, 14*(4), 269–275.

Garcia, J.A., & Rini, B.I. (2007). Recent progress in the management of advanced renal cell carcinoma. *CA: A Cancer Journal for Clinicians, 57*(2), 112–125.

Goldstein, I. (1985). Impotence. In B. Taylor (Ed.), *Difficult diagnosis* (pp. 300–309). Philadelphia: Saunders.

Goldstein, I., Lue, T.F., Padma-Nathan, H., Rosen, R.C., Steers, W.D., Wicker, P.A., et al. (1998). Oral sildenafil in the treatment of erectile dysfunction. *New England Journal of Medicine, 338*(20), 1397–1404.

Goldstein, I., Meston, C., Davis, S., & Traish, A. (Eds.). (2006). *Women's sexual function and dysfunction.* London: Taylor & Francis.

Goldstein, I., Newman, I., & Baum, N. (1997). Safety and efficacy outcome of mentor alpha-1 inflatable prosthesis implantation for impotence treatment. *Journal of Urology, 157*(3), 833–839.

Gordon, D., Groutz, A., Sinai, T., Wiezman, A., Lessing, J., David, M., et al. (1999). Sexual function in women attending a urogynecology clinic. *International Urogynecology Journal and Pelvic Floor Dysfunction, 10*(5), 325–328.

Gott, M., Galena, E., Hinchliff, S., & Elfor, H. (2004). "Opening a can of worms": GP and practice nurse barriers to talking about sexual health in primary care. *Family Practice, 21*(5), 528–536.

Govier, F.E. (1998). Mechanical reliability, surgical complications, and patient and partner satisfaction of the modern three-piece inflatable penile prosthesis. *Urology, 52*(2), 282–286.

Guay, A., Munarriz, R., Spark, R., Goldstein, I., Jacobson, J., & Talakoub, L. (2001). *Serum androgen and androgen precursor hormone levels in women with and without sexual dysfunction.* Boston: Female Sexual Function Forum.

Haboubi, N.H.J., & Lincoln, N. (2003). Views of health professionals on discussing sexual issues with patients. *Disability and Rehabilitation, 25*(6), 291–296.

Hafron, J., & Kaouk, J.H. (2007a). Ablative techniques for the management of kidney cancer. *Nature Clinical Practice Urology, 4*(5), 261–269.

Hafron, J., & Kaouk, J.H. (2007b). Cryosurgical ablation of renal cell carcinoma. *Cancer Control, 14*(3), 211–217.

Hampel, C., Weinhold, D., Benken, N., Eggersmann, C., & Thuroff, J.W. (1997). Definition of overactive bladder and epidemiology of urinary incontinence. *Urology, 501*(Suppl. 6A), S4–S14.

Hatfield, E. (1982). Passionate love, companionate love, and intimacy. In M. Fisher & G. Stricker (Eds.), *Intimacy* (pp. 267–292). New York: Plenum.

Hatzichristou, D.G., Apostolidis, A., Tzortzis V., Ioannides, E., Yannakoyorgos, K., & Kalinderis, A. (2000). Sildenafil versus intracavernous injection therapy: Efficacy and preference in patients on intracavernous injection for more than 1 year. *Journal of Urology, 164*(4), 1197–1200.

Hatzichristou, D., Rosen, R.C., Broderick, G., Clayton, A., Cuzin, B., Derogatis, L., et al. (2004). Clinical evaluation and management strategy for sexual dysfunction in men and women. *Journal of Sexual Medicine, 1*(1), 49–57.

Hellstrom, W., Gittelman, M., Karlin, G., Segerson,T., Thibonnier, M., Taylor, T., et al. (2002). Vardenafil for treatment of men with erectile dysfunction: Efficacy and safety in a randomized, double-blind, placebo-controlled trial. *Journal of Andrology, 23*(26), 763–771.

Hensley, P.L., & Nurnberg, G. (2006). Depression. In I. Goldstein, C. Meston, S. Davis, & A. Traish (Eds.), *Women's sexual function and dysfunction* (pp. 619–626). London: Taylor & Francis.

Herman, S. (2000). *Interstitial cystitis: Impact on female sexual function.* Toronto, Canada: Society for the Scientific Study of Sex Annual Meeting.

Jemal, A., Siegel, R., Ward, E., Hao, Y., Xu, J., Murray, T., et al. (2008). Cancer statistics, 2008. *CA: A Cancer Journal for Clinicians, 58*(2), 71–96.

Jensen, P.T., Groenvold, M., Klee, M.C., Thranov, I., Petersen, M.A., & Machin, D. (2003). Longitudinal study of sexual function and vaginal changes after radiotherapy for cervical cancer. *International Journal of Radiation Oncology, Biology, Physics, 56*(4), 937–949.

Johnson, J., & Klein, L. (1994). *I can cope: Staying healthy with cancer* (2nd ed.). Minneapolis, MN: Chronimed Publishing.

Kandeel, F., Koussa, V., & Swerdloff, R. (2001). Male sexual function and its disorders: Physiology, pathophysiology, clinical investigation, and treatment. *Endocrine Reviews, 22*(3), 342–388.

Katz, A. (2004). Androgen replacement therapy in aging men. *Nurse Practitioner, 29*(10), 58–64.

Katz, A. (2005). The sounds of silence: Sexuality information for cancer patients. *Journal of Clinical Oncology, 22*(10), 238–241.

Kellogg-Spadt, S. (2002). *Listening to the voices of women diagnosed with vulvodynia*. Ann Arbor, MI: Proquest Press.

Kellogg-Spadt, S., & Albaugh, J. (2002). Intimacy and bladder pain: Helping women reclaim sexuality. *Urologic Nursing, 22*(5), 355–356.

Kellogg-Spadt, S., & Whitmore, K. (2006). Role of the urologist/urogynecologist. In I. Goldstein, C. Meston, S. Davis, & A. Traish (Eds.), *Women's sexual function and dysfunction* (pp. 708–714). London: Taylor & Francis.

Kloner, R.A. (2000). Cardiovascular risk and sildenafil. *American Journal of Cardiology, 86*(2A), 57F–61F.

Krebs, L.U. (2005). Sexual and reproductive dysfunction. In C.H. Yarbro, M.H. Frogge, M. Goodman, & S. Groenwald (Eds.), *Cancer nursing: Principles and practice* (6th ed., pp. 841–869). Sudbury, MA: Jones and Bartlett.

Krebs, L.U. (2006). What should I say? Talking with patients about sexuality issues. *Clinical Journal of Oncology Nursing, 10*(3), 313–315.

Krebs, L.U. (2008). Sexual assessment in cancer care: Concepts, methods and strategies for success. *Seminars in Oncology Nursing, 24*(2), 80–90.

Lampe, H., Horwich, A., Norman, A., Nicholls, J., & Dearnaley, D. (1997). Fertility after chemotherapy for testicular germ cell cancers. *Journal of Clinical Oncology, 15*(1), 239–245.

Lally, R.M. (2006). Sexuality: Everything you might be afraid to ask but patients need to know. *ONS News, 21*(9), 1, 4–5.

Laumann, E.O., Gagnon, J.H., Michael, R.T., & Michaels, S. (2000). *The social organization of sexuality: Sexual practices in the United States*. Chicago: University of Chicago Press.

Leiblum, S. (1993). Libido and lubrication: Tips for sexual counseling. *Menopause Management, 2*(2), 16–19.

LeCroy, C. (2006). Urinary incontinence occurring during intercourse: Effect on sexual function in women. *Urologic Nursing, 26*(1), 53–56.

Levine, S.B. (1976). Marital sexual dysfunction: Introductory concepts. *Annals of Internal Medicine, 84*(4), 448–453.

Levy, B.S. (2002). Break the silence: Discuss sexual dysfunction. *OBG Management, 14*(3), 70–83.

Linet, O.I., & Ogring, F.G. (1996). Efficacy and safety of intracavernosal alprostadil in men with erectile dysfunction. *New England Journal of Medicine, 334*(14), 873–877.

Lue, T.F., Giuliano, F., Montorsi, F., Rosen, R.C., Andersson, K.E., Althof, S., et al. (2004). Summary of the recommendations on sexual dysfunctions in men. *Journal of Sexual Medicine, 1*(1), 6–23.

Lukban, J.C., & Whitmore, K.E. (2000). Pelvic floor muscle re-education: Treatment of the overactive bladder and painful bladder syndrome. *Clinical Obstetrics and Gynecology, 45*(1), 273–280.

Magelssen, H., Haugen, T., von During, V., Melve, K., Sandstad, B., & Fossa, S. (2005). Twenty years experience with semen cryopreservation in testicular cancer patients: Who needs it? *European Urology, 48*(5), 779–785.

Magnan, M.A., & Reynolds, K. (2006). Barriers to addressing patient sexuality concerns across five areas of specialization. *Clinical Nurse Specialist, 20*(6), 285–292.

Magnan, M., Reynolds, K.E., & Galvin, E.A. (2005). Barriers to addressing patient sexuality in nursing practice. *Medical-Surgical Nursing, 14*(5), 282–289.

Maliski, S.L., Heilemann, M.V., & McCorkle, R. (2001). Mastery of postprostatectomy incontinence and impotence: His work, her work, our work. *Oncology Nursing Forum, 28*(6), 985–992.

Margo, K., & Winn, R. (2006). Testosterone treatments: Why, when and how? *American Family Physician, 73*(9), 1591–1598.

Martis, G., D'Elia, G., Massimo, D., Ombres, M., & Mastrangeli, B. (2005). Prostatic capsule and nerve-sparing cystectomy in organ-confined bladder cancer: Preliminary results. *World Journal of Surgery, 29*(10), 1277–1281.

Masters, W., & Johnson, V. (1970). *Human sexual inadequacy*. Boston: Little, Brown & Co.

Masters, W., & Johnson, V. (1986). *Sex and human loving*. Boston: Little, Brown & Co.

Maurice, W.L. (1999). *Sexual medicine in primary care* (pp. 153–191). St. Louis, MO: Mosby.

Mayo Clinic. (2007). *Cancer treatment for women: Possible sexual side effects*. Retrieved February 22, 2009, from http://www.mayoclinic.com/health/cancer-treatment/SA00071

McKay, M. (1991). Vulvitis and vulvovaginitis: Cutaneous considerations. *American Journal of Obstetrical Gynecology, 165*(4, Pt. 2), 1176–1182.

McLaren, R.H., & Barrett, B.M. (1992). Patient and partner satisfaction with AMS 700 penile prosthesis. *Journal of Urology, 147*(1), 62–65.

Mick, J., Hughes, M., & Cohen, M.Z. (2004). Using the BETTER model to assess sexuality. *Clinical Journal of Oncology Nursing, 8*(1), 84–86.

Montague, D.K., & Angermeier, K.W. (2006). Predicting penile length after penile prosthesis implantation. *Journal of Sexual Medicine, 3*(Suppl. 1), 102.

Montague, D.K., Jarow, J.P., Broderick, G.A., Dmochowski, R.R., Heaton, J.P.W., Lue, T.F., et al. (2006). *The American Urological Association Erectile Dysfunction Clinical Guidelines Panel report on the treatment of erectile dysfunction*. Baltimore: American Urological Association.

Nappi, R.E., Ferdeghini, F., & Polatti, F. (2006). Mechanisms involved in desire and arousal dysfunction. In I. Goldstein, C. Meston, S. Davis, & A. Traish (Eds.), *Women's sexual function and dysfunction* (pp. 203–209). London: Taylor & Francis.

National Institutes of Health Consensus Development Panel on Impotence. (1993). NIH consensus conference: Impotence. NIH consensus development panel on impotence. *JAMA, 270*(1), 83–90.

Neal, M.S., Nagel, K., Duckworth, J., Bissessar, H., Fischer, M.A., Portwine, C., et al. (2007). Effectiveness of sperm banking in adolescents and young adults with cancer: A regional experience. *Cancer, 110*(5), 1125–1129.

Nehra, A., Blute, M.L., Barrett, D.M., & Moreland, R.B. (2002). Rationale for combination therapy of intraurethral prostaglandin E1 and sildenafil in the salvage of erectile dysfunction patients desiring noninvasive therapy. *International Journal of Impotence Research, 14*(Suppl. 1), S38–S42.

Nusbaum, M.R.H., Lanahan, P., & Sadovsky, R. (2005). Addressing the physiologic and psychological sexual changes that occur with age. *Geriatrics, 60*(9), 18–23.

Ohl, D.A., & Quallich, S.A. (2006). Clinical hypogonadism and androgen replacement therapy: An overview. *Urologic Nursing, 26*(4), 253–269.

Padma-Nathan, H., Hellstrom, W.J., Kaiser, F.E., Labasky, R.F., Lue, T.F., Nolten, W.E., et al. (1997). Treatment of men with erectile dysfunction with transurethral alprostadil, Medicated Urethral System for Erection (MUSE) Study Group. *New England Journal of Medicine, 336*(1), 1–7.

Padma-Nathan, H., Tam, P.Y., & Place, V.A. (1997). Improved erectile response to transurethral alprostadil by use of a novel, adjustable penile band [Abstract]. *Journal of Urology, 157*(Suppl.), 181A.

Park, S., & Cadeddu, J.A. (2007). Outcomes of radiofrequency ablation for kidney cancer. *Cancer Control, 14*(3), 205–210.

Parker, W.H., Rosenman, A.E., & Parker, R. (2002). Sexuality. In W.H. Parker, A.E. Rosenman, & R. Parker (Eds.), *The incontinence solution* (pp. 94–110). New York: Simon & Schuster.

Petersen, M.L., Skakkebaek, N.E., Vistisen, K., Rorth, M., & Giwercman, A. (1999). Semen quality and reproductive hormones before and after orchiectomy in men with testicular cancer. *Journal of Urology, 161*(3), 822–826.

Pharmacia. (2002). Caverject impulse [Package insert]. Kalamazoo, MI: Pharmacia and UpJohn.

Pfizer Inc. (2007). Viagra [Package insert]. New York: Author.

Poirier, S.M., & Rawl, S.M. (2000). Testicular germ cell cancer. In C.H. Yarbro, M.H. Frogge, M. Goodman, & S. Groenwald (Eds.), *Cancer nursing: Principles and practice* (5th ed., pp. 1494–1510). Sudbury, MA: Jones and Bartlett .

Pow-Sang, J.M. (2007). Minimally invasive procedures in urologic oncology: When less becomes more. *Cancer Control, 14*(3), 202–203.

Process of Care Consensus Panel. (1999). Process of care model: The process of care model for evaluation and treatment of erectile dysfunction. *International Journal of Impotence Research, 11*(2), 59–74.

Renshaw, D. (1996). Profile of a sex therapy clinic in 1996. *Journal of Women's Health, 5*(5), 481–487.

Riedner, C.E., Rhoden, E.L., Ribeiro, E.P., & Fuchs, S.C. (2006). Central obesity is an independent predictor of erectile dysfunction in older men. *Journal of Urology, 176*(4, Pt. 1), 1519–1523.

Ries, L.A.G., Harkins, D., Krapcho, M., Mariotto, A., Miller, B.A., Feuer, E.J., et al. (Eds.). (2006). *SEER cancer statistics review, 1975–2003*. Bethesda, MD: National Cancer Institute. Retrieved August 5, 2007, from http://seer.cancer.gov/csr/1975_2003

Rioux, J.E., Devlin, M.C., Gelfand, M.M., Steinberg, W.M., & Hepburn, D.S. (2000). 17 ß-estradiol vaginal tablet versus conjugated equine estrogen vaginal cream to relieve menopausal atrophic vaginitis. *Menopause, 7*(3), 156–161.

Rini, B.I., & Campbell, S.C. (2007). The evolving role of surgery for advanced renal cell carcinoma in the era of molecular targeted therapy. *Journal of Urology, 177*(6), 1978–1984.

Roe, B., & May, C. (1999). Incontinence and sexuality: Findings from a qualitative prospective. *Journal of Advanced Nursing, 30*(2), 573–579.

Romero, F.R., Romero, K.R., Mattos, M.A., Garcia, C.R., Fernandes Rde, C., & Perez, M.D. (2005). Sexual function after partial penectomy for penile cancer. *Urology, 66*(6), 1292–1295.

Rosen, R.C., Friedman, M., & Kostis, J.B. (2005). Lifestyle management of erectile dysfunction: The role of cardiovascular and concomitant risk factors. *American Journal of Cardiology, 96*(12B), 76M–79M.

Rosen, R.C., Lane, R.M., & Menza, M. (1999). Effects of SSRIs on sexual function: A comprehensive review. *Journal of Clinical Psychopharmacology, 19*(1), 67–85.

Rosen, R.C., Wing, R.R., Schneider, S., Wadden, T.A., Foster, G.D., West, D.S., et al. (2009). Erectile dysfunction in type 2 diabetic men: Relationship to exercise fitness and cardiovascular risk factors in the Look AHEAD Trial. *Journal of Sexual Medicine, 6*(5), 1414–1422.

Saenz de Tejada, I., Angulo, J., Cuevas, P., Fernandez, A., Moncada, I., Allona, A., et al. (2001). The phosphodiesterase inhibitory selectivity and the in vitro and in vivo potency of the new PDE5 inhibitor vardenafil. *International Journal of Impotence Research, 13*(5), 282–290.

Santen, R.J., Pinkerton, J.V., Conaway, M., Ropka, M., Wisniewski, L., Demer, L., et al. (2002). Treatment of urogenital atrophy with low-dose estradiol: Preliminary results. *Menopause, 9*(3), 179–187.

Sarrell, P.M. (1990). Sexuality and menopause. *Obstetrics and Gynecology, 75*(Suppl. 4), 26S–30S.

Sarwer, D.B., & Durlak, J.A. (1997). A field trial of the effectiveness of behavioral treatment for sexual dysfunctions. *Journal of Sex and Marital Therapy, 23*(2), 87–97.

Schover, L. (2006). *Sexuality and cancer: For the woman who has cancer and her partner*. Atlanta, GA: American Cancer Society.

Schover, L.R. (1998). Sexual dysfunction. In J.C. Holland (Ed.), *Psycho-oncology* (pp. 494–499). New York: Oxford University Press.

Schover, L.R., Brey, K., Lichtin, A., Lipshultz, L.I., & Jeha, S. (2002). Knowledge and experience regarding cancer, infertility, and sperm banking in younger male survivors. *Journal of Clinical Oncology, 20*(7), 1880–1889.

Schrader, M., Muller, M., Sofikitis, N., Straub, B., Krause H., & Miller, K. (2003). "Onco-tese": Testicular sperm extraction in azoospermic cancer patients before chemotherapy-new guidelines? *Urology, 61*(2), 421–425.

Schuster, T.G. (2006). Premature ejaculation. *Urologic Nursing, 26*(4), 245–249.

Schwarz Pharma. (2004). Edex [Package insert]. Milwaukee, WI: Author.

Shabsigh, R., Padma-Nathan, H., Gittleman, M., McMurray, J., Kaufman, J., & Goldstein, I. (2000). Intracavernous alprostadil alfadex is more efficacious, better tolerated, and preferred over intraurethral alprostadil plus optional Actis: A comparative, randomized, crossover, multicenter study. *Urology, 55*(1), 109–113.

Shabsigh, R., Perelman, M.A., Laumann, E.O., & Lockhart, D.C. (2004). Drivers and barriers to seeking treatment for erectile dysfunction: A comparison of six countries. *BJU International, 94*(7), 1055–1065.

Shah, K., & Montoya, C. (2007). Do testosterone injections increase libido for elderly hypogonadal patients? *Journal of Family Practice, 56*(4), 301–305.

Shinohara, N., Harabayashi, T., Sato, S., Hioka, T., Tsuchiya, K., & Koyanagi, T. (2001). Impact of nephron-sparing surgery on quality of life in patients with localized renal cell carcinoma. *European Urology, 39*(1), 114–119.

Sidi, A.A., & Lewis, J.H. (1992). Clinical trial of a simplified vacuum erection device for impotence treatment. *Urology, 39*(6), 526–528.

Srinivasan, A.K., Kaye, J.D., & Moldwin, R. (2007). Myofascial dysfunction associated with chronic pelvic floor pain: Management strategies. *Current Pain and Headache Reports, 11*(5), 359–364.

Stewart, E., & Spencer, P. (2002). *The v book: A doctor's guide to complete vulvovaginal health*. New York: Bantam Books.

Thiele, G.H. (1963). Coccygodynia: Cause and treatment. *Diseases of the Colon and Rectum, 6,* 422–426.

Thompson, C.A., Shanafelt, T.D., & Loprinzi, C.L. (2003). Andropause: Symptom management for prostate cancer patients treated with hormonal ablation. *Oncologist, 8*(5), 474–487.

Thompson, I.M., Tangen, C.M., Goodman, P.J., Probstfield, J.L., Moinpour, C.M., & Coltman, C.A. (2005). Erectile dysfunction and subsequent cardiovascular disease. *JAMA, 294*(23), 2996–3002.

Tobisu, K. (2006). Function-preserving surgery for urologic oncology. *International Journal of Clinical Oncology, 11*(5), 351–356.

Trant, A.S., & Polan, M.L. (2000). *Clinical study on a nutraceutical supplement for the enhancement of female sexual function*. Boston: Female Sexual Function Forum.

Travell, J., & Simons, D.G. (1992). *Myofascial pain and dysfunction: The trigger point manual: Vol. 2, The lower extremities*. Baltimore: Lippincott Williams & Wilkins.

Travison, T.G., Shabsigh, R., Araujo, A.B., Kupelian, V., O'Donnell, A.B., & McKinlay, J.B. (2007). The natural progression and remission of erectile dysfunction: Results from the Massachusetts Male Aging Study. *Journal of Urology, 177*(1), 241–246.

Turner, L.A., Althof, S.E., Levine, S.B., Bodner, D.R., Kursh, E.D., & Resnick, M.I. (1992). Twelve-month comparison of two treatments for erectile dysfunction: Self-injection versus external vacuum devices. *Urology, 39*(2), 139–144.

United Press International. (2007). *Nurses top list of trusted professions*. Retrieved June 5, 2008, from: http://www.upi.com/Odd_News/2007/01/08/Nurses_top_list_of_trusted_professions/UPI-36251168288943/

UpToDate. (2008). *Intravesical therapy* [version 16.1]. Retrieved July 9, 2008, from http://www.uptodate.com/online/content/topic.do?topicKey=gucancer/7957&selectedTitle=1~88&source=search_result

Vivus, Inc. (2003). *MUSE prescribing information*. Mountain View, CA: Author.

Webb, D.J., Muirhead, G.J., Wulff, M., Sutton, J.A., Levi, R., & Dinsmore, W.W. (2000). Sildenafil citrate potentiates the hypotensive effects of nitric oxide donor drugs in male patients with stable angina. *Journal of the American College of Cardiology, 36*(1), 25–31.

Webster, D., & Brennan, T. (1995). Use and effectiveness of sexual self-care strategies for interstitial cystitis. *Urologic Nursing, 15*(1), 14–18.

Weiss, C., Wolze, C., Engehausen, D.G., Ott, O.J., Krause, F.S., Schrott, K.M., et al. (2006). Radiochemotherapy after transurethral resection for high-risk T1 bladder cancer: An alternative to intravesical therapy or early cystectomy? *Journal of Clinical Oncology, 24*(15), 2318–2324.

Whitmore, K., Kellogg-Spadt, S., & Fletcher, E. (1998, Fall). Comprehensive assessment of the pelvic floor. *Issues in Incontinence*, pp. 1–10.

Wilkes, G.M., & Barton-Burke, M. (2007). *2007 oncology nursing drug handbook*. Sudbury, MA: Jones and Bartlett.

Williams, J.E., & Lloyd, L.K. (1998). Pelvic pain of urinary origin. In R.E. Blackwell & D.L. Olive (Eds.), *Chronic pelvic pain: Evaluation and management* (pp. 19–42). New York: Springer.

Wilmoth, M.C. (2006). Life after cancer: What does sexuality have to do with it? *Oncology Nursing Forum, 33*(5), 905–910.

Windahl, T., Skeppner, E., Andersson, S.O., & Fugl-Meyer, K.S. (2004). Sexual function and satisfaction in men after laser treatment for penile carcinoma. *Journal of Urology, 172*(2), 648–651.

Zippe, L.D., Kedia, A.W., Kedia, K., Nelson, D.R., & Agarwal, A. (1998). Treatment of erectile dysfunction after radical prostatectomy with sildenafil citrate (Viagra). *Urology, 52*(6), 963–966.

CHAPTER 10

Evidence-Based Practice for Urology Oncology Nursing Care

Frances Crighton, RN, PhD

Introduction

Evidence-based practice (EBP) in oncology nursing involves taking the best scientific evidence, whether derived from meta-analyses, randomized studies, or a consortium of clinical experts, to develop nursing interventions that improve patient care. The definition of EBP frequently used in nursing is from Rutledge and Grant (2002), who stated that EBP "defines care that integrates best scientific evidence with clinical expertise, knowledge of pathophysiology, knowledge of psychosocial issues, and decision-making preference of patients" (p. 1). Our colleagues in medicine identify EBP as "the integration of best research evidence, clinical expertise, and patient values in making decisions about the care of individualized patients" (Institute of Medicine [IOM], 2003, p. 56). It is important to note that both of these definitions identify the importance of scientific findings as they apply to patients' individual preferences. The professional community recognizes that one requirement of EBP is scientific rigor in conducting the research; however, they acknowledge that a consensus of expert opinions has a role when practice guidelines are needed and the science is not fully developed. In such cases, the guidelines can be revised when sufficient science is reported.

Historical Perspective

Nursing is both an art and science. The focus of the art in nursing is the compassionate care nurses have delivered since the era of Florence Nightingale in the mid-1850s, beginning with the Crimean War. Additionally, the early years of scientific work in nursing was begun by Florence Nightingale. She collaborated with other scientists and played the central role in the establishment of the Royal Commission on the Health of the Army (Attewell, 1998).

In the 1970s, Cochrane, a British epidemiologist and medical researcher, argued for the use of randomized con-trolled trials to ensure patients received the best possible therapeutic care while maintaining health resources (Milton, 2007; Traynor, 2002). In 1993, The Cochrane Collaboration, an international network of reviewers, was established and is recognized as the center of the worldwide EBP movement in medicine. Traynor reported that in the 1990s the term *evidence-based medicine* was first used by a small group of practitioners at McMaster University in Canada. This gave birth to the development of EBP in many other professional groups, including nursing.

Traynor (2002) explained that the development of the current emphasis on EBP emerged from three societal factors. The first factor is risk. During the 1990s, society worldwide became concerned with scientific integrity, death statistics of babies, teen pregnancy, and other epidemiology variables. In addition, patients wanted more information about and challenged the status quo of health care. The medical community became acutely aware of documentation and the threat of legal consequences of malpractice.

The second factor is a rise in the *managerialism* or oversight by hospital accrediting agencies. This movement increased hospital monitoring and reporting of patient outcomes. For example, patient safety results that are reported include patient falls, nosocomial infections, medication errors, and hospital-acquired decubitus ulcers. The media regularly publishes safety deviations incurred by hospitals and health providers. Particularly, younger consumers are critical of agencies that do not meet the safety standards (Traynor, 2002).

The third element Traynor (2002) discussed is information technology. Although an abundance of scientific studies are available for regular review, physicians and nurses struggle to keep up with the rapid pace of discovery and the burdening number of publications and research articles. Patients, on the other hand, are consumers of health care, and may spend hours on the Internet studying their diagnosis. It is difficult for many patients to understand why their providers are unaware of specific information or studies.

The Oncology Nursing Society (ONS) joined the EBP movement in 1998 and focused on the oncology interventions nurses deliver. The historical review of this undertaking is outlined by Given and Sherwood (2005). The contention is that patient outcomes, such as quality of life (QOL), symptom experience, physical function, performance status, patient satisfaction, resource utilization, and healthcare costs, are directly affected by oncology nursing interventions. To further clarify the ONS stance on EBP, the term *nursing-sensitive patient outcome* (NSPO) was coined. Given and Sherwood reported that NSPOs have special significance for nursing, the public, and policymakers for three reasons. First, they posited that nursing interventions make a difference in the outcomes of patients' recovery from cancer or their journey through the cancer experience. Outcomes of the care delivered are measurable as defined by the practice guidelines, which are developed through scientific study. Second, NSPOs provide a means to measure the quality of care that nurses deliver. For example, performance improvement projects evaluate NSPOs and present results for patients to review. Third, Given and Sherwood stated, "the quality of patient healthcare outcomes has become a priority for legislators, healthcare agencies, purchasers, regulators, insurers, providers, and consumers as decisions are being made regarding the quality of, access to, and reimbursement of healthcare services" (p. 1). Oncology nurses are accountable for the service they provide. ONS has accepted the challenge to develop NSPOs through research and collaboration with other nursing organizations and health professional disciplines. Furthermore, they strive to implement NSPOs by developing the ONS Putting Evidence Into Practice (PEP) Resources (Gobel, Beck, & O'Leary, 2006). This is the latest movement in EBP among oncology nurses. The PEP resources focus on the utilization of scientific findings in easily accessible format. Thus far, ONS has developed recommendations for practice on the following topics: chemotherapy-induced nausea and vomiting, fatigue, prevention of infection, sleep-wake disturbances, constipation, caregiver strain and burden, depression, dyspnea, mucositis, peripheral neuropathy, pain, prevention of bleeding, anorexia, anxiety, diarrhea, and lymphedema.

Evidence-Based Practice Process

EBP focuses on utilization of the research findings. The EBP movement stemmed from the underutilization of research in practice. Burns and Grove (2007) identified two nursing projects that pushed the EBP movement forward. The first project was the Western Interstate Commission for Higher Education Regional Nursing Research Development Project, which was initiated in the mid-1970s to help nurses to critique research as applied to theory (Krueger, 1978; Krueger, Nelson, & Wolanin, 1978). This project was impeded by the lack of studies that could be implemented for practice. The second

project was the Conduct and Utilization of Research in Nursing Project (Horsley, Crane, Crabtree, & Wood, 1983). It was conducted over five years during the early 1980s. The project involved identifying the steps for the development of protocols to evaluate and implement research findings for practice.

The first step for the development and implementation of EBP is to identify the problem or process that requires improvement. At first, nurses may be stumped by this question. However, while nurses sit in a breakroom talking about patients and how the day is going, they discuss problems, which need to be studied. Several important issues have emerged concerning the development of the patient problem into a researchable project. Craig (2002) succinctly stated, "It is the clinical question that drives each step of the process" (p. 29). The clinical question should be important to patient outcomes, narrowly focused, measurable, and clearly defined. The issue that most nurses face during the step of problem identification is undertaking too much and not focusing on one aspect of the problem. Time is a huge resource that nurses in the clinical area rarely have the luxury to spend on research. In addition, the research process should be feasible with the time and financial resources available. The question or process to improve is derived out of issues with assessment, diagnosis, treatment, patients' learning needs, and systems problems that nurses identify with their patients.

The following example of rash will be used to describe the development of the problem statement. Skin rash is a common side effect for patients with kidney cancer who are receiving biologic therapies. Nurses have limited resources for the assessment, diagnosis, treatment, and learning needs of patients who experience targeted therapy–induced rash. The research question might be, "What is the incidence of rash among patients treated with a particular drug?" The current patient problem with skin rash can be studied easily in the clinical area through chart review. After a thorough understanding of the problem with skin rash, further development and testing of assessment criteria and interventions can be established.

After the problem is identified, and the problem statement agreed upon, the second step is to review the current sources of research evidence. Mitchell and Friese (2007) outlined seven levels of evidence to evaluate interventions for nursing practice that were adapted for ONS's development of NSPOs (see Figure 10-1). The weight-of-evidence level given to the intervention is one of the following (Mitchell, Beck, Hood, Moore, & Tanner, 2007).
- Recommended for practice
- Likely to be effective
- Benefits balanced with harms
- Effectiveness not established
- Effectiveness unlikely
- Not recommended for practice
- Expert opinion

The strongest level of evidence is a meta-analysis or systematic reviews of multiple well-designed, randomized,

Figure 10-1. Weight-of-Evidence Categories

Recommended for Practice

Interventions for which effectiveness has been demonstrated by strong evidence from rigorously conducted studies, meta-analyses, or systematic reviews, and for which expectation of harm is small compared with the benefits

Interventions that are recommended for practice are those with strong evidence from

- At least two well-conducted randomized controlled trials each with a sample size of at least 100 participants, and each performed at more than one institutional site. In studies with fewer than 100 participants and a large effect size, observed power of greater than or equal to 80% should be reported or evident.
- A meta-analysis of research studies that included a total of 100 participants or more in its estimate of effect size and confidence intervals for the size of the effect
- A systematic review or practice guidelines from a panel of experts that derive from an explicit literature search strategy and include thorough analysis, quality rating, and synthesis of the evidence.

Likely to Be Effective

Interventions for which effectiveness has been demonstrated by supportive evidence from a single rigorously conducted controlled trial, consistent supportive evidence from two well-designed controlled trials using small samples, or guidelines developed from evidence and supported by expert opinion

Interventions that are likely to be effective are those with consistent supportive evidence from

- A single well-conducted randomized controlled trial that included at least 100 participants. In a study with fewer than 100 participants and a large effect size, observed power of greater than or equal to 80% should be reported or evident.
- Several rigorously conducted controlled trials using small samples (N < 100)
- A meta-analysis that does not include a total of 100 participants or more in its estimate of effect size and confidence intervals for the size of the effect
- A systematic review that derives from an explicit literature search strategy and includes thorough analysis, quality rating, and synthesis of the evidence from rigorously conducted controlled trials using small samples (N < 100)
- Guidelines or recommendations that include both expert opinion that an intervention is effective and positive findings from studies that were critically reviewed by a panel of experts.

Benefits Balanced With Harms

Interventions for which clinicians and patients should weigh the beneficial and harmful effects according to individual circumstances and priorities

- Supportive evidence from one or more randomized trials, meta-analyses, or systematic reviews, where the intervention has been associated with adverse effects in certain patient populations. Such adverse effects include those that contribute or potentially contribute to mortality, significant morbidity or functional disability, hospitalization, or excess length of stay.

Effectiveness Not Established

Interventions for which insufficient or conflicting data currently exist, or data of inadequate quality, with no clear indication of harm

Interventions where effectiveness has not been established are those with supportive evidence that is insufficient, conflicting, or of poor quality, such as from

- A single well-conducted randomized controlled trial with a sample size of less than 100 participants
- A well-conducted case control study
- Conflicting evidence concerning the efficacy of an intervention with no clear indication of harm
- Supportive or conflicting evidence from a poorly controlled or uncontrolled study
  - Evidence from randomized clinical trials with one or more major, or three or more minor, methodologic flaws that could invalidate the results
  - Evidence from nonexperimental studies with high potential for bias (such as case series with comparison to historical controls)
  - Evidence from case series or case reports

Effectiveness Unlikely

Interventions for which a lack of effectiveness has been demonstrated by negative evidence from a single rigorously conducted controlled trial, consistent negative evidence from well-designed controlled trials using small samples, or guidelines developed from evidence and supported by expert opinion

Interventions unlikely to be effective are those where there is consistent evidence of ineffectiveness from

- A single well-conducted randomized controlled trial that included at least 100 participants and was conducted at more than one institution
- Several rigorously conducted randomized controlled trials using small samples
- A well-conducted case control study, a poorly controlled or uncontrolled study, a randomized trial with major methodologic flaws, or an observational study (e.g., case series with historical controls) together with a prominent and unacceptable pattern of adverse events and serious toxicities (Common Terminology Criteria for Adverse Events [CTCAE] grade III/IV)
- Guidelines or recommendations that are supported both by expert opinion that an intervention lacks effectiveness and by negative findings from studies that were critically reviewed by a panel of experts.

(Continued on next page)

Figure 10-1. Weight-of-Evidence Categories *(Continued)*

Not Recommended for Practice

Interventions for which lack of effectiveness or harmfulness has been demonstrated by strong evidence from rigorously conducted studies, meta-analyses, or systematic reviews, or interventions where the costs, burdens, or harm associated with the intervention exceed anticipated benefits

Interventions not recommended for practice are those where there is strong evidence of ineffectiveness or harmfulness based on

- Two or more well-conducted randomized controlled trials with at least 100 participants, conducted at more than one site, which showed no benefit for the intervention and that excessive costs, burdens, or harm may accrue from the intervention
- A single trial that attributed a prominent and unacceptable pattern of life-threatening adverse events and toxicities (CTCAE grade IV/V) to the intervention
- A meta-analysis of research studies that included a total of 100 participants or more in its estimate of effect size and that demonstrated lack of benefit or prominent and unacceptable toxicities
- Systematic review or practice guidelines from a panel of experts that discourage use of the intervention based on an explicit literature search strategy and include thorough analysis, quality rating, and synthesis of the evidence.

Expert Opinion

Low-risk interventions that are (1) consistent with sound clinical practice, (2) suggested by an expert in a peer-reviewed publication (journal or book chapter), and (3) for which limited evidence exists. An expert is an individual with peer-reviewed journal publications in the domain of interest.

Note. Based on information from Mitchell & Friese, n.d.

From "Putting Evidence Into Practice: Evidence-Based Interventions for Fatigue During and Following Cancer and Its Treatment," by S.A. Mitchell, S.L. Beck, L.E. Hood, K. Moore, and E.R. Tanner, 2007, *Clinical Journal of Oncology Nursing, 11*(1), p. 101. Copyright 2007 by Oncology Nursing Society. Adapted with permission.

controlled clinical trials. These studies are a powerful source of evidence (Smyth, 2002). The strength of the meta-analysis is providing a collection of smaller, well-controlled studies, which alone do not provide enough power to justify making practice changes. Some meta-analyses include a statistical analysis and, when possible, describe the *effect size* (the name given to a family of indices that measure the magnitude of a treatment effect of the evidence). Also included in the first level of evidence recognized by ONS are well-controlled, randomized, clinical trials with adequate power. Interventions derived from systematic review or practice guidelines from a panel of experts that are thoroughly analyzed and given a quality rating may be categorized as recommended for practice.

The second level of evidence includes interventions considered likely to be effective. These are interventions derived from scientific studies that lack the power of the interventions studied and recommended for practice. Examples of evidence likely to be effective are a single well-conducted, randomized, controlled trial with a sample of at least 100 subjects, several studies with a sample size less than 100, or a meta-analysis with less than 100 subjects. In addition, systematic reviews conducted that include studies with less than 100 subjects and guidelines reviewed by a panel of experts are in the second level of evidence.

Interventions given an unfavorable weight-of-evidence rating are those where the benefit of the intervention is outweighed by its harmfulness. Interventions not established for use in practice (Mitchell et al., 2007)

- Lack scientific findings from studies with a sample size of at least 100 subjects

- Include findings from studies conducted with conflicting evidence
- Lack scientific rigor
- Are flawed.

An intervention where effectiveness is unlikely includes evidence from well-conducted, randomized, controlled trials or guidelines, and supported by expert opinion that determined that the intervention lacks sufficient efficacy to be recommended for practice. Interventions not recommended for practice include those that lack scientific evidence or efficacy, and where harmfulness from the interventions has been demonstrated. The last weight-of-evidence category is expert opinion, which includes evidence suggested by an expert in a peer-reviewed publication when limited evidence exists.

The next step in the development of EBP includes a comprehensive review of the literature. Several databases are available to assist in this process, as outlined by Cope (2003). The most relevant for nursing studies is the Cumulative Index of Nursing and Allied Health Literature® (CINAHL). This database includes both research and practice review journal articles. The electronic version is available as part of the Ovid online service and is user friendly and easily accessible. Hospital or college librarians are helpful for nurses who have not used a large search engine to gather information. Other databases useful to nurses are MEDLINE®, available either through PubMed or Ovid search engines, the Cochrane Collaboration, clinical evidence from British Medical Journal Publishing, and the Agency for Healthcare Research and Quality. Many other databases are available to facilitate the literature acquisition. The National Guideline Clearinghouse (www.guideline.gov) lists more than 2,164 guidelines that include individual summaries.

The literature search begins by entering some limiting qualification for the search such as language, type of evidence, and publication year. This process is easy in most databases. Next, identify the key terms needed for study. For this chapter, the author focused on bladder, kidney, penile, and testicular cancer and symptoms frequently seen in this group of patients. Another important step is to review the type and peer-reviewed journals. After nurses have critiqued various studies, they can recognize the value of peer review and scholarly publications.

The next step in the EBP process is evaluating the evidence. LoBiondo-Wood (2006) outlined the rigor required for quantitative studies. Experimental studies require control through sampling, data collection methods, manipulation of independent variables, and randomization. It is important for nurses who are developing clinical guidelines to practice doing several research critiques by following a critique guide with the help of an experienced nurse scientist (see Table 10-1). Mitchell et al. (2007) outlined the systematic process to develop the fatigue guideline. They developed a tracking worksheet to categorize the intervention categories and subcategories. Mitchell et al. then ranked each study

according to the ONS levels of evidence outlined in Figure 10-1 and summarized the major and minor flaws of each study. The studies were ranked from one to six with benefits and harms outlined. The fifth and sixth categories reflected those studies that described interventions unsuitable for the practice guideline.

The final and probably most difficult step is the implementation of EBP into clinical practice. This step requires changing the practice habits of many nurses and helping them to understand that old trial-and-error methods are outdated and that newer evidence-based practices will benefit patients. The process is challenging to the EBP team who have studied the research and are deeply ingrained with the new evidence. Robinson et al. (2007) outlined the steps for change after developing an EBP guideline to reduce urinary catheter usage in their hospital. Their steps included
- Presenting the guideline to unit-based councils
- Organizing the evidence in poster format for display in all the nursing units
- Presenting the guideline and outcomes of the pilot project to nursing grand rounds.

EBP implementation requires that nurses be educated to the new findings, shown how the proposed change will benefit patients, and how the guideline is used. The education

Table 10-1. Quantitative Research Criteria	
Critique Criteria	**Questions**
Research design	Is there an interrelationship between the research question, purpose, literature review, theoretical framework, hypothesis, and research design? Is the design appropriate based on the research questions asked? Is it reasonable in the research setting? Is the sample size stated? Are the independent and dependent variables stated and appropriate to the problem studied? Are there controls for threats to internal and external validity? Is the design linked to levels of evidence?
Research question and/or hypotheses	Is the research question stated early in the study? Is the research question clearly stated? Does the research question state a relationship between an independent and dependent variable?
Review of the literature	Is the literature review written critically, is sufficient literature reviewed, and does it address the research question? Is the theoretical framework identified? Is the literature reviewed current? Is the literature reviewed organized, and does it give direction for the study?
Data collection and analysis	Are the steps for data collection clearly outlined? Are the reliability and validity of the data collection instruments stated, and were the instruments previously used with the study sample for this study? Are the statistical tests used for analysis of the data appropriate? Are the results clearly stated, and do they answer the research question? Do the tables and figures used to present the findings stand alone without further explanation?
Discussion	Are the results of this study linked to the review of the literature and theoretical framework? Does the researcher identify recommendations for research, clinical practice, and education?

Note. Based on information from Heermann & Craft, 2006.

process can be accomplished through planned in-services, video development for easy access, learning models that are self-paced, and posters displayed as reminders of the change in procedure. After the initial implementation process is completed, reevaluation should be planned to determine if the EBP guideline is being used, if patients are more satisfied with their care, if nurses follow the guideline, and if the guideline is cost effective. In addition, outcome measures should be evaluated. A postimplementation meeting between guideline stakeholders, such as the designated committee or group to do the literature research and write the nursing guidelines, and nurses will allow open dialogue concerning various advantages and disadvantages of the EBP guideline. Basic tenets of EBP guideline implementation include

- Open lines of communication
- Ability and willingness to accept change
- Ownership in the process and enthusiasm for making a difference.

Genitourinary Cancer Research

Identification of scientific evidence related to the genitourinary cancers covered in this chapter began with an extensive search of the literature. The author searched the CINAHL, MEDLINE, Cochrane Library Reviews, and PsyLIT. The qualifier of the searches focused on English language, 1992–2007, adults, and research. Few research articles were identified; therefore, the search was expanded to include review articles. The terms searched included cancer or neoplasm of the bladder, kidney, penis, and testicles, as well as nursing, and various symptoms frequently seen in these patients such as sexual issues, coping, QOL, and body image. A total of 2,134 research articles from 1992 to 2007 were identified searching MEDLINE. This included 862 bladder cancer studies, 958 kidney cancer studies, 38 penile cancer studies, and 275 testicular cancer studies. Of the 2,134 studies, 796 were published during 2002–2007. Far fewer scientific studies concerning nursing issues were identified in the CINAHL literature search. A total of 264 research studies were published during 1992–2007, with about half of them published since 2002. These studies were mostly small case studies or qualitative studies. Very few nursing scientific studies of non-prostate genitourinary cancers were found. No penile cancer scientific studies were identified related to nursing. Because the research literature was sparse, well-described expert opinion articles on delivery of nursing care to this genitourinary cancer population were reviewed and reported, as well as applicable issues found in the medical literature. After an extensive search of the literature, the following four major categories evolved: risk factors for genitourinary cancers, delivery of care, QOL, and survivorship. A summary of the studies can be found in Table 10-2.

Research Regarding Genitourinary Cancer Risk Factors

Several authors explored the relationships between physical activity and the risk of renal and testicular cancer. Srivastava and Kreiger (2000) examined the data from the Enhanced Cancer Surveillance Study conducted in all but two Canadian provinces. They reported on physical activity data of 212 men who had testicular cancer and 251 controls between the ages of 20 and 74 years. Questions asked on the survey pertained to the frequency and degree of exercise, ranging from moderate to strenuous levels; in addition, the intensity of occupational activity was assessed. Different life periods also were examined. It is interesting that participants who had a relatively high frequency of moderate and strenuous recreational activity during their teens and moderate or strenuous occupational demands during their 20s had an increased risk of testicular cancer compared to controls.

Two studies were reviewed that examined risk associated with either smoking or use of performance-enhancing supplements. The evidence reported from these studies is weak but provides examples for the need to carefully examine the risk factors for bladder, kidney, and testicular cancer for the development of EBP. Nieder, Seeniann, Messina, Granek, and Adler (2006) distributed questionnaires seeking the level of knowledge of smoking related to cancer to several groups of patients with cancer in four clinics, including patients with bladder and kidney cancers. They found that approximately one-third of the subjects stated that smoking was related to bladder or kidney cancers, whereas nearly all subjects stated that smoking was related to lung cancer. Subjects who are female or those with more education were more likely to perceive smoking as a risk factor for bladder cancer. In addition, the scientists reported that smoking status, whether as a former smoker or current smoker, was associated with the knowledge of smoking as a risk factor for kidney cancer. A small descriptive study of 129 patients with testicular cancer who completed questionnaires that gathered information on the use of exercise performance-enhancing supplements was conducted to determine the risk of these supplements (Chang, Ivey, Smith, Roth, & Cookson, 2005). They found a 20% use of performance-enhancing supplements among the people studied. Furthermore, the mean age of supplement users was 8.8 years younger than the patients without supplement use.

To solve the mysteries of the etiology of kidney cancer, Tavani et al. (2007) and Chiu et al. (2006) studied physical activity. Tavani's group found an inverse association between risk for kidney cancer and occupational physical activity consistent for sex, body mass index, smoking habits, alcohol use, and age at diagnosis among 767 patients with kidney cancer and 1,534 matched controls. However, they did not identify a significant association for leisure-time physical activity and kidney cancer among the subjects studied. Likewise, Chiu et al. reported a

Table 10-2. Summary of Bladder, Kidney, Penile, and Testicular Evidence Reviewed

Author and Publication Year	Cancer Studied	Topic Studied	Outcome
Taub et al., 2006	Bladder	Length of hospitalization from 1988 to 2000	Decreased length of stay from 13 days to 9 days and increased use of home health agencies were noted.
Baumgartner et al., 2002	Bladder	Evaluation of bladder cancer treatment clinical pathway	Approximately three-fourths of patients treated met the targeted length of stay of 8 days.
Beitz & Zuzelo, 2003	Bladder	Phenomenology study of patients' experience of bladder cancer treatment	Six themes emerged from diagnosis through treatment, with patients' relationship to provider being a constant.
Perimenis & Koliopanou, 2004	Bladder	Expert clinician's report of nurses' role in teaching self-care	Self-care included metabolic/laboratory, catheter care, bladder re-training, prevention, and surveillance for recurrence.
Faithfull, 1999	Bladder	Satisfaction with care and economic cost	Increased satisfaction and 31% decrease in cost of care among patients was seen in the treatment group.
Karvinen et al., 2007	Bladder	Exercise and quality of life (QOL)	Survivors who reported meeting the public health exercise guidelines had a significantly ($p < 0.001$) better QOL.
Bjerre et al., 1998	Bladder	Sexual problems and type of urinary diversion (Kock reservoir or ileal conduit)	Only 9% of 76 patients studied where able to achieve an erection; 38% were able to achieve orgasm regardless of type of diversion. Patients with an ileal conduit were more likely to lose coitus sensitivity (96%) compared to patients with a Kock reservoir (77%).
Hilton & Henderson, 2003	Bladder	Phenomenology study of women's lived experiences with bladder cancer	Lived experiences among survivors were unknowing, suffering, loss of self, insider view, metamorphosis, and restoration.
Nieder et al., 2006	Bladder and kidney	Cancer incidence and smoking	In this assessment of the subjects' views on smoking and cancer, all subjects in the study were smokers. One-third of the subjects attributed smoking as a cause of bladder or kidney cancer. Subjects who were female and had more education were more likely to associate smoking with bladder and kidney cancer.
Tavani et al., 2007	Kidney	Risk and occupational physical activity	Inverse relationship exists between risk for kidney cancer and occupational physical activity.
Chiu et al., 2006	Kidney	Risk and nonoccupational physical activity	Inverse relationship exists between risk for kidney cancer and non-occupational physical activity among women.
Romero et al., 2005	Penile	Qualitative study of QOL and sexual function after partial penectomy	Only 33.3% of the 18 men studied maintained their preoperative sexual intercourse frequency and were satisfied with their sex life.
Incrocci et al., 2002	Testicular	QOL and erectile dysfunction	No difference was found between patients and matched controls on sexual interest, erectile difficulty, and sex life satisfaction.
Fleer et al., 2004	Testicular	Review of 23 studies	Three domains of QOL were identified: physical well-being, psychological well-being, and social well-being.
Srivastava, 2000	Testicular	Risk and physical exercise and occupational activity	Increased risk of testicular cancer among teens who reported moderate and strenuous recreational activity and in men in their 20s reporting moderate or strenuous occupational demands.
Chang et al., 2005	Testicular	Use of exercise performance-enhancing supplements	20% of the participants with testicular cancer used exercise performance-enhancing supplements.

(Continued on next page)

Table 10-2. Summary of Bladder, Kidney, Penile, and Testicular Evidence Reviewed *(Continued)*			
Author and Publication Year	**Cancer Studied**	**Topic Studied**	**Outcome**
McCullagh et al., 2005	Testicular	Program to teach testicular self-examination	Subjects in the intervention group reported increased knowledge of testicular cancer and use of self-examination.
Girasole et al., 2006	Testicular	Sperm banking among testicular cancer survivors	Survivors who banked sperm were younger, childless at the time of treatment, and less likely to have children after treatment.
Meinardi et al., 2000	Testicular	Survivors' risk of cardiovascular morbidity	Five survivors of 87 patients studied experienced some type of myocardial event; one had a fatal outcome.
Zoltick et al., 2005	Testicular	Expert opinion on cardiovascular risk factors and prevention teaching techniques for nurses	Teaching included risk of cardiovascular disease, smoking cessation, diet modification, and weight control.
Thorsen et al., 2002	Testicular	Testicular cancer survivors and physical activity	Testicular cancer survivors were significantly more highly active compared to a comparison group of men from the population.
Tuinman et al., 2006	Testicular	Survivors' relationships and support	Survivors who were single during treatment reported more dissatisfaction with support and worse mental health than survivors who were in a relationship or married.
Rudberg et al., 2002	Testicular	Testicular cancer survivors and self-perceived physical, psychological, and general symptoms	Patients treated with chemotherapy reported more Raynaud symptoms, sexual problems, infertility, and feelings of unattractiveness.

significant inverse association for nonoccupational physical activity and the risk of kidney cancer among women. They studied 406 people with kidney cancer and matched controls. In addition, they reported that compared to controls, patients with kidney cancer consumed more red meat, ate fewer vegetables, weighed more during specified life time periods, had a history of hypertension; and had a family history of kidney cancer. Female patients were more likely to be current smokers.

Research Regarding Nursing Care Delivery

Literature surrounding the delivery of care to patients with bladder, testicular, kidney, or penile cancer focused on hospital care strategies and patient education. Outcome measures to study changes in the delivery of care often are analyses of variance from large databases. Taub, Dunn, Miller, Wei, and Hollenbeck (2006) analyzed outcome variables among patients who were treated with either a partial or radial cystectomy. The target variables included in-hospital postoperative mortality, length of stay, discharge status (home versus subacute care facility), and the use of home healthcare services. Length of stay was operationalized as total number of days in the hospital, and greater than 21 days was ranked as prolonged. Data were analyzed during four time periods between 1988 and 2000. The outcomes of this analysis showed a decrease in treatment with radical cystectomy and partial cystectomy; although, the incidence of bladder cancer increased over the same period.

The length of hospitalization for surgery decreased from 13 days to 9 days, and the use of intermediate care facilities and home health agencies increased. This study indicates the shift of care responsibility from the hospital to the patients and their caregivers. In addition, these findings indicate the need for nursing guidelines related to telephone assessment and patient teaching of self-care. Baumgartner, Wells, Chang, Cookson, and Smith (2002) reported on an evaluation of a clinical pathway for patients who underwent radical cystectomy. This was a 300-patient retrospective chart review according to the pathway guidelines with a targeted hospital length of stay of eight days. Variables were divided into minor and major complications. Minor complications included such events as the need for a blood transfusion, ileus, deep vein thrombosis, and other similar events, whereas major complications included life-threatening events such a cardiovascular event, sepsis, pulmonary embolus, and respiratory failure. Overall, 233 patients (74%) met the targeted length of stay. The contributing variables experienced by the 77 patients who had an extended length of stay up to 12 days were ethnic minority, ileus, other minor complications, major complications, and blood transfusion.

A phenomenologic qualitative study was conducted by Beitz and Zuzelo (2003). They reported and identified the patients' experience of being treated for bladder cancer with a neobladder. All participants were interviewed during one session lasting one to two hours. Six major themes emerged from these data concerned with three time periods from diagnosis to living with the neobladder. During the diagnosis stage, participants described the experience of receiving the diagnosis and initially detesting the idea of wearing a bag. The intermediate themes were divided into three phases, including

- Phase I: the acute perioperative experience of dealing with surgery and postoperative pain
- Phase II: early discharge from the hospital. Concerns were tube management, incontinence, and change in physical self.
- Phase III: self-catheterization, training the neobladder, urination with a neobladder, and change in urine characteristics.

The third time period reflected acceptance of the neobladder as a new normal and focused on issues such as adapting to new toileting needs, keeping the neobladder healthy, changes in bowel movements, changes in sex, consideration of the impact of smoking, realization that cancer was a lifelong threat, and reflection on the neobladder choice. One theme was present across all time periods regarding the patients' relationships with healthcare providers and experiences with ongoing stressful events.

One expert clinician report was reviewed to outline the care of patients treated surgically for bladder cancer that documented the importance of nurses' role in teaching patient self-care. Perimenis and Koliopanou (2004) outlined the rehabilitation of patients treated with ileal orthotopic bladder diversion, including both acute surgical care and long-term care. *Acute nursing care* involves monitoring for fluid and electrolyte imbalance, changes in hemoglobin, wound and catheter care, catheter irrigation, early ambulation, nasogastric tube management, and other self-care strategies. Ambulatory nurses managed late postoperative care, which was about 10 days through 30 days after surgery. The care and teaching during the late postoperative period involved voiding retraining and metabolic management. The long-term nursing EBP guidelines needed for patients with bladder cancer focus on prevention and monitoring for urinary tract infection, identification of urinary retention related to stricture formation at the neobladder neck, and surveillance for cancer recurrence.

Nurses in a radiation therapy department at a specialist cancer center conducted a study to determine if a nursing care intervention decreased emotional and physical discomfort among 115 men who were treated for either bladder cancer or prostate cancer with radiation therapy (Faithfull, 1999). Patients' satisfaction and economic cost also were evaluated. Patients in the nursing care intervention group received an initial clinic visit with a nurse, telephone contact, two weekly clinic visits during treatment, and a clinic visit at the end of treatment. The intervention group had a weekly clinic visit during treatment. The intervention focused on (a) the meaning of the diagnosis of cancer, symptoms, and health, (b) information of symptom recognition, events that occur during treatment, and management of problems, and (c) advice on how to prevent urinary problems. The control group had the standard of care teaching at the beginning of treatment. Data were collected from patients at three times, at weeks 1, 6, and 12, from completion of three questionnaires concerning functional status, global health status, and symptoms. Faithfull reported that men in the intervention group reported significantly less urinary frequency and associated symptoms than the control group. Symptoms reported as problematic were nocturia, fatigue, and urinary frequency. Patient satisfaction and treatment cost also were significantly different ($p < 0.002$) between the intervention group and control group. Patients in the intervention group were significantly more satisfied ($p < 0.002$) with their care and appreciated the continuity of care. Overall, the cost of the care received by the intervention group was reduced by 31%.

McCullagh, Lewis, and Warlow (2005) studied a method to increase the awareness and practice of testicular self-examination among males. These researchers conducted a quasi-experimental, pre- and post-test design study of 835 men to evaluate the efficacy of a program titled "Check 'Em Out," an intervention to improve men's awareness of testicular cancer and self-examination. Self-administered questionnaires were distributed to men at 10 study sites before and after the intervention, and to men who did not receive the intervention at four control sites. These results showed a difference in knowledge of testicular cancer among the intervention group compared to the control group as evaluated on the post-test scores. In addition, men in the intervention group scored significantly higher on the use of self-examination compared to men in the control group on post-test scores.

Research Regarding Patients' Quality of Life

Various QOL studies were found among patients treated either for testicular cancer or bladder cancer. Karvinen, Courneya, North, and Venner (2007) studied the effects of exercise and QOL among patients with bladder cancer. The survivors were identified through the Canadian Provincial Cancer Registry and were mailed the Godin Leisure Time Exercise Questionnaire, the Functional Assessment of Cancer Therapy–Bladder Scale, and the Fatigue Symptom Inventory. A total of 525 survivors were mailed questionnaires. Karvinen et al. reported that more than half of the 51% of the subjects who responded were completely sedentary, 22.3% had met the public health exercise guidelines over the past month, and 16% were insufficiently active. A significant difference in QOL existed among those meeting the public health exercise guidelines and those who were completely sedentary, with the subjects meeting the public health guidelines reporting better QOL.

Fleer, Hoekstra, Sleijfer, and Hoekstra-Weebers (2004) conducted an extensive review of 23 studies of men with testicular cancer and QOL. The following methodologic and treatment-related criteria were followed in sampling studies that were reviewed: design, sample size, use of comparison groups, measurement instruments, type of treatment, and time since diagnosis. They identified three domains of QOL. The first domain was physical well-being, which was for patients with testicular cancer who were concerned with health perception, fatigue, and body image. The second domain was psychological well-being, which involved psychological distress, health worries, fertility distress, and psychological well-being. The third domain was social well-being, which involved marital functioning, social support, and functional life.

Bjerre, Johansen, and Steven (1998) studied QOL in relation to sexual problems among patients with bladder cancer who had either a Kock reservoir or an ileal conduit diversion. A convenience sample of 76 patients, 49 of whom had a Kock reservoir and 27 of whom had an ileal conduit diversion, completed a questionnaire. Overall, only 9% of patients in either group could achieve an erection at least every second time of attempted sexual activity, in comparison to 82% who had achieved an erection preoperatively. Thirty-eight percent of all patients were able to achieve orgasm, and 26% were coitally active to some degree. Loss of coitus sensitivity was related to loss of potency among 77% of patients who had a Kock pouch diversion and 96% of patients who had an ileal conduit diversion. There were no between-group differences on decreased libido, partner refusal, and feeling less sexually attractive. In the regression analysis, patients older than 68 years did predict orgasmic ability and coital activity; however, type of operation did not influence either variable. Radiation treatment influenced whether the patient felt less sexually attractive than before surgery.

Romero et al. (2005) studied 18 men after partial penectomy for penile cancer. Patients completed the International Index of Erectile Function questionnaire, reporting their pre-surgical and post-surgical sexual function. In addition, each had a 45-minute phone interview. The researchers reported that 55.6% of the patients reported erections firm enough for penetration and intercourse. Those patients who did not resume sexual intercourse reported reasons of diminished penis size and absence of the glans penis. Sexual desire was maintained by 66.7% of the patients to the same degree as before surgery. Ejaculation and orgasm occurred every time they had sexual stimulation or intercourse for 72.2% of the patients. However, 33.3% of the patients maintained their preoperative sexual intercourse frequency and were satisfied with their sexual relationship with their partners and their overall sex life. Incrocci, Hop, Wijnmaalen, and Slob (2002) conducted a retrospective chart review of 166 patients with testicular cancer who were treated with radiotherapy for testicular seminoma. A questionnaire regarding symptoms at presentation, treatment side effects, satisfaction with the information received from the radiation oncologist, concerns about fertility, testicular implants, body image, and current sexual functioning was mailed to 157 patients of the total 166 patients (6 patients were lost to follow-up and 3 had died). Of this total, 123 patients responded. In addition, 185 age-matched controls were identified, and a questionnaire to determine prevalence of erectile dysfunction and its influence on QOL was mailed to them. Interest in sex, erectile difficulties, and satisfaction with sexual life did not differ for patients treated for testicular cancer and their age-matched control group. There was evidence for concern about fertility in 20% of the patients, body image change in 52% of the patients, and negative influence on sexual life in 32% of the patients.

Research Regarding Survivorship Issues

Seven articles focusing on survivorship issues of patients with bladder or testicular cancer were selected to report. These included five research studies, one case study, and one expert opinion review. Hilton and Henderson (2003) reported on a phenomenologic study of women's lived experiences of chronic bladder cancer. The lived experiences identified were unknowing, suffering, loss of self, insider view, metamorphosis, and restoration. Hilton and Henderson concluded that qualitative research methods give nurses information otherwise unavailable to them on patients' perspective of their disease and allows nurses to better design care plans that can meet these patients' needs.

Girasole et al. (2006) studied sperm banking in 330 patients with testicular cancer. Men who were treated during 1994–2004 at a large medical center were mailed a questionnaire seeking answers to questions regarding the use of sperm banking at the time of their treatment. Of the 330 men who were sent questionnaires, 129 (39%) men responded. The men who chose to bank sperm at the time of treatment were significantly younger, childless at the time of treatment, and less likely to have children after treatment. In addition, 2 of the 31 of the men who banked sperm used their sperm to conceive a child, 1 indicated that he intended to use his sperm in the future, and 28 men indicated that they either had not used their banked sperm or that they did not intend to use it. Of these 28 men, 12 men had conceived children naturally without using their banked sperm.

Meinardi et al. (2000) conducted a survey of long-term survivors of metastatic testicular cancer to determine the risk of cardiovascular morbidity among men more than 10 years after chemotherapy treatment compared with a comparison group of patients with stage I testicular cancer who were in a surveillance follow-up treatment plan. Of the 87 patients with metastatic testicular cancer who were treated with chemotherapy, 5 men experienced some type of myocardial event, including 2 men who reported a myocardial infarction (1 with a fatal outcome) and 3 men who developed angina pectoris with ischemia. In addition, one of the following cardiovascular risk factors was identified in 97% of the men surveyed: hypertension, hypercholesterolemia, smoking history, or positive family history for cardiovascular event. Furthermore, 36% of the men treated with chemotherapy reported Raynaud phenomenon and 22% had microalbuminuria. Zoltick, Jacobs, and Vaughn (2005) reported an expert opinion review of the cardiovascular risk factors among testicular cancer survivors who were treated with chemotherapy and suggested nursing interventions to reduce the cardiovascular risk factor within this patient group. The interventions included informing patients at the beginning of treatment of the known risk factor for cardiovascular disease, smoking cessation counseling, diet modification, and weight control.

Thorsen et al. (2002) conducted a cross-sectional study to determine the level of physical activity among men treated for testicular cancer as compared to men from the general population. The researchers hypothesized that patients treated with chemotherapy would be less active. Questionnaires were mailed to a total of 1,643 men treated for testicular cancer who were 20–59 years of age. The comparison group consisted of 20,391 men also ages 20–59. Men were mailed questionnaires seeking information about physical activity. Level of physical activity was subdivided into two levels of physical activity. Low level of physical activity included walking, and high level of physical activity included activities that led to sweating and breathlessness. Depending on the level of activity and frequency of activity, men were divided into one of three groups:

- Group 1 included inactive or no low-level activity or low-level activity less than one hour per week and no high-level activity.
- Group 2 included men who were minimally active as identified by doing low-level activity more than one hour per week and either no high-level activity or high-level activity less than one hour per week.
- Group 3 included the highly active group who did more than one high-level activity per week.

Other variables in the analysis were age, body mass index, education, living as a couple, comorbidity, and daily smoking. Thorsen et al. found that long-term testicular cancer survivors were significantly more highly active as compared to the comparison group of men from the general population. In addition, the logistic regression analysis showed that level of activity was higher for those patients with testicular cancer who had more education and less comorbidity.

Two descriptive studies described physical and psychosocial factors. Rudberg, Carlsson, Nilsson, and Wikblad (2002) conducted a study of long-term survivors of testicular cancer to seek answers to two research questions. The first question was to determine the self-perceived physical, psychological, and general symptoms in men treated for testicular cancer as compared to men from the general population. The second question sought to determine the self-perceived physical, psychological, and general symptoms in relation to secondary Raynaud phenomenon, sexual dysfunction, infertility, and self-perceived attractiveness among men treated with different treatment modalities for testicular cancer. Testicular cancer treatment groups were surveillance, radiation therapy, chemotherapy plus radiation, or retroperitoneal lymph node dissection. Overall, patients with testicular cancer reported significantly less frequency of backache, leg pain, cough, and eye problems than the comparison group. Men treated with chemotherapy or chemotherapy plus radiation therapy or surgery reported significantly more Raynaud phenomenon symptoms, lower sexual interest and ability to enjoy sex, more erectile difficulties, and infertility than the comparison group. Likewise, patients with testicular cancer who were treated with chemotherapy, or chemotherapy plus either radiation therapy or surgery, reported the feeling of being less attractive. Men who perceived themselves as being as attractive as before treatment had fathered children significantly more often than those assessing themselves as more attractive or less attractive than before treatment.

Tuinman et al. (2006) studied relationships among men treated for testicular cancer. Men were either single, with the same partner as they were at the diagnosis of cancer, or with a partner they met after completion of treatment. Patients who were single reported significantly more dissatisfaction with support and worse mental health than patients who were in a relationship during treatment or had a relationship after treatment. Single patients who reported more self-esteem and satisfaction with their support team also reported significantly better mental health. In the regression analysis, a low level of mental health among single patients was predicted by dissatisfaction with support.

Summary

The review of the literature of bladder, kidney, penile, and testicular cancer reveals that more research is required to develop EBP guidelines for the nursing care of these patients. Although a number of studies were reported, researchers other than nurses did most of this work. The studies, except for a few, were descriptive studies and did not focus on nurses' delivery of care. A number of studies were conducted among patients with bladder or testicular cancer, whereas only a few studies were reported among patients with kidney or penile cancer. Penile cancer is a rare cancer in the United States and comprises less than 1% of all cancers diagnosed; nevertheless, the unique issues within this patient group require study. Likewise, few studies were concerned with the issues that patients with kidney cancer experience. Patients with kidney cancer who were treated with the newer targeted treatments have many problems that also warrant study (Wood & Manchen, 2007).

Directions for the Future

A number of issues have impeded the nursing research needed to develop EBP guidelines for bladder, kidney, penile, and testicular cancer. Molassiotis et al. (2006) outlined these after conducting a systematic review of worldwide cancer nursing research. These issues include but are not limited to the following.

- Lack of funding to conduct research among patients with cancer
- Need for collaboration with multidisciplinary teams of researchers
- Lack of infrastructure to support nursing research
- Dearth of senior cancer nursing researchers who hold program grants
- Lack of focus on research methodology
- Focus of scientifically rigorous studies in a small number of high-quality research publications
- Lack of publications of scientific findings published in the general news for patients to identify the contributions nurses are making to improve patient care

These issues are complicated and will not be resolved easily; however, investigators should begin to resolve some of the issues so that evidence-based nursing can continue. To address a few of these issues, nurses should begin looking for creative sources for research funding such as contributors to community hospitals. In most instances, nurses have made a large contribution to the care and well-being of the family members of contributors. Academic professors frequently receive support for research projects. Families often ask what they can do to show their appreciation for the outstanding service nurses provide. Nurses need to inform patients and their families about the difference nurses make for patients and encourage families to support nursing research. This also can be accomplished through more nursing research coverage by the news media. For example, after the spring meeting of the American Society of Clinical Oncology, multiple scientific findings are published in the media. Nurses need to follow this example and share findings presented at the annual ONS Congress.

In determining a future direction for nursing research, three sources were examined to determine where nurses should focus their research efforts. Ropka et al. (2002) reported on the ONS research priorities survey; Molassiotis et al. (2006) identified areas of nursing research needed; and the Joint Commission (2009) identified patient safety goals for hospitals and ambulatory care facilities. Molassiotis et al. pointed out that most nursing research had focused on patients with breast and hemologic malignancies and that there was a need for further research among patients with bladder and testicular cancer. Furthermore, they stressed the need for intervention studies among these and all cancers. Ropka et al. reviewed the high-priority research studies recommended by oncology nurses. The recommendations identified here support the agenda of research needs of both of these groups. An urgent need exists for nurses to study interventions to direct patients in determining which urinary diversion will work best for them. Physicians present the surgical options to the patient, and nurses play a huge role in helping patients to make treatment decisions. Guidelines developed from a body of research evi-

dence will help nurses in giving patients accurate information in a systematic format. The next need for this patient group is intervention studies to determine the best methods to care for various types of urinary diversions. No intervention studies could be found to develop EBP. Another priority regarding patients with bladder, penile, or testicular cancer is developing interventions to help them to manage sexual dysfunction. These studies should focus on interventions to restore erectile and coitial functions, as well as psychosocial studies to help patients adjust to altered sexual function. Symptom management studies needed include interventions for helping patients with kidney cancer who experience skin rash. No nursing interventions studies were reported that addressed issues regarding skin rash and new targeted agents used to treat kidney cancer. Skin rash impedes QOL, and more patients with various cancers are receiving targeted agent treatments. Also, diet, fatigue, pain, anorexia, diarrhea, nausea, and vomiting among patients with kidney cancer need study. Diet and metabolic imbalance also should be studied among patients with bladder cancer. As more robotic-assisted surgeries are done, nurses need to focus on intervention studies designed to assist patients in treatment decisions, preparation for surgery, postoperative care, and teaching self-care. As patients are discharged earlier from the hospital, ambulatory nurses are faced with bigger challenges with telephone nursing. Studies to evaluate telephone assessments and patient self-care education are needed to determine the best practice for the delivery of nursing care. Patients with advanced cancer experience end-of-life issues, and nurses are primary caregivers either in the patients' home environment or hospice care facilities. These patients' problems include suffering, pain, depression, fatigue, and QOL. Nurses need to focus research studies on Joint Commission safety recommendations. A venue for this research is encouraging staff nurses to conduct performance improvement studies and to encourage all the nurses in the clinic or hospital unit to take part in the study. Some of these studies might include interventions to decrease nosocomial urinary tract infection, methods to effectively communicate patient transfer information to another unit or department, interventions to decrease medication errors, and interventions to improve patient self-care. A tremendous amount of nursing research is needed for bladder, kidney, penile, and testicular cancer. Nurses have only begun to focus research among these patients. Oncology and urologic nurses need to work together to develop an impressive body of evidence to develop practice guidelines for the delivery of care.

Conclusions

EBP nursing practice is the future of nursing. Trial and error, clinicians' opinions, or "this is the way we have always done it" are no longer acceptable standards for nurses to follow in determining practice guidelines and standards of practice. Nurses now recognize the need to develop a body of knowledge that is evidence-based to determine best practice. In this chapter, historical events in the development of EBP, and a model to follow in gathering and evaluating research evidence to develop guidelines for practice were presented. An overview of the current research in bladder, kidney, penile, and testicular cancer included four major categories of research: cancer risk factors, delivery of care, QOL, and survivorship issues. Finally, directions for future development of EBP were reviewed.

References

Attewell, A. (1998). Florence Nightingale's relevance to nurses. *Journal of Holistic Nursing, 18*(2), 281–291.

Baumgartner, R.G., Wells, N., Chang, S.S., Cookson, M.S., & Smith, J.A., Jr. (2002). Causes of increased length of stay following radical cystectomy. *Urologic Nursing, 22*(5), 319–339.

Beitz, J.M., & Zuzelo, P.R. (2003). The lived experience of having a neobladder. *Western Journal of Nursing Research, 25*(3), 292–316.

Bjerre, B.D., Johansen, C., & Steven, K. (1998). Sexological problems after cystectomy: Bladder substitution compared with ileal conduit diversion. A questionnaire study of male patients. *Scandinavian Journal of Urology and Nephrology, 32*(3), 187–193.

Burns, N., & Grove, S.K. (2007). *Understanding nursing research: Building an evidence-based practice* (7th ed.). St. Louis, MO: Saunders.

Chang, S.S., Ivey, B., Smith, J.A., Roth, B.J., & Cookson, M.S. (2005). Performance-enhancing supplement use in patients with testicular cancer. *Urology, 66*(2), 242–245.

Chiu, B.C.H., Gapstur, S.M., Chow, W.H., Kirby, K.A., Lynch, C.F., & Cantor, K.P. (2006). Body mass index, physical activity, and risk of renal cell carcinoma. *International Journal of Obesity, 30*(6), 940–947.

Cope, D. (2003). Evidence-based practice: Making it happen in your clinical setting. *Clinical Journal of Oncology Nursing, 7*(1), 97–98.

Craig, J.V. (2002). How to ask the right question. In J.V. Craig & R.L. Smyth (Eds.), *The evidence-based practice manual for nurses* (2nd ed., pp. 29–47). Philadelphia: Elsevier.

Faithfull, S. (1999). Randomized trial, a method of comparisons: A study of supportive care in radiotherapy nursing. *European Journal of Oncology Nursing, 3*(3), 176–184.

Fleer, J., Hoekstra, H.J., Sleijfer, D.T., & Hoekstra-Weebers, J.E. (2004). Quality of life of survivors of testicular germ cell cancer: A review of the literature. *Supportive Care in Cancer, 12*(7), 476–486.

Girasole, C.R., Cookson, M.S., Smith, J.A., Ivey, B.S., Roth, B.J., & Chang, S.S. (2006). Sperm banking: Use and outcomes in patients treated for testicular cancer. *BJU International, 99*(1), 33–36.

Given, B., & Sherwood, P.R. (2005). Nursing-sensitive patient outcomes—A white paper. *Oncology Nursing Forum, 32*(4), 773–784.

Gobel, B.H., Beck, S.I., & O'Leary, C. (2006). Nursing-sensitive patient outcomes: The development of the putting evidence into practice resources for nursing practice. *Clinical Journal of Oncology Nursing, 10*(5), 621–624.

Heermann, J.A., & Craft, B.J. (2006). Evaluating quantitative research. In G. LoBiondo-Wood & J. Haber (Eds.), *Nursing research: Methods and critical appraisal for evidence-based practice* (6th ed., pp. 400–420). St. Louis, MO: Mosby.

Hilton, E.L., & Henderson, L.J. (2003). Lived female experience of chronic bladder cancer: A phenomenologic case study. *Urologic Nursing, 23*(5), 349–353.

Horsley, J.A., Crane, J., Crabtree, M.K., & Wood, D.J. (1983). *Using research to improve nursing practice: A guide.* New York: Grune & Stratton.

Incrocci, L., Hop, W.C., Wijnmaalen, A., & Slob, A.K. (2002). Treatment outcome, body image, and sexual functioning after orchiectomy radiotherapy for stage I–II testicular seminoma. *International Journal of Radiation Oncology, Biology, Physics, 33*(5), 1165–1173.

Institute of Medicine. (2003). *Health professions education: A bridge to quality.* Washington, DC: National Academies Press.

Joint Commission. (2009). *The Joint Commission national patient safety goals.* Retrieved April 2, 2009, from http://www.jointcommission.org/patientsafety/nationalpatientsafetygoals

Karvinen, K.H., Courneya, K.S., North, S., & Venner, P. (2007). Associations between exercise and quality of life in bladder cancer survivors: A population-based study. *Cancer Epidemiology, Biomarkers and Prevention, 16*(5), 984–990.

Krueger, J.C. (1978). Utilization of nursing research: The planning process. *Journal of Nursing Administration, 8*(1), 6–9.

Krueger, J.C., Nelson, A.H., & Wolanin, M.O. (1978). *Nursing research: Development collaboration and utilization.* Germantown, MD: Aspen.

LoBiondo-Wood, G. (2006). Introduction to quantitative research. In G. LoBiondo-Wood & J. Haber (Eds.), *Nursing research: Methods and critical appraisal for evidence-based practice* (6th ed., pp. 201–219). St. Louis, MO: Mosby.

McCullagh, J., Lewis, G., & Warlow, C. (2005). Promoting awareness and practice of testicular self-examination. *Nursing Standard, 19*(51), 41–49.

Meinardi, M.T., Gietema, J.A., Van Der Graaf, W.T.A., Van Veidhuisen, D.J., Runne, M.A., Sluiter, W.J., et al. (2000). Cardiovascular morbidity in long-term survivors of metastatic testicular cancer. *Journal of Clinical Oncology, 18*(8), 1725–1732.

Milton, C.L. (2007). Evidence-based practice: Ethical questions for nursing. *Nursing Science Quarterly, 20*(2), 123–126.

Mitchell, S.A., Beck, S.L., Hood, L.E., Moore, K., & Tanner, E.R. (2007). Putting evidence into practice: Evidence-based interventions for fatigue during and following cancer and its treatment. *Clinical Journal Oncology Nursing, 11*(1), 99–113.

Mitchell, S.A., & Friese, C.R. (n.d.). *Weight of evidence.* Retrieved November 25, 2007, from http://www.ons.org/outcomes/volume1/fatigue/fatigue_woe.shtml

Molassiotis, A., Gibson, F., Kelly, D., Richardson, A., Dabbour, R., Ahmad, A.M.A., et al. (2006). A systematic review of worldwide cancer nursing research. *Cancer Nursing, 29*(6), 431–440.

Nieder, A.M., Seeniann, J., Messina, C.R. Granek, I.A., & Adler, H.L. (2006). Are patients aware of the association between smoking and bladder cancer? *Journal of Urology, 176*(6, Pt. 1), 2405–2408.

Perimenis, P., & Koliopanou, E. (2004). Postoperative management and rehabilitation of patients receiving an ileal orthotopic bladder substitution. *Urologic Nursing, 24*(5), 383–386.

Robinson, S., Allen, L., Barnes, M.R., Berry, R.A., Foster, R.A., Friedrich, L.A., et al. (2007). Development of an evidence-based protocol for reduction of indwelling urinary catheter usage. *MedSurg Nursing, 16*(3), 157–161.

Romero, F.R., Romero, K.R., Mattos, M.A., Garcia, C.R., Fernandes Rde, C., & Perez, M.D. (2005). Sexual function after partial penectomy for penile cancer. *Urology, 66*(6), 1292–1295.

Ropka, M.E., Guterbock, T.A., Krebs, L.U., Murphy-Ende, K., Stetz, K.M., Summers, B.L., et al. (2002). Year 2000 Oncology Nursing Society research priorities survey. *Oncology Nursing Forum, 29*(3), 481–491.

Rydberg, L., Carlsson, M., Nilsson, S., & Wikblad, K. (2002). Self-perceived physical, psychologic, and general symptoms in survivors of testicular cancer 3 to 13 years after treatment. *Cancer Nursing, 25*(3), 187–195.

Rutledge, D.N., & Grant, M. (2002). Evidence-based practice in cancer nursing. Introduction. *Seminars in Oncology Nursing, 18*(1), 1–2.

Smyth, R.L. (2002). Systematic reviews: What are they and how can they be used? In J.V. Craig & R.L. Smyth (Eds.), *The evidence-based practice manual for nurses* (2nd ed., pp. 185–207). Philadelphia: Elsevier's Health Sciences.

Srivastava, A., & Kreiger, N. (2000). Relation of physical activity to risk of testicular cancer. *American Journal of Epidemiology, 151*(1), 78–87.

Taub, D.A., Dunn, R.L., Miller, D.C., Wei, J.T., & Hollenbeck, B.K. (2006). Discharge practice patterns following cystectomy for bladder cancer: Evidence for the shifting of the burden of care. *Journal of Urology, 176*(6, Pt. 1), 2612–2617.

Tavani, A., Zucchetto, A., Dal Maso, L., Montella, M., Ramazzotti, V., Talamini, R., et al. (2007). Lifetime physical activity and the risk of renal cell cancer. *International Journal of Cancer, 120*(9), 1977–1980.

Thorsen, L., Nystad, W., Dahl, O., Klepp, O., Bremnes, R.M., Wist, E., et al. (2002). The level of physical activity in long-term survivors. *European Journal of Cancer, 39*(9), 1216–1221.

Traynor, M. (2002). The oil crisis, risk and evidence-based practice. *Nursing Inquiry, 9*(3), 162–169.

Tuinman, M.A., Hoekstra, H.J., Fleer, J., Sleijfer, D.T., & Hoekstra-Weebers, J.E. (2006). Self-esteem, social support, and mental health in survivors of testicular cancer: A comparison based on relationship status. *Urologic Oncology, 24*(4), 279–286.

Wood, L.S., & Manchen, B. (2007). Sorafenib: A promising new targeted therapy for renal cell carcinoma. *Clinical Journal of Oncology Nursing, 11*(5), 649–656.

Zoltick, B.H., Jacobs, L.A., & Vaughn, D.J. (2005). Cardiovascular risk in testicular cancer survivors treated with chemotherapy: Incidence, significance, and practice implications. *Oncology Nursing Forum, 32*(5), 1005–1009.

Systemic Chemotherapy Agents Used in the Management of Genitourinary Malignancies

Jeanne Held-Warmkessel, MSN, RN, AOCN®, ACNS-BC

Systemic Chemotherapy Agents Used in the Management of Genitourinary Malignancies	
Agent	**Nursing Implications**
Bleomycin	• Lifetime cumulative dose must not exceed 400 units or 30 units per dose if given IV, SC, or IM once or twice per week. • Drug-drug interactions with cisplatin, phenothiazines, digoxin, and phenytoin. Administer bleomycin prior to cisplatin. • Life-threatening risk for pulmonary toxicity in the form of interstitial pneumonitis that progresses to fatal pulmonary fibrosis. May result from a single low dose or cumulative doses. Monitor PFTs, including DLCO at baseline, prior to each cycle and periodically after treatment is completed. Discontinue drug if PFTs decrease by more than 15%, and hold drug with onset of pulmonary signs and symptoms. Monitor chest x-ray at baseline, prior to each cycle, and routinely (every 1–2 weeks) between cycles. Risk factors for pulmonary toxicity include exceeding lifetime cumulative dose of 400 units, patient's age older than 70 years, smoking, impaired renal function, radiation therapy to the chest, and inspiration of high concentrations of O_2. Limit O_2 exposure to 25% O_2 and for as short a time period as possible. Assess lung sounds and ask patient about respiratory signs and symptoms such as SOB or DOE prior to each drug dose. Listen for end-inspiratory crackles, which are a sign of pulmonary toxicity. Administer as little supplemental O_2 as possible. Provide patient education, including avoiding smoking, telling all healthcare providers about bleomycin therapy, wearing a medical alert bracelet, limiting supplemental O_2 use and exposure, and avoiding scuba diving where high concentrations of O_2 are used. The risk for pulmonary toxicity persists for life after therapy has been completed (Sleijfer, 2001). • Drug administration alert: Risk for anaphylaxis. Monitor patient for hypotension. Monitor vital signs at baseline, at 15 minutes, and as needed. Monitor patient for mental confusion, fever, chills, and wheezing. Be prepared to manage anaphylaxis by taking vital signs prior to drug administration, providing emergency treatment, and maintaining IV access while obtaining emergency medical care. Pressor agents, volume expanders, antihistamines, and corticosteroids may be used to treat individual symptoms. • Drug administration alert: Risk for drug-induced fevers, as high as 40.6°C (105°F). Premedicate patient with acetaminophen to reduce risk of febrile episodes, and repeat every 4 hours for 24 hours. • Drug administration alert: Pain at tumor site. Possible pain at tumor site requires baseline pain assessment and as-needed pain medications. Provide comfort measures. • Drug administration issue: Renal impairment. Drug excretion is through the kidneys; therefore, bleomycin should be administered *prior* to any renal toxic agents and must be given prior to cisplatin. Dose is reduced in presence of renal impairment. Monitor BUN and SCr prior to each dose; use bleomycin with caution in presence of renal impairment. Do not administer if CrCl is < 10 ml/minute. Encourage the patient to consume at least 2 liters of fluid per day. • Risk for altered skin integrity such as rash, peeling skin, thickening of skin, edema, and hyperpigmentation. Educate the patient to avoid sun exposure. Manage rash and dry skin with topical preparations such as unscented lotions and creams. • Risk for nausea, vomiting, anorexia, and weight loss. Premedicate patient with antiemetic, as needed. Monitor weight. Educate the patient to try to eat frequent, small portions of cool, bland foods. Educate the patient to call healthcare provider for persistent symptoms. • Risk for bone marrow depression. Check CBC with differential prior to each dose and periodically during nadir. Educate the patient to recognize signs and symptoms of anemia (e.g., increasing fatigue, SOB, chest pain, headaches) to report to healthcare provider. Educate the patient to recognize signs and symptoms of infection and thrombocytopenia as well, including fever higher than 40.6°C (100.5°F), chills, bruising, or bleeding. • Risk for altered sexuality and fertility. Patients should not breast-feed while receiving this agent. Encourage sperm banking before beginning therapy. Effective contraception required during drug therapy.

(Continued on next page)

Systemic Chemotherapy Agents Used in the Management of Genitourinary Malignancies *(Continued)*	
Agent	**Nursing Implications**
Carboplatin	• Drug is dosed using AUC.
	• Drug-drug interactions with taxanes. Administer taxanes prior to carboplatin.
	• Drug-drug interaction with warfarin. Monitor INR and adjust warfarin dose as needed. Other drug-drug interactions include phenytoin and aminoglycosides.
	• Drug administration alert: Do not use with products containing aluminum.
	• Drug administration alert: Administer prior to any renal toxic agents.
	• Risk for bone marrow depression. Check CBC with differential prior to each dose and periodically during nadir. Educate the patient to recognize signs and symptoms of anemia (e.g., increasing fatigue, SOB, chest pain, headaches) to report to healthcare provider. Also educate the patient to recognize signs and symptoms of infection and thrombocytopenia, including fever, chills, bruising, or bleeding.
	• Risk for renal toxicity requires monitoring of BUN and SCr prior to each dose. Use cautiously in patients with renal impairment. Use other nephrotoxic agents with caution. Encourage patient to consume at least 2 liters of fluid per day.
	• Risk for nausea, vomiting, anorexia, and weight loss. Premedicate patient with 5-HT$_3$ antiemetic and steroid. Monitor weight. Educate the patient to try to eat frequent, small portions of cool, bland foods. Educate the patient to call healthcare provider for persistent symptoms.
	• Risk for hepatotoxicity requires routine LFTs. Dose modifications of drug may be needed. Avoid use in patients with impaired liver function. Educate the patient to avoid alcohol consumption.
	• Risk for diarrhea requires patient education to notify healthcare provider at onset. Educate the patient regarding use of antidiarrheal medication, hydration, diet modifications such as low-residue diet, elimination of dairy products, and electrolyte replacement. Send stool for *Clostridium (C.) difficile* testing.
	• Risk for allergic reactions/anaphylaxis increases after cycle 6. Monitor patient for hypotension. Monitor vital signs at baseline, at 15 minutes, and as needed. Monitor patient for mental confusion, fever, chills, and wheezing. Be prepared to manage anaphylaxis by taking vital signs prior to drug administration, providing emergency treatment, and maintaining IV access while obtaining emergency medical care. Pressor agents, volume expanders, antihistamines, and corticosteroids may be used to treat individual symptoms.
	• Risk for peripheral neuropathy; may affect motor and sensory peripheral nerves and is cumulative (Hausheer et al., 2006). Assess for signs and symptoms (e.g., numbness, tingling, loss of deep tendon reflexes, difficulty walking) at baseline and routinely during therapy. Educate the patient about safety measures in the home (e.g., furniture placement, avoiding use of throw rugs), to use caution when operating machinery, and to notify healthcare provider of signs and symptoms indicating onset or worsening of peripheral neuropathy (Wickham, 2007).
	• Risk for ototoxicity. Monitor patient for high-frequency hearing loss. Risk may be increased by use of other ototoxic agents. Audiogram at baseline and during treatment may be needed. Avoid use of other ototoxic agents such as aminoglycosides. Contraindicated in patients with hearing deficit.
	• Risk for altered sexuality and fertility. Patients should not breast-feed while receiving this agent. Encourage sperm banking before beginning therapy. Effective contraception required during drug therapy.
Cisplatin	• Multiple drug-drug interactions with other antineoplastic agents because of cisplatin-induced impaired renal clearance. Interactions occur with other drugs such as phenytoin, and other nephrotoxic agents such as aminoglycosides and furosemide.
	• Drug administration alert: Do not use with products containing aluminum.
	• Drug administration alert: Administer cisplatin after methotrexate, bleomycin, taxanes, ifosfamide, and etoposide. Renal toxicity of cisplatin is increased by other nephrotoxic agents.
	• Life-threatening risk of nephrotoxicity requires mandatory pre- and post-treatment hydration and diuresis. Electrolyte replacement is frequently required, especially potassium and magnesium. Monitor BUN and Cr, magnesium, and electrolyte levels prior to therapy. Closely monitor I&O. Patient must be voiding at least 100 ml of urine per hour for 3 hours prior to and 8 hours after cisplatin infusion. Notify prescriber if urine output inadequate; hold infusion for inadequate urine output. Educate the patient to drink fluids after discharge (at least 2 liters per day, more in hot weather) and to call a healthcare provider if nausea and vomiting interfere with fluid consumption. Other nephrotoxic agents increase renal toxicity. Use with extreme caution and in reduced doses in patients with renal insufficiency.
	• High risk for severe acute and delayed emesis requires mandatory pretreatment with 5-HT$_3$ antiemetics, steroids, neurokinin-1 receptor antiemetics, and post-treatment antiemetic prophylaxis. Monitor weight. Educate the patient to try to eat frequent, small portions of cool, bland foods. Educate the patient to call healthcare provider for persistent symptoms.
	• Risk for allergic reactions/anaphylaxis increases after cycle 6. Monitor patient for hypotension. Monitor vital signs at baseline, at 15 minutes, and as needed. Monitor patient for mental confusion, fever, chills, and wheezing. Be prepared to manage anaphylaxis by taking vital signs prior to drug administration, providing emergency treatment, and maintaining IV access while obtaining emergency medical care. Pressor agents, volume expanders, antihistamines, and corticosteroids may be used to treat individual symptoms.

(Continued on next page)

Systemic Chemotherapy Agents Used in the Management of Genitourinary Malignancies *(Continued)*	
Agent	**Nursing Implications**
Cisplatin *(cont.)*	• Risk for ototoxicity. Monitor patient for high-frequency hearing loss. Risk may be increased by use of other ototoxic agents. Audiogram at baseline and during treatment may be needed. Avoid use of other ototoxic agents such as aminoglycosides. Contraindicated in patients with hearing deficit. • Risk for peripheral neuropathy that may affect motor and sensory peripheral nerves and is cumulative (Sul & DeAngelis, 2006). Assess for signs and symptoms (e.g., numbness, tingling, loss of deep tendon reflexes, difficulty walking) at baseline and routinely during therapy. Educate the patient about safety measures in the home (e.g., furniture placement, avoiding use of throw rugs), to use caution when operating machinery, and to notify healthcare provider of signs and symptoms indicating onset or worsening of peripheral neuropathy. • Risk for cardiovascular toxicity such as MI or Raynaud phenomenon (Chaudhary & Haldas, 2003), especially when administered concomitantly with other chemotherapeutic agents or radiation therapy. Replace electrolytes and ions to keep levels in normal range. Educate the patient to immediately report any cardiovascular side effects and to go to an emergency room. • Risk of premature atherosclerosis (Carver et al., 2007). Educate patient on long-term risk and need for lifelong monitoring. • Risk for bone marrow depression, especially anemia, which is common. Patient may need pRBC transfusions. Check CBC with differential prior to each dose and periodically during nadir. Educate the patient to recognize signs and symptoms of anemia (e.g., increasing fatigue, SOB, chest pain, headaches) to report to healthcare provider. Also, educate the patient to recognize signs and symptoms of infection and thrombocytopenia, including fever higher than 40.6°C (100.5°F), chills, bruising, or bleeding. • Risk for hepatotoxicity requires routine LFTs. Dose modifications may be needed. Avoid use in patients with impaired liver function. Educate the patient to avoid alcohol consumption. • Risk for altered sexuality and fertility. Patients should not breast-feed while receiving this agent. Encourage sperm banking before beginning therapy. Effective contraception required during drug therapy. • Risk for taste alteration. Educate the patient to use spices and seasonings to improve food flavor. Refer patient to nutritionist for additional counseling as needed.
Doxorubicin	• Lifetime cumulative dose not to exceed 550 mg/m²; 450 mg/m² in patients with any chest irradiation or those receiving cyclophosphamide or other cardiotoxic agents. • Drug colors urine an orange-red color; educate the patient to anticipate changes. • Multiple drug-drug interactions, including other chemotherapeutic agents such as cyclophosphamide, which increases risk of cardiac toxicity and hemorrhagic cystitis, and nonchemotherapeutic agents such as digoxin. • Life-threatening risk for cardiac toxicity requires patient assessment and determination of %EF prior to and during treatment. Avoid drug use in patients with a %EF < 30%. Test %EF at baseline and repeat at 250–300 mg/m² and at 450 mg/m². Stop therapy if %EF falls 10%, falls to < 50%, or if test result was between 30%–50% and falls to ≤ 30%. Educate the patient to report signs and symptoms of cardiac toxicity such as edema or dyspnea. Late cardiotoxicity may occur. May be contraindicated in patients with a history of heart disease. • Drug administration issue: Potent vesicant. Administer using vesicant administration precautions via side arm of a rapidly infusing IV with frequent assessments of IV site. Be prepared to treat and manage extravasation per institutional policy. Antidote is dexrazoxane IV (Totect®, TopoTarget). • Risk for bone marrow depression. Check CBC with differential prior to each dose and periodically during nadir. Educate the patient to recognize signs and symptoms of anemia (e.g., increasing fatigue, SOB, chest pain, headaches) to report to healthcare provider. Educate the patient to recognize signs and symptoms of infection and thrombocytopenia as well, including fever, chills, bruising, or bleeding. • Risk for nausea and vomiting requires administration of antiemetics prior to therapy. Monitor weight. Educate the patient to try to eat frequent, small portions of cool, bland foods. Educate the patient to call healthcare provider for persistent symptoms. • Risk for radiation recall in prior sites of radiation therapy. Educate the patient as to the possibility, along with need to notify healthcare provider. Educate the patient to avoid sun exposure. • Risk for hepatotoxicity requires routine LFTs. Dose modifications may be needed. Avoid use in patients with impaired liver function. • Risk for alopecia. Educate the patient to keep head warm with wig, hat, or other coverings and to not expose scalp to the sun, as it will burn easily. • Risk for mucositis and esophagitis. Educate the patient about oral care and to report these symptoms to healthcare provider. If patient is unable to swallow liquids, parenteral hydration and replacement of electrolytes may be needed. • Risk for diarrhea requires patient education to notify healthcare provider at onset. Educate the patient regarding use of antidiarrheal medication, hydration, diet modifications (e.g., low-residue diet, elimination of dairy products), and electrolyte replacement. Send stool for *C. difficile* testing. • Risk for altered sexuality and fertility. Patients should not breast-feed while receiving this agent. Encourage sperm banking before beginning therapy. Effective contraception required during drug therapy. • Risk for hyperpigmentation. Encourage patient to avoid sun exposure. Risk may decrease with time.

(Continued on next page)

Systemic Chemotherapy Agents Used in the Management of Genitourinary Malignancies *(Continued)*	
Agent	**Nursing Implications**
Etoposide	• Multiple drug-drug and herb interactions, including warfarin. Monitor INR and adjust warfarin doses as needed. St. John's wort, which interferes with drug effect, is not to be used in patients receiving etoposide. • Drug administration alert: Administer with caution, as drug is a known irritant. Be prepared to treat and manage extravasation per institutional policy. • Drug administration alert: Administer over a minimum of 60 minutes to avoid risk for hypotension and bronchospasm. • Risk for anaphylaxis, respiratory distress, and blood pressure changes (both hypo- and hypertension). Monitor vital signs at baseline, at 15 minutes, and as needed. Monitor patient for mental confusion, fever, chills, and wheezing. Be prepared to manage anaphylaxis by taking vital signs prior to drug administration, providing emergency treatment, and maintaining IV access while obtaining emergency medical care. Pressor agents, volume expanders, antihistamines, and corticosteroids may be used to treat individual symptoms. • Risk for bone marrow depression. Check CBC with differential prior to each dose and periodically during nadir. Educate the patient to recognize signs and symptoms of anemia (e.g., increasing fatigue, SOB, chest pain, headaches) to report to healthcare provider. Also, educate the patient to recognize signs and symptoms of infection and thrombocytopenia, including fever, chills, bruising, or bleeding. • Risk for alopecia. Educate the patient to keep head warm with wig, hat, or other coverings and to not expose scalp to the sun, as it will burn easily. • Risk for peripheral neuropathy; may affect motor and sensory peripheral nerves and is cumulative. Assess for signs and symptoms (e.g., numbness, tingling, loss of deep tendon reflexes, difficulty walking) at baseline and routinely during therapy. Educate the patient about safety measures in the home (e.g., furniture placement, avoiding use of throw rugs), to use caution when operating machinery, and to notify healthcare provider of signs and symptoms indicating onset or worsening of peripheral neuropathy. • Risk for radiation recall, especially if administered with cisplatin, in prior sites of radiation therapy. Educate the patient as to the possibility, along with need to notify healthcare provider. Educate the patient to avoid sun exposure. • Risk for altered sexuality and fertility. Patients should not breast-feed while receiving this agent. Encourage sperm banking before beginning therapy. Effective contraception required during drug therapy. • Risk for hepatotoxicity requires routine LFTs. Dose modifications may be needed. Avoid use in patients with impaired liver function. • Risk for renal toxicity requires monitoring of BUN and SCr. Dose modifications may be needed. Avoid use in patients with impaired renal function. • Risk for secondary malignancies such as AML requires ongoing monitoring of CBC with differential for life.
5-fluorouracil	• Multiple drug-drug interactions including warfarin. Monitor INR and adjust warfarin doses as needed. Increased 5-fluorouracil toxicity when given with leucovorin. • Drug administration issue: Administer with caution, as drug is a known irritant. Be prepared to treat and manage extravasation per institutional policy. • Risk for potentially life-threatening diarrhea requires patient education to notify healthcare provider at onset. Educate the patient regarding use of antidiarrheal medication, hydration, diet modifications (e.g., low-residue diet, elimination of dairy products), and electrolyte replacement. Educate the patient to notify healthcare provider if unable to consume liquids because of nausea or vomiting, if urine output decreases or becomes dark in color, or if the patient feels dizzy or lightheaded. Send stool for *C. difficile* testing. • Risk for cardiotoxicity requires prompt interruption of medication with onset of chest pain or other cardiac symptoms, which may be caused by arterial vasoconstriction. Monitor vital signs. Notify prescriber. Required cardiac assessments include ECG, pulse oximetry, troponin blood tests, and chest x-ray. Risk factors include preexisting cardiac and renal disease (Jensen & Sorensen, 2006). • Risk of mucositis is high. Assess oral cavity for ulcers prior to drug administration. Consider using ice chip oral prophylaxis during bolus administration. Start 10–15 minutes before and after administration. • Educate the patient regarding good oral care and to call healthcare provider if unable to eat or drink bland liquids and water because of risk of dehydration. • Risk for renal toxicity requires monitoring of BUN and SCr. May require dose modifications. Avoid use in patients with impaired renal function. • Risk for hepatotoxicity requires routine LFTs. Dose modifications may be needed. Avoid use in patients with impaired liver function. Educate the patient to avoid alcohol consumption. • Risk for bone marrow depression. Check CBC with differential prior to each dose and periodically during nadir. Educate the patient to recognize signs and symptoms of anemia (e.g., increasing fatigue, SOB, chest pain, headaches) to report to healthcare provider. Also educate the patient to recognize signs and symptoms of infection and thrombocytopenia, including fever, chills, bruising, or bleeding. • Risk of photosensitivity and hyperpigmentation along veins used for drug administration and in skinfolds. Educate the patient to avoid sun exposure. Hyperpigmentation from drug should fade with time.

(Continued on next page)

Systemic Chemotherapy Agents Used in the Management of Genitourinary Malignancies *(Continued)*

Agent	Nursing Implications
5-fluoroura-cil *(cont.)*	• Monitor glucose levels closely in patients with diabetes. • Risk of neurotoxicity requires monitoring patient for ataxia and other signs of cerebellar toxicity. Educate the patient about safety measures in the home (e.g., furniture placement, avoiding use of throw rugs), to use caution when operating machinery, and to notify healthcare provider of signs and symptoms indicating onset or worsening of cerebellar toxicity.
Gemcitabine	• Drug-drug interactions with other chemotherapeutic agents. Infuse gemcitabine prior to cisplatin and after paclitaxel. • Drug-drug interactions including warfarin. Monitor INR closely and adjust warfarin doses as needed. • Drug administration alert: Risk of peripheral vein irritation. Administer over 30 minutes through a large peripheral vein. Longer infusion times increase drug toxicity. If patient complains of discomfort, apply warm soak to site or add NSS to run concurrently with drug for additional dilution. If long-term therapy is possible, a central line is recommended for drug administration. Infusion reactions have occurred. • Risk for bone marrow depression. Check CBC with differential prior to each dose and periodically during nadir. Reduce or hold dose for lowered counts. Educate the patient to recognize signs and symptoms of anemia (e.g., increasing fatigue, SOB, chest pain, headaches) to report to healthcare provider. Educate the patient to recognize signs and symptoms of infection and thrombocytopenia as well, including fever, chills, bruising, or bleeding. • Risk for renal toxicity requires monitoring of BUN and SCr. May require dose modifications. Avoid use in patients with impaired renal function. May cause proteinuria or hematuria. • Risk for hepatotoxicity requires routine LFTs. Dose modifications may be needed. Avoid use in patients with impaired liver function. Educate the patient to avoid alcohol consumption. • Risk of flu-like symptoms such as fever, chills, and myalgia, which can be managed with acetaminophen. Educate the patient to report fever to healthcare provider, as cultures may be indicated. • Risk for nausea and vomiting requires administration of antiemetics prior to therapy. Monitor weight. Educate the patient to try to eat frequent, small portions of cool, bland foods. Educate the patient to call healthcare provider for persistent symptoms. • Risk for diarrhea requires patient education to notify healthcare provider at onset. Educate the patient regarding use of antidiarrheal medication, hydration, diet modifications (e.g., low-residue diet, elimination of dairy products), and electrolyte replacement. Send stool for *C. difficile* testing. • Risk for rash. Educate the patient to use skin lotions and topical antihistamines to manage rash and itching. • Risk for pulmonary toxicity requires monitoring respiratory function and PFTs, if indicated at baseline and during therapy. Assess breath sounds. Educate the patient to report any difficulty breathing and to avoid smoking. • Risk for edema. Educate the patient to report any difficulty breathing and the development of any edema to healthcare provider. • Risk for cardiotoxicity requires prompt interruption of medication with onset of chest pain or other cardiac symptoms. Monitor vital signs. Notify prescriber. Cardiac assessment required includes ECG, pulse oximetry, troponin blood tests, and chest x-ray. Risk factors include preexisting cardiac and renal disease. Educate the patient to seek emergency medical care if outside of clinical setting. • Risk of mucositis. Assess oral cavity for ulcers prior to drug administration. Educate the patient regarding good oral care and to call healthcare provider if unable to eat or drink bland liquids and water because of risk of dehydration. • Risk for sedation. Educate the patient not to drive a car, operate mechanical equipment, or attempt to perform any activities that may endanger himself or others. • Risk for altered sexuality and fertility. Patients should not breast-feed while receiving this agent. Encourage sperm banking before beginning therapy. Effective contraception required during drug therapy.
Ifosfamide with mesna	• Multiple drug-drug interactions increase risk of toxicity. Monitor INR in patients receiving warfarin. Dose adjustments may be needed during therapy and three to four days after ifosfamide therapy. Educate patient to avoid grapefruit and its juice. • Drug administration alert: Administer with caution, as drug is a known irritant. Be prepared to treat and manage extravasation per institutional policy. • Drug administration alert: Administer hydration prior to starting therapy, continuously through therapy, and after therapy. • Drug administration alert: Send urine to lab to test for blood prior to starting therapy and at least daily, and also dipstick urine at bedside for blood. Encourage frequent urination. • Risk of hemorrhagic cystitis from metabolite, acrolein, requires mandatory concurrent administration of mesna, which binds acrolein for excretion in urine. Mesna may be administered by a variety of schedules including bolus and continuous infusion, and may be mixed with the ifosfamide in the same bag or run as a separate infusion. Mesna bolus doses should be 60% of ifosfamide dose divided into three doses before ifosfamide administration, then at four hours and at eight hours after administration. After the ifosfamide is completed, a 12-hour infusion of mesna is administered. • Risk for renal toxicity requires monitoring of BUN and SCr prior to starting therapy and daily while receiving therapy. May require dose modifications. Monitor I&O. Avoid use in patients with impaired renal function. • Risk of SIADH requires monitoring of electrolytes at baseline and daily. Monitor patient for signs and symptoms such as change in mental status.

(Continued on next page)

Systemic Chemotherapy Agents Used in the Management of Genitourinary Malignancies *(Continued)*	
Agent	**Nursing Implications**
Ifosfamide with mesna *(cont.)*	• Risk of central nervous system toxicity from metabolite, chloracetaldehyde, which may cause encephalopathy. Assess for risk factors such as low serum albumin, young or old age, first cycle of therapy, poor performance status, impaired liver or renal function, and pelvic disease (Brunello et al., 2007; David & Picus, 2005; Meanwell et al., 1986; Rieger et al., 2004). A wide range of signs and symptoms may occur, including changes in orientation, cognition, word finding, agitation, coma, ataxia, hand flapping, and tremor (Lokiec, 2006). Assess patient for neurotoxicity prior to each dose of drug and at least each shift and as needed. Stop drug and notify prescriber for changes in mental status and other signs and symptoms of neurotoxicity. Neurotoxicity may respond to IV methylene blue (Patel, 2006). Drug that has been interrupted for neurotoxicity may be restarted at the discretion of the prescriber if patient becomes more oriented or toxicity subsides. • Risk for nausea and vomiting is high and requires administration of antiemetics prior to therapy and as needed for breakthrough nausea and vomiting. Monitor weight. Educate the patient to try to eat frequent, small portions of cool, bland foods. Educate the patient to call healthcare provider for persistent symptoms. • Risk for diarrhea requires patient education to notify healthcare provider at onset. Educate the patient regarding use of antidiarrheal medication, hydration, diet modifications (e.g., low-residue diet, elimination of dairy products), and electrolyte replacement. Send stool for *C. difficile* testing. • Risk for hepatotoxicity requires routine LFTs. Dose modifications may be needed. Avoid use in patients with impaired liver function. Educate the patient to avoid alcohol consumption. • Risk for bone marrow depression. Check CBC with differential prior to each dose and periodically during nadir. Reduce or hold dose for lowered counts. Educate the patient to recognize signs and symptoms of anemia (e.g., increasing fatigue, SOB, chest pain, headaches) to report to healthcare provider. Also, educate the patient to recognize signs and symptoms of infection and thrombocytopenia, including fever, chills, bruising, or bleeding. • Risk for alopecia. Educate the patient to keep head warm with wig, hat, or other coverings and to not expose scalp to the sun, as it will burn easily. • Risk for altered sexuality and reproduction as drug is a carcinogen, mutagen, and teratogen. Patients should not breastfeed while receiving this agent. Encourage sperm banking before beginning therapy. Effective contraception required during drug therapy.
Methotrexate (standard dose)	• Multiple drug-drug interactions. Increases INR in patients taking warfarin. Dose adjustments may be needed. Educate the patient to avoid use of aspirin, nonsteroidal anti-inflammatory agents, folic acid, and several other commonly used drugs. • Drug causes urine to be bright yellow in color; educate the patient to anticipate changes. • Risk for renal toxicity. Monitor BUN and SCr. Reduce dose for impaired renal function and use with caution. Drug is excreted extensively by the kidneys. Educate the patient to consume fluids (at least 2 liters per day or more in warm weather) and notify healthcare provider of reduced urine output or reduced fluid consumption. Monitor for acute renal failure. Use with caution in patients with urinary diversions, ascites, pleural effusion, or other third-spaced fluid. • Risk for rash. Educate the patient to use skin lotions and topical antihistamines to manage rash and itching. Educate the patient to avoid sun exposure. • Risk for radiation recall in prior sites of radiation therapy. Educate the patient as to the possibility, along with need to notify healthcare provider. Educate the patient to avoid sun exposure. • Risk of photosensitivity. Educate the patient to avoid sun exposure. • Risk of hepatotoxicity requires routine LFTs. Dose modifications may be needed. Avoid use in patients with impaired liver function. Educate the patient to avoid alcohol consumption. • Risk of mucositis. Assess oral cavity for ulcers prior to drug administration. Educate the patient regarding good oral care and to call healthcare provider if unable to eat or drink bland liquids and water because dehydration may result. • Risk for bone marrow depression. Check CBC with differential prior to each dose and periodically during nadir. Reduce or hold dose for lowered counts. Educate the patient to recognize signs and symptoms of anemia (e.g., increasing fatigue, SOB, chest pain, headaches) to report to healthcare provider. Educate the patient to recognize signs and symptoms of infection and thrombocytopenia as well, including fever, chills, bruising, or bleeding. • Risk for diarrhea requires patient education to notify healthcare provider at onset. Educate the patient regarding use of antidiarrheal medication, hydration, diet modifications (e.g., low-residue diet, elimination of dairy products), and electrolyte replacement. Send stool for *C. difficile* testing. • Risk of neurotoxicity requires monitoring patient for confusion, changes in mental status, and ataxia. Educate the patient about safety measures in the home (e.g., furniture placement, avoiding use of throw rugs), to use caution when operating machinery, and to notify healthcare provider of signs and symptoms indicating onset or worsening of neurotoxicity. • Rarely causes pulmonary toxicity. Educate the patient to report any breathing symptoms to healthcare provider.

(Continued on next page)

Systemic Chemotherapy Agents Used in the Management of Genitourinary Malignancies *(Continued)*	
Agent	**Nursing Implications**
Paclitaxel	• Multiple drug-drug interactions: Metabolized by P450 liver enzymes. Educate the patient to not use St. John's wort. • Drug administration alert: Always administer prior to cisplatin and carboplatin, as clearance of paclitaxel is impaired by renal toxicity caused by platinum compounds. • Drug administration alert: Administer after doxorubicin. • Drug administration alert: Use only non-PVC bags and tubing, and filter using < 0.22 micron in-line filter. • Drug administration alert: Administer with caution, as drug is a known vesicant/irritant. Be prepared to treat and manage extravasation per institutional policy. • Drug administration alert: Risk for life-threatening anaphylaxis, most common with the first dose. Premedicate patient with diphenhydramine, dexamethasone, and a histamine-2 blocker such as ranitidine. Stay at bedside for first 15 minutes, and be prepared to stop infusion if necessary. Monitor patient for hypotension and cardiac arrhythmias. Monitor vital signs at baseline, at 15 minutes, and as needed. Monitor patient for mental confusion, fever, chills, and wheezing. Be prepared to manage anaphylaxis by taking vital signs prior to drug administration, providing emergency treatment, and maintaining IV access while obtaining emergency medical care. Pressor agents, volume expanders, antihistamines, and corticosteroids may be used to treat individual symptoms. • Risk for bone marrow depression. Check CBC with differential prior to each dose and periodically during nadir. Reduce or hold dose for lowered counts. Educate the patient to recognize signs and symptoms of anemia (e.g., increasing fatigue, SOB, chest pain, headaches) to report to healthcare provider. Also educate the patient to recognize signs and symptoms of infection and thrombocytopenia, including fever, chills, bruising, or bleeding. • Risk for hepatotoxicity requires routine LFTs. Dose modifications may be needed. Avoid use in patients with impaired liver function. Educate the patient to avoid alcohol consumption. • Risk for alopecia. Educate the patient to keep head warm with wig, hat, or other coverings and to not expose scalp to the sun, as it will burn easily. • Risk for peripheral neuropathy. May affect motor and sensory peripheral nerves and is cumulative. Assess for signs and symptoms (e.g., numbness, tingling, loss of deep tendon reflexes, difficulty walking) at baseline and routinely during therapy. Educate the patient about safety measures in the home (e.g., furniture placement, avoiding use of throw rugs), to use caution when operating machinery, and to notify healthcare provider of signs and symptoms indicating onset or worsening of peripheral neuropathy. • Risk for myalgia and arthralgia. May be managed with a mild, over-the-counter analgesic. • Risk of mucositis. Assess oral cavity for ulcers prior to drug administration. Educate the patient regarding good oral care and to call healthcare provider if unable to eat or drink bland liquids and water because of dehydration risk. • Risk for nausea and vomiting may require administration of an antiemetic prior to therapy and as needed for breakthrough nausea and vomiting. Monitor weight. Educate the patient to try to eat frequent, small portions of cool, bland foods. Educate the patient to call healthcare provider for persistent symptoms. • Risk for cardiotoxicity requires prompt interruption of medication with onset of chest pain or other cardiac symptoms. Transient bradycardia, which typically does not produce symptoms, may occur. Monitor vital signs. Notify prescriber. Required cardiac assessments include baseline and periodic multigated acquisition scans in patients with a cardiac history, as well as ECG, pulse oximetry, troponin blood tests, and chest x-ray, as needed. Risk factors include preexisting cardiac and renal disease.
Vinblastine	• Multiple drug-drug interactions, including grapefruit juice, St. John's wort, drugs metabolized by CYP3A4 isoenzyme (e.g., dexamethasone), methotrexate, phenytoin, and many other drugs. • High medication error alert: Do not confuse vinblastine with vincristine. Severe toxicity has occurred when these drugs have been confused. Follow facility policy related to reduction of vinblastine medication errors. • Drug administration alert: Must only be administered by IV route. **Fatal if administered intrathecally.** • Drug administration alert: Administer with caution, as drug is a known vesicant. Administer according to institution's vesicant drug administration policy. Be prepared to treat and manage extravasation per institutional policy. • Risk for cardiovascular toxicity in form of Raynaud phenomenon, especially when administered concomitantly with bleomycin. • Risk for bone marrow depression. Check CBC with differential prior to each dose and periodically during nadir. Reduce or hold dose for lowered counts. Educate the patient to recognize signs and symptoms of anemia (e.g., increasing fatigue, SOB, chest pain, headaches) to report to healthcare provider. Also educate the patient to recognize signs and symptoms of infection and thrombocytopenia, including fever, chills, bruising, or bleeding. • Risk for peripheral neuropathy. May affect motor and sensory peripheral nerves and is cumulative. Assess for signs and symptoms (e.g., numbness, tingling, loss of deep tendon reflexes, difficulty walking) at baseline and routinely during therapy. Educate the patient about safety measures in the home (e.g., furniture placement, avoiding use of throw rugs), to use caution when operating machinery, and to notify healthcare provider of signs and symptoms indicating onset or worsening of peripheral neuropathy. • Constipation often occurs and requires a prophylactic bowel regimen with stool softener and laxative.

(Continued on next page)

Systemic Chemotherapy Agents Used in the Management of Genitourinary Malignancies *(Continued)*	
Agent	**Nursing Implications**
Vinblastine *(cont.)*	• Risk for altered sexuality and fertility. Patients should not breast-feed while receiving this agent. Encourage sperm banking before beginning therapy. Effective contraception required during drug therapy. • Risk of SIADH requires monitoring electrolytes at baseline and daily. Monitor patient for signs and symptoms such as change in mental status. • Risk for alopecia. Educate the patient to keep head warm with wig, hat, or other coverings and to not expose scalp to the sun, as it will burn easily. • Risk for hepatotoxicity requires routine LFTs. Dose modifications may be needed. Avoid use in patients with impaired liver function. Educate the patient to avoid alcohol consumption. • Risk of mucositis. Assess oral cavity for ulcers prior to drug administration. Educate the patient regarding good oral care and to call healthcare provider if unable to eat or drink bland liquids and water, because dehydration may result. • Risk for nausea and vomiting requires administration of antiemetics prior to therapy and as needed for breakthrough nausea and vomiting. Monitor weight. Educate the patient to try to eat frequent, small portions of cool, bland foods. Educate the patient to call healthcare provider for persistent symptoms.
Vincristine	• Maximum drug dose of 2 mg per week. Question any prescription for doses that exceed this limit. • Multiple drug-drug interactions including grapefruit juice, St. John's wort, drugs metabolized by CYP3A4 isoenzyme (e.g., dexamethasone), methotrexate, phenytoin, and many other drugs. • High medication error alert: Do not confuse vincristine with vinblastine. Severe toxicity has occurred when these drugs have been confused. Follow facility policy related to reduction of vincristine medication errors. • Drug administration alert: Must only be administered by IV route. **Fatal if administered intrathecally.** • Drug administration alert: Administer with caution, as drug is a known vesicant. Administer according to institution's vesicant drug administration policy. Be prepared to treat and manage extravasation per institutional policy. • Risk of ascending peripheral neuropathy (cumulative) in stocking-and-glove distribution is expected and requires baseline neurologic assessment and ongoing assessments prior to each drug dose. Assess patient for numbness, tingling, loss of deep tendon reflexes, difficulty walking, and jaw pain. Acute neurotoxicity may present as abdominal pain, urinary retention, postural hypotension, and loss of deep tendon reflexes. Educate the patient to notify healthcare provider of peripheral neuropathy. Worsening neuropathy often requires dose adjustment or delays. Cranial nerve neuropathy may also occur. Educate the patient as to safety precautions in the home and safety with mechanical devices. Affects autonomic, sensory, and motor nerves. Erectile dysfunction may occur from neurotoxicity and may resolve after treatment completed. • High risk of constipation requires a prophylactic bowel regimen with stool softener and laxative while the patient is on therapy and as long as constipation persists. Assess bowel function. Educate the patient to consume fluids and a high-fiber diet and to notify provider if signs or symptoms of paralytic ileus occur. • Risk for altered sexuality and fertility. Patients should not breast-feed while receiving this agent. Encourage sperm banking before beginning therapy. Effective contraception required during drug therapy. • Risk of SIADH requires monitoring of electrolytes at baseline and daily. Monitor patient for signs and symptoms such as change in mental status. • Risk for alopecia. Educate the patient to keep head warm with wig, hat, or other coverings and to not expose scalp to the sun, as it will burn easily. • Risk for hepatotoxicity requires routine LFTs. Dose modifications may be needed. Avoid use in patients with impaired liver function. Educate the patient to avoid alcohol consumption. • Risk for bone marrow depression is rare. Educate the patient to recognize signs and symptoms of anemia (e.g., increasing fatigue, SOB, chest pain, headaches) to report to healthcare provider. Also educate the patient to recognize signs and symptoms of infection and thrombocytopenia, including fever, chills, bruising, or bleeding.

AML—acute myeloid leukemia; AUC—area under curve; BUN—blood urea nitrogen; CBC—complete blood count; Cr—creatinine; CrCl—creatinine clearance; DLCO—diffusion lung capacity for carbon monoxide; DOE—dyspnea on exertion; ECG—electrocardiogram; %EF—ejection fraction; 5-HT$_3$—5-hydroxytryptamine-3; IM—intramuscular; INR—international normalized ratio; I&O—intake and output; IV—intravenous; LFTs—liver function tests; MI—myocardial infarction; ml—milliliter; NSS—normal saline solution; O$_2$—oxygen; PFTs—pulmonary function tests; pRBC—packed red blood cell; PVC—polyvinyl chloride; SC—subcutaneous; SCr—serum creatinine; SIADH—syndrome of inappropriate antidiuretic hormone; SOB—shortness of breath

Note. Based on information from Brunello et al., 2007; Carver et al., 2007; Chanan-Khan et al., 2004; Chaudhary & Haldas, 2003; Chu & DeVita, 2007; David & Picus, 2005; Gullatte, 2007; Hausheer et al., 2006; Jensen & Sorensen, 2006; Lokiec, 2006; Meanwell et al., 1986; Patel, 2006; Rieger et al., 2004; Sleijfer, 2001; Sudhoff et al., 2004; Uzel et al., 2005; Wilkes & Barton-Burke, 2008.

References

Brunello, A., Basso, U., Rossi, E., Stefani, M., Ghiotto, C., Marino, D., et al. (2007). Ifosfamide-related encephalopathy in elderly patients: Report of five cases and review of the literature. *Drugs and Aging, 24*(11), 967–973.

Carver, J.R., Shapiro, C.L., Ng, A., Jacobs, L., Schwartz, C., Virgo, K.S., et al. (2007). American Society of Clinical Oncology clinical evidence review of the ongoing care of adult cancer suvirors: Cardiac and pulmonary late effects. *Journal of Clinical Oncology, 25*(25), 3991–4008.

Chanan-Khan, A., Srinivasan, S., & Czuczman, M.S. (2004). Prevention and management of cardiotoxicity from antineoplastic therapy. *Journal of Supportive Oncology, 2*(3), 251–256.

Chaudhary, U.B., & Haldas, J.R. (2003). Long-term complications of chemotherapy for germ cell tumours. *Drugs, 63*(15), 1565–1577.

Chu, E., & DeVita, V.T. (2007). *Physicians' cancer chemotherapy drug manual.* Sudbury, MA: Jones and Bartlett.

David, K.A., & Picus, J. (2005). Evaluating risk factors for the development of ifosfamide encephalopathy. *American Journal of Clinical Oncology, 28*(3), 277–280.

Gullatte, M.M. (Ed.). (2007). *Clinical guide to antineoplastic therapy: A chemotherapy handbook* (2nd ed.). Pittsburgh, PA: Oncology Nursing Society.

Hausheer, F.H., Schilsky, R.L., Bain, S., Berghorn, E.J., & Lieberman, F. (2006). Diagnosis, management, and evaluation of chemotherapy-induced peripheral neuropathy. *Seminars in Oncology, 33*(1), 15–49.

Jensen, S.A., & Sorensen, J.B. (2006). Risk factors and prevention of cardiotoxicity induced by 5-fluorouracil or capecitabine. *Cancer Chemotherapy and Pharmacology, 58*(4), 487–493.

Lokiec, F. (2006). Ifosamide: Pharmacokinetic properties for central nervous system metastasis prevention. *Annals of Oncology, 17*(Suppl. 4), iv33–iv36.

Meanwell, C.A., Blake, A.E., Kelly, K.A., Honigsberger, L., & Blackledge, G. (1986). Prediction of ifosfamide/mesna associated encephalopathy. *European Journal of Cancer and Clinical Oncology, 22*(7), 815–819.

Patel, P.N. (2006). Methylene blue for management of ifosfamide-induced encephalopathy. *Annals of Pharmacotherapy, 40*(2), 299–303.

Rieger, C., Fiegl, M., Tischer, J., Ostermann, H., & Schiel, X. (2004). Incidence and severity of ifosfamide-induced encephalopathy. *Anti-Cancer Drugs, 15*(4), 347–350.

Sleijfer, S. (2001). Bleomycin-induced pneumonitis. *Chest, 120*(2), 617–624.

Sudhoff, T., Enderle, M.D., Pahlke, M., Petz, C., Teschendorf, C., Graeven, U., et al. (2004). 5-fluorouracil induces arterial vasocontractions. *Annals of Oncology, 15*(4), 661–664.

Sul, J.K., & DeAngelis, L.M. (2006). Neurologic complications of cancer chemotherapy. *Seminars in Oncology, 33*(3), 324–332.

Uzel, I., Ozguroglu, M., Uzel, B., Kaynak, K., Demirhan, O., Akman, C., et al. (2005). Delayed onset bleomycin-induced pneumonitis. *Urology, 66*(1), 195e.23–195e.25.

Wickham, R. (2007). Chemotherapy-induced peripheral neuropathy: A review and implications for oncology nursing practice. *Clinical Journal of Oncology Nursing, 11*(3), 361–376.

Wilkes, G.M., & Barton-Burke, M. (2008). *Oncology nursing drug handbook 2008.* Sudbury, MA: Jones and Bartlett.

Index

The letter f after a page number indicates that relevant content appears in a figure; the letter t, in a table.